Elma D. Baron
Editor

Light-Based Therapies for Skin of Color

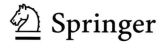 Springer

Editor
Elma D. Baron
Department of Dermatology
Case Western Reserve University
Veterans Affairs Medical Center
Cleveland, OH 44106
USA

ISBN 978-1-84882-327-3   e-ISBN 978-1-84882-328-0
DOI 10.1007/978-1-84882-328-0
Springer Dordrecht Heidelberg London New York

British Library Cataloguing in Publication Data
A catalogue record for this book is available from the British Library

Library of Congress Control Number: 2009927589

Printed on acid-free paper

Springer is part of Springer Science+Business Media (www.springer.com)

I wish to dedicate this book to my husband, John Carl Baron, and our wonderful children, John Christopher and Joanna Katrina.

Preface

The science and practice of photodermatology has been largely based on knowledge derived from white skin. Therapeutic modalities based on lasers and light sources are often based on protocols that have been utilized in Caucasian populations. The biologic effects of light in pigmented skin are not as well understood. Consequently, we are just beginning to elucidate mechanisms and develop treatment strategies that are more specifically tailored to darker skin types. The writing of this book has been a challenge primarily because there is not yet sufficient information in the literature to arrive at concrete recommendations as far as treating pigmented skin with lasers and light sources. The information presented here represents what is currently known, as well as what needs to be further investigated. Although this book aims to discuss therapy, it is important to not overlook some basic foundations in photobiology, such as principles of optics, biology of photodamage and photoaging, protection afforded by endogenous pigmentation, and the issues surrounding the use of photoprotective agents in nonwhite skin. These topics are discussed in the first part of the book. Practical information on the use of specific treatment modalities and the approach to specific dermatologic conditions, which are either more common or more problematic in dark-skinned patients, such as vitiligo, follicular disorders, pigmentation, among others, are then provided in the second part of the book. It is our hope that this book would help dermatologists and other health care providers in understanding and managing patients with pigmented skin.

Cleveland, OH   Elma D. Baron

Contents

1 Principles of Light–Skin Interactions 1
Marjorie F. Yang, Valery V. Tuchin, and Anna N. Yaroslavsky

2 Photoaging in Skin of Color 45
Mary F. Bennett and Kevin D. Cooper

3 Endogenous Protection by Melanin 83
Bernhard Ortel, Mark Racz, Deborah Lang,
and Pier G. Calzavara-Pinton

4 Photoprotection in Non-Caucasian Skin 111
Diana Santo Domingo and Mary S. Matsui

5 Light Treatment of Follicular Disorders in Dark Skin 135
Bassel H. Mahmoud and Iltefat H. Hamzavi

6 Phototherapy for Vitiligo 171
Camile L. Hexsel, Richard H. Huggins, and Henry W. Lim

7 Lasers and Light Therapies for Pigmentation 189
Malcolm S. Ke

8 Light Therapies for Cutaneous T-Cell Lymphoma 205
Katalin Ferenczi and Elma D. Baron

**9 Light Treatment and Photodynamic Therapy in
Acne Patients with Pigmented Skin** 249
Vicente Torres and Luis Torezan

10 Clinical Application of Intense Pulsed Light in Asian Patients 263
Yuan-Hong Li, Yan Wu, and Hong-Duo Chen

Index 277

Contributors

Elma D. Baron, MD
Department of Dermatology, Case Western Reserve University, Veterans Affairs Medical Center, Cleveland, OH, USA

Mary F. Bennett, MD, MRCPI
Department of Dermatology, University Hospital Case Medical Center, Cleveland, OH, USA

Piergiacomo Calzavara-Pinton, MD
Dermatology Department, University of Brescia, Brescia, Italy

Hong-Duo Chen, MD
Dermatology, No. 1 Hospital of China Medical University, Shenyang, China

Kevin D. Cooper
Department of Dermatology, Case Western Reserve University, Veterans Affairs Medical Center, Cleveland, OH, USA

Diana Santo Domingo
Department of Dermatology, University Hospitals Case Medical Center, Cleveland, OH, USA

Katalin Ferenczi, MD
Department of Dermatology, Case Western Reserve University, Cleveland, OH, USA

Iltefat H. Hamzavi, MD
Dermatology, Henry Ford Hospital, Detroit, MI, USA

Camile L. Hexsel, MD
Dermatology, Henry Ford Hospital, Detroit, MI, USA

Richard H. Huggins, MD
Department of Dermatology, Multicultural Dermatology Center, Henry Ford Hospital, Detroit, MI, USA

Malcolm S. Ke, MD
Division of Dermatology, David Geffen School of Medicine,
University of California, Los Angeles, CA, USA

Deborah Lang, PhD
Biological Sciences Division, University of Chicago, Chicago, IL, USA

Yuanhong Li, MD, PhD
Dermatology, Institute of Dermatology and Cosmetic Dermatology,
Shenyang, China

Henry W. Lim, MD
Dermatology, Henry Ford Hospital, Detroit, MI, USA

Bassel H. Mahmoud, MD, PhD
Dermatology, Henry Ford Hospital, Detroit, MI, USA

Mary S. Matsui
External Research R&D, The Estee Lauder Companies, Melville, NY, USA

Bernhard Ortel, MD
Dermatology, University of Chicago, Chicago, IL, USA

Mark Racz, MD
Pathology, The Vancouver Clinic, Vancouver, WA, USA

Luis A. Torezan
Dermatology Department, Hospital de las Cinicas – Facultad de Medicina
Universidad de São Paulo – Brasil, Sao Paulo, Brazil

Vicente R. Torres Lozada, MD
Department of Dermatology, Juarez Hospital Mexico City, Atizapan, Mexico

Valery V. Tuchin, DSc
Department of Optics and Biomedical Physics, Institute of Optics and
Biophotonics, Saratov State University, Saratov, Russia

Yan Wu, MD, PhD
Dermatology, No. 1 Hospital of China Medical University, Shenyang, China

Marjorie F. Yang
Department of Dermatology, Indiana University, Indianapolis, IN, USA

Anna N. Yaroslavsky, PhD
Dermatology, Wellman Center for Photomedicine and Department of
Dermatology, Harvard Medical School and Massachusetts General Hospital,
Boston, MA, USA

Chapter 1
Principles of Light–Skin Interactions

Marjorie F. Yang, Valery V. Tuchin, and Anna N. Yaroslavsky

1.1 Introduction

Skin is the largest human organ. It covers between 1.5 and 2 m², comprising about one-sixth of total body weight. Skin performs a complex role in human physiology. It serves as a barrier to the environment and acts as a channel for communication to the outside world. For example, skin protects us from water loss, ultraviolet (UV) rays of the sun, friction, and impact wounds. It also helps in regulating body temperature and metabolism. All photobiological responses are influenced heavily by the optical properties of skin. Therefore, for the successful development of photomedicine, in-depth knowledge and understanding of light-skin interactions, specifically known as skin optics, is required. The transfer of optical radiation into human skin depends on the absorption and scattering properties of three functional skin layers: epidermis, dermis, and hypodermis. The structures and component chromophores of these layers determine the attenuation of radiation in skin. The enhanced penetration of optical radiation as well as selective targeting of pathology can be achieved by studying and analyzing the wavelength-dependent interactions of light with skin. For example, considering that melanin exhibits maximum absorption in the UV and blue spectral ranges, whereas blood preferentially absorbs blue and yellow light, the treatment protocol have been devised that target pigmented and vascular lesions, respectively.[1] The chromophores, such as melanin, blood, water, and lipid determine skin absorption.

M.F. Yang
Department of Dermatology, Indiana University School of Medicine, Indianapolis, IN, USA
e-mail: mfyang@hotmail.com

V.V. Tuchin
Department of Optics and Biomedical Physics, Institute of Optics and Biophotonics, Saratov State University, Saratov, Russia

A.N. Yaroslavsky(✉)
Wellman Center for Photomedicine and Department of Dermatology, Harvard Medical School and Massachusetts General Hospital, Boston, MA, USA
e-mail: yaroslav@helix.mgh.harvard.edu

E.D. Baron (ed.), *Light-Based Therapies for Skin of Color*,
DOI: 10.1007/ 978-1-84882-328-0_1, © Springer-Verlag London Limited 2009

Scattering largely determines the depths to which light penetrates through skin, as it dominates absorption in the visible and near-infrared (NIR) spectral ranges by at least one order of magnitude. It has also been shown that light scattering from dermal collagen significantly modifies skin color.[2] Thus, detailed information on scattering is required for the accurate estimation of the light penetration through skin. An optical "window" between 600 and 1300 nm offers the possibility of treating large tissue volumes[3] and using exogenous chromophores/fluorophores for contrast-enhancing.[4-6] Optical imaging and spectroscopy allow for noninvasive assessment of skin pathology and treatment efficacy.[7-9] In particular, reflectance imaging and spectroscopy provide information on the distribution and quantities of the scatterers and chromophores,[10] whereas fluorescence responses determine the biochemical composition of the interrogated biotissue.[11,12] The development of lasers and light-based medical devices has been stimulated by the achievements of diagnostic and therapeutic photomedicine.[13-15] This chapter provides a brief summary and description of the properties of light, its interaction with human skin, the list of the medical light sources, and the diagnostic and/or therapeutic uses of currently available light-based devices within the visible to NIR spectral range in dermatology.

1.2   Fundamental Properties of Light

Light can be described as the energy that is carried in the form of traveling wave composed of electric and magnetic fields. Electric and magnetic fields vary in intensity and are at right angles to each other and to the direction that the wave is propagating (Fig. 1.1a). These fields propagate until energy of wave is converted into other form of energy. The electromagnetic (EM) wave is characterized by its wavelength, λ, period, T, frequency, f, and speed of propagation, v. The distance between neighboring crests is called the wavelength, λ (Fig. 1.1b). The time that is required for a crest to travel distance λ is called the period, T. The number of completed periods per unit time (or the number of crests that pass by per unit time)

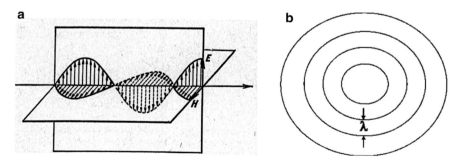

Fig. 1.1 (a) Propagating electromagnetic wave. Arrow points toward the direction of the propagation. (b) The wavelength, λ, is the distance between neighboring crests

is called the frequency, $f = 1/T$. The speed of propagation of the electromagnetic wave is calculated as $v = \lambda/T = f\lambda$. In vacuum, the electromagnetic waves propagate with the speed of $c = 299{,}792$ km/s. In the media, such as skin, the speed of light is lower, $v = c/n$, where n is the absolute refractive index of the medium. Polarization is yet another important property of any transverse wave. It describes the orientation of the oscillations in the plane perpendicular to the wave's direction of travel. Polarization characterizes electromagnetic waves, such as light, by specifying the direction of the wave's electric field. Natural light is not polarized. When the electric field vector of the electromagnetic radiation (EMR) oscillates in a single, fixed plane all along the beam, the light is said to be linearly polarized; when the plane of the electric field rotates, the light is said to be elliptically polarized because the electric field vector traces out an ellipse at a fixed point in space as a function of time; and when the ellipse happens to be a circle, the light is said to be circularly polarized (Fig. 1.2). Electromagnetic waves in the wavelength range from 400 to 750 nm are visually perceived as different colors, including violet, 400–450 nm; blue, 450–480 nm; green, 510–560 nm; yellow, 560–590 nm; orange, 590–620 nm; and red, 620–750 nm (Fig. 1.3). Initially, light was defined as the electromagnetic waves in the visible spectral range. At present, however, light is defined as electromagnetic radiation between 100 and 10,000 nm. In photomedicine, this spectral range is subdivided in the following ways: UV light: UVC, 100–280 nm; UVB, 280–315 nm; and UVA, 315–400 nm; visible: 400–780 nm (violet, 400–450 nm;

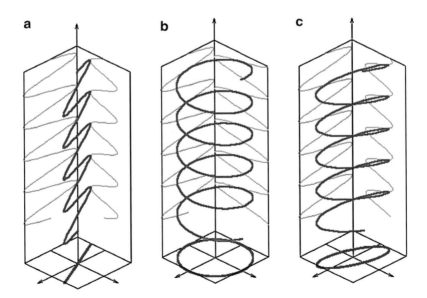

Fig. 1.2 The evolution of the electric field vector (blue), with time (the vertical axes), as a particular point in space, along with its x and y components (red/left and green/right), and the path traced by the tip of the vector in the plane (purple). (**a**) Linearly polarized light. (**b**) Circularly polarized light. (**c**) Elliptically polarized light

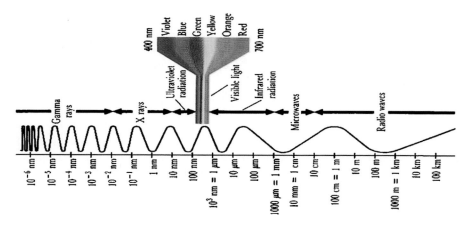

Fig. 1.3 Electromagnetic spectrum

blue, 450–480 nm; green, 510–560 nm; yellow, 560–590 nm; orange, 590–620 nm; and red, 620–780 nm); infrared (IR) light: IRA, 0.78–1.4 μm; IRB, 1.4–3.0 μm; and IRC, 3–1000 μm. In physics, the light is classified as UV, 100–400 nm; visible, 400–800 nm; NIR, 0.8–2.5 μm; middle-IR (MIR), 2.5–50 μm; and far-infrared (FIR), 50–2000 μm.

Simultaneously, light can also be described as a stream of particles, photons, which have a rest mass of zero, are electrically neutral, and carry certain amount of energy. In other words, the energy that is transported by EM wave is not continuously distributed over the wave front defined by crests. Energy is located at discrete points, photons, along the wave front. Photons are created inside the atoms of radiating body from which they receive their energy content. Photons move with velocity of light. When photons are absorbed by atoms of the matter, they lose their identity by transferring their energy to an atom. Energy content in photon is inversely proportional to its wavelength: $E_{photon} = hc/\lambda$, where c is the velocity of light, λ the photon wavelength, $h = 6.626 \times 10^{34}$ Js the Planck's constant. Energy is measured in joules (J). Energy characterizes the ability of light to produce some work. Power is the rate of the energy delivery. It is normally measured in watts (W), that is, joules (J) per second (s). The efficiency of light–tissue interaction depends on the energy density, also called fluence. Light fluence is the energy, which propagates through a unit area, which is perpendicular to direction of light propagation. Fluence is measured in J/m². Power density is power of light wave, which propagates through a unit area which is perpendicular to direction of propagation of light wave. A power density or intensity is measured in W/m². Fluence (F_1) and intensity (I_1) are proportional: $F = I \cdot \tau_p$, where τ_p is the length of pulse (pulse width) or exposure time. Another important parameter that characterizes light is its fluence rate that is defined as the sum of the radiance over all angles at a point $\bar{r}$ and is measured in W/m².

1.3 Interactions of Light with Skin

1.3.1 Optical Interactions

When the light is incident on the turbid medium, such as skin, it can be reflected or refracted. After that the light propagates through the medium, being elastically and inelastically scattered and absorbed along the way (Fig. 1.4). Reflection is the change in direction of the light propagation at an interface between two media with different indices of refraction, so that it returns into the medium from which it originated. Light can be reflected specularly (mirror-like) and diffusely. Skin exhibits a combination of specular and diffuse reflection. If the skin is rough and uneven, it has a higher proportion of diffuse reflection. Smooth and polished skin has a greater proportion of specular reflection. According to the law of the specular reflection, the angle of incidence equals to the angle of reflection (Fig. 1.5a).

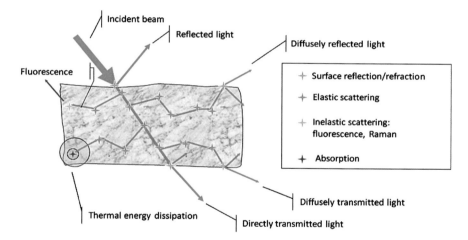

Fig. 1.4 Light propagation in skin

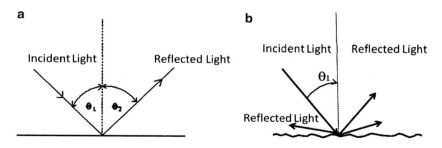

Fig. 1.5 (a) Specular reflection of light, $\theta_1 = \theta_2$. (b) Diffuse reflection of light

In contrast, the diffuse reflection happens in a broad range of directions (Fig. 1.5b). In the most general case, a certain fraction of the light is reflected from the interface, and the remainder is refracted. The light refraction is the change in direction of a ray of light in passing obliquely from one medium into another in which light speed is different. Light refraction is characterized by index of refraction, n, indicating the speed of light in a given medium as either the ratio of the speed of light in a vacuum to that in the given medium (absolute index of refraction) or the ratio of the speed of light in a specified medium to that in the given medium (relative index of refraction), $m = n_1/n_2$. For different human skin components, refractive index in the visible/NIR wavelength range varies from a value a little bit higher than for water due to influence of some organic components ~1.35 for interstitial fluid to 1.55 for the stratum corneum. Snell's law, also known as Descartes' law or the law of refraction, is used to describe the relationship between the angles of incidence and refraction. It states that the ratio of the sines of the angles of incidence and refraction is equivalent to the ratio of the light velocities in the two media, or equivalent to the opposite ratio of the indices of refraction: $(\sin\theta_1 / \sin\theta_2) = v_1/v_2 = n_2/n_1$, where θ_1 and θ_2, v_1 and v_2, n_1 and n_2 are the angles, the velocities of light, the refractive indices of incidence and refraction, respectively. The Snell's law demonstrates that when light moves from a medium with a higher refractive index (dense medium) into the medium with the lower refractive index (less dense medium), the resolved sine value can be higher than 1. At this point, light is reflected in the incident medium. This phenomenon is known as the total internal reflection (Fig. 1.6). Before the ray totally internally reflects, the light refracts at the critical angle, θ_{crit} = $\sin^{-1} (n_2 /n_1)$, when it travels directly along the surface between the two media.

When the light propagates in the turbid medium, it is being absorbed and scattered. The energy of absorbed photons is thermally dissipated. However, in most cases in the optical wavelength range, scattering dominates absorption by at least one order

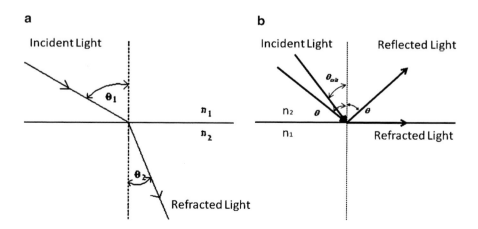

Fig. 1.6 (**a**) Refraction of light, $n_2 > n_1$. (**a**) Total internal reflection of light, $n_2 > n_1$, θ_{crit}-critical angle of incidence when the light is propagating along the boundary of the two media

of magnitude. More than 99% of light is scattered elastically or without the change of wavelength (or frequency). The lifetime, τ_e, of the elastic scattering process is usually very short on the order of 10^{-15} s. A small fraction is scattered inelastically, that is, with the change of wavelength. Inelastic scattering includes fluorescence, phosphorescence, and Raman. The cross sections of the inelastic processes are generally very low. For example, the cross section of fluorescence is approximately 1×10^{-16}, whereas the Raman cross section is approximately 1×10^{-30}, which means that the probability of these processes is much lower, as compared to elastic scattering. The fluorescence and phosphorescence processes are illustrated in the Jablonksi diagram (Fig. 1.7). Once a photon has transferred its energy to the molecule of the medium, there are a number of routes by which it can return to ground state, the statistically most populated energy state for room temperature. If the photon emission (shown in blue in the diagram) occurs between states of the same spin state, for example, $S_1 \rightarrow S_0$, the process is termed fluorescence. If the spin state of the initial and final energy levels is different, for example, $T_1 \rightarrow S_0$, the emission is called phosphorescence (shown in red). Since fluorescence is statistically much more likely than phosphorescence, the lifetimes of fluorescent states, τ_f, are very short (1×10^{-6} to 10^{-10} s) and phosphorescence, τ_p, somewhat longer (1×10^{-4} s to min or even hours). Three nonradiative deactivation processes are also significant: internal conversion (IC), intersystem crossing (ISC), and vibrational relaxation. Examples of the first two can be seen in the diagram. Internal conversion is the radiationless transition between energy states of the same spin state. Intersystem crossing is a radiationless transition between different spin states. Raman scattering is yet another type of inelastic scattering process (Fig. 1.8). In Raman scattering,

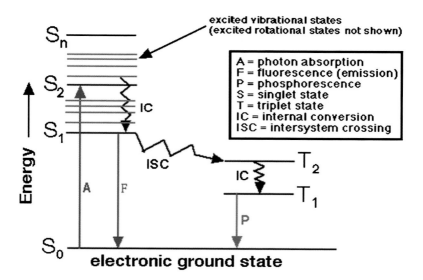

Fig. 1.7 Jablonski diagram

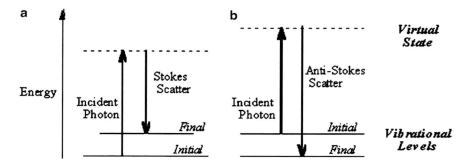

Fig. 1.8 (**a**) Stokes Raman scattering. (**b**) Anti-Stokes Raman scattering. The energy difference between the incident and scattered photons is represented by the arrows of different lengths

the incident photon energy excites vibrational modes of the molecules, yielding scattered photons that are diminished in energy by the amount of the vibrational transition energies (Stokes lines). If there is significant excitation of vibrational excited states of the scattering molecules, then the scattering at frequencies above the incident frequency are observed, as the vibrational energy is added to the incident photon energy. These lines are called anti-Stokes lines. The lifetime of Raman scattering, τ_R, is less than 1×10^{-14}.

1.3.1.1 The Structure and Optical Properties of Skin

Light propagation in and interaction with turbid media, such as skin, is determined by their intrinsic optical properties.[16] Those are the absorption coefficient μ_a, the scattering coefficient μ_s, the scattering phase function $f(\mu)$ (μ is the cosine of the scattering angle), and the refractive index. In the cases when multiple light scattering is of importance, the reduced or transport scattering coefficient is considered. It is determined as $\mu'_s = \mu_s (1-\overline{\mu})$, where $\overline{\mu}$ is the average cosine of the scattering angle. Absorption and scattering coefficients are defined as the probability for the photon to be absorbed and scattered per unit length, respectively. They are measured in 1/m. The angular distribution of the scattered light is called the scattering phase function. The information on the light propagation and interaction with turbid media is imperative for accurate dosimetry of light treatments, as well as for the evaluation of treatment efficacy. Therefore, the optical properties of skin have been studied extensively over the last 30 years.[17-28]

Skin consists of three functional layers: epidermis, dermis, and hypodermis. In all three layers, the epidermal appendages, such as nails, hair, and glands, can be found (Fig. 1.9a). As the outermost skin layer, the epidermis forms the actual protective covering against environmental influences. The average thickness of epidermis is approximately 0.1 mm (Fig. 1.9b). However, on the face it maybe as thin as 0.02 mm, while on the soles of the feet it is as thick as 1–5mm. The epidermis consists

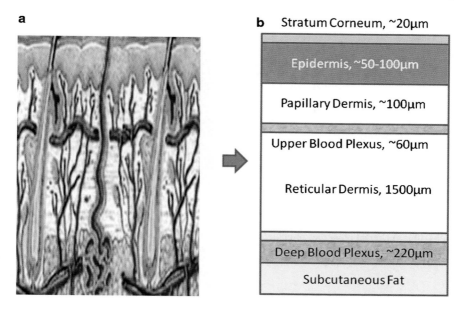

Fig. 1.9 (**a**) Human skin. (**b**) The model of human skin

of up to 90% keratinocytes, which functions as a barrier, keeping harmful substances out and preventing water and other essential substances from escaping the body. The other 10% of epidermal cells are melanocytes, which manufacture and distribute melanin, the protein that adds pigment to skin and protects the body from UV rays. Melanin is one of the strongest skin chromophores with the absolute refractive index of 1.7. Absorption and scattering of epidermis in the visible and NIR spectral ranges are defined almost exclusively by its melanin and water contents, respectively. Dermis is composed of gel-like and elastic materials, water, and, primarily, collagen. Embedded in this layer are systems and structures common to other organs such as lymph channels, blood vessels, nerve fibers, and muscle cells, but unique to the dermis are hair follicles, sebaceous glands, and sweat glands. Blood and water content define the absorptive properties of dermis in the visible and NIR spectral ranges, respectively. The hypodermis consists of spongy connective tissue interspersed with energy-storing adipocytes (fat cells). Fat cells are grouped together in large cushion-like clusters held in place by collagen fibers called connective tissue septa or sheaths. The hypodermis is heavily interlaced with blood vessels, ensuring a quick delivery of stored nutrients as needed.

Absorption and scattering coefficients of skin layers are shown in Figs. 1.10–1.13.[24] The graphs demonstrate that the scattering of skin layers decreases with the increasing wavelength. The scattering of epidermis is noticeably higher than the scattering of dermis and subcutaneous fat in the entire wavelength range. It is known that optical properties of epidermis in the range 370–1200 nm are determined by melanin

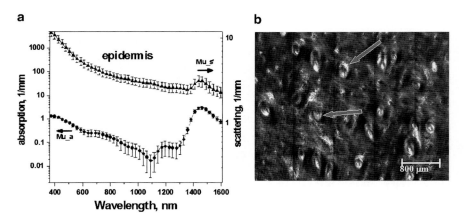

Fig. 1.10 (**a**) Optical properties of epidermis, *Triangles* – reduced scattering coefficients, *circles* absorption coefficients, *bars* – standard errors. Averaged over 7 samples. (**b**) Typical confocal image of epidermis; arrows point to hair follicles

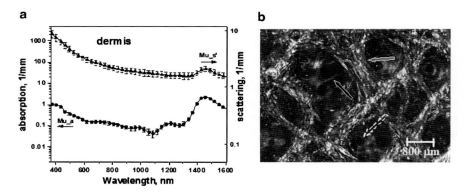

Fig. 1.11 (**a**) Optical properties of dermis. *Triangles* – reduced scattering coefficients, *bars* – standard errors. Averaged over eight samples. (**b**) Typical confocal image of dermis; gray arrow points to collagen-elastin bundle, black arrow points to sebaceous gland, dashed arrow points to hair shaft

content (Fig. 1.10),[2] which exhibits high relative refractive index of approximately 1.3 with respect to the surrounding medium.[29] Therefore, light scattering in the epidermis is significantly higher as compared to the other skin layers. In the dermis, scattering is predominantly caused by collagen fibers and their associated small structures.[24] The bundles of thick collagen and elastin fibers can be clearly seen in the confocal image of the dermis (Fig.1.11, the gray arrow points toward the fibers). The scattering properties of subcutaneous fat are also affected by the presence of connective tissue septa composed of collagen and elastin. In the confocal image of subcutaneous fat (Fig. 1.12), the septum separating conglomerates

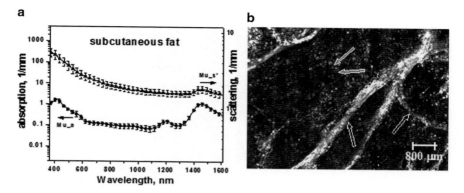

Fig. 1.12 (**a**) Optical properties of subcutaneous fat. *Triangles* – reduced scattering coefficients, *circles* – absorption coefficients, bars – standard errors. Averaged over ten samples. (**b**) Typical confocal image of subcutaneous fat; gray arrows point to fat cells–adipocytes, black arrow points to connective tissue septum

of fat cells – adipocytes – is shown with black arrows. Scattering properties of fat differed depending on the body area. The collagen–elastin net appears thicker and denser in the subcutaneous fat samples obtained from the facial or scalp area (Fig. 1.13a), collagen bundles are shown with black arrows. The presence of collagen and elastin resulted in increased scattering coefficients (Fig. 1.13c). Skin excisions taken from the back of the subjects revealed fat with large multilocular adipocytes and very thin connective tissue septa (Fig. 1.13b). In this case, scattering was much lower (Fig. 1.13c).

The knowledge of the skin optical properties allows for the estimation of the light-effective penetration depth, μ_{eff}, which depends on the wavelength, the absorption and the transport scattering coefficients. In the diffusion approximation, it is given by the formula:

In the Appendix we present the summary of the optical properties of human skin layers together with the corresponding effective penetration depths for the visible and NIR spectral ranges.[24]

1.3.1.2   Skin Chromophores

In the visible wavelength range, melanin determines absorption in the epidermis. Absorption of melanin is monotonously decreasing with the increase of the wavelength. Therefore, the effect of melanin on epidermis absorption properties is more pronounced at shorter wavelengths. Hemoglobin dominates absorption properties of dermis and fat in the visible spectral range. Hemoglobin absorption peaks around 410 and 540 nm appear. Absorption of the epidermis, dermis, and fat in the

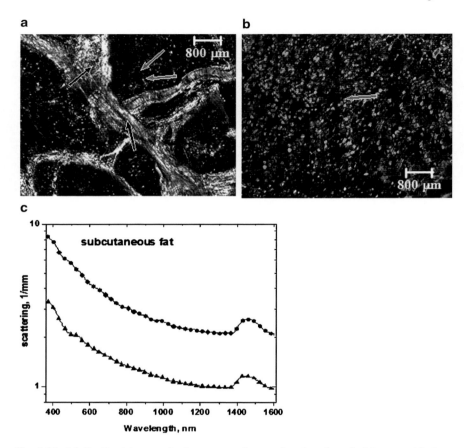

Fig. 1.13 (**a**) Confocal image of subcutaneous fat sample taken from facial area, with dense connective tissue septa separating multilocular adipocytes. (**b**) Confocal image of subcutaneous fat sample, taken from the back, without the septa. Gray arrows point to fat cells–adipocytes, black arrows point to connective tissue septum. (**c**) Scattering properties of subcutaneous fat. Circles – reduced scattering coefficient of fat with dense connective tissue septa, triangles – reduced scattering coefficient of fat without the septa

NIR region is determined by water and lipid content. In the proximity of 1200 nm, water and lipid absorption bands overlap. Therefore, this peak is more pronounced for the subcutaneous fat as compared to the epidermis and dermis. At the same time, the epidermis and dermis exhibit stronger absorption in the range from 1350 to 1600 nm.

The spectral ranges of the major skin chromophores are summarized in Fig. 1.14.[2,12,15,30-35] In skin, the strongest chromophores in the visible spectral range are melanin and hemoglobin. In the IR spectral range, water and lipids are the main absorbers (Fig. 1.15). Chromophores exhibit characteristic bands of absorption at

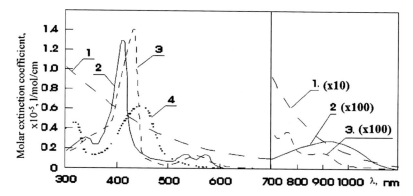

Fig. 1.14 Absorption spectra of major skin chromophores. (1) DOPA – melanin (in H_2O), (2) oxyhemoglobin (in H_2O), (3) deoxyhemoglobin (in H_2O), (4) bilirubin (in $CHCl_3$). *Source:* Anderson RR, Parrish JA. *The optics of human skin*

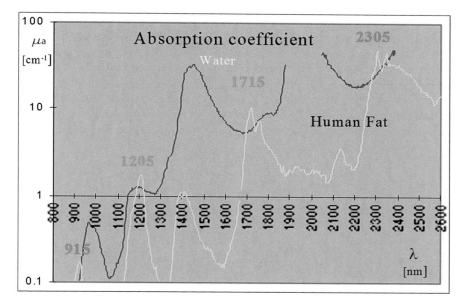

Fig. 1.15 Absorption of water and human fat

specific wavelengths. Melanin is located in the epidermis, occupying the top 50–100 μm of the skin. Oxy- and deoxyhemoglobins are present in the microvascular network of the dermis, typically 50–500 μm below the epidermal surface. Other chromophores may be present in the skin in pathological conditions such as bilirubin (Fig. 1.14), giving the skin the characteristic yellow color of jaundice, which has a broad absorption band at 460 nm.[36]

Melanin synthesis occurs in the melanosomes, which are organelles found in the melanocytes. Human skin is characterized by variable concentration of melanin, ranging from very low in fair-skinned individuals (skin type I) to very high in black African skin individuals (skin type VI). Although absorption of epidermal melanin is highest in the UV spectrum, it is also significant in the visible and NIR regions.[37] At 600–1100 nm range, together with a decrease in dermal scattering and decreased absorption by both hemoglobin and melanin, there is markedly increased skin penetration. The major cutaneous chromophore within the highly penetrating 600–1100 nm region is melanin. The Q-switched 532 nm (green), 694 nm (red), and 1064 nm (NIR) regions have been used to treat pigmented lesions.

Blood, more specifically oxy-, deoxy-, carboxy-, and methemoglobins, is absorbed in the blue, green, and yellow bands (Fig. 1.16).[38] Methemoglobin (met-Hb) has an additional maximum around 630 nm. Oxy- and met-Hbs also exhibit a weaker absorption band in the NIR spectral range, with the maximum around 940 nm. Despite the higher extinction coefficient at the Soret absorption band around 415 nm, the penetration of photons into the dermis at this wavelength is insufficient, because of the high attenuation of the incident light by the melanin of epidermis. At 577–595 nm, melanin absorption and scattering are reduced and tissue penetration is increased. In addition, the epidermal damage is less at this wavelength and more energy is transmitted to the blood vessels. Beyond 600 nm, there is a steep decrease in the absorption by hemoglobins, except met-Hb, which comprise 0.5% of the total hemoglobins content. Heating of blood to 50–54°C causes partial oxidation of oxy-hemoglobin, which leads to met-Hb formation. Optical absorption of met-Hb in the NIR spectral range is much higher than that of either hemoglobin or oxyhemoglobin.[39] Several in vitro studies have demonstrated that when blood is photocoagulated by

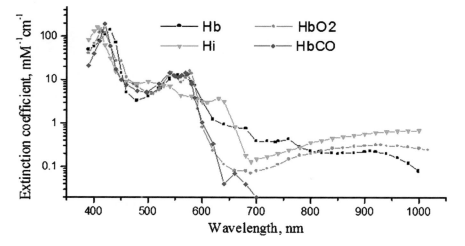

Fig. 1.16 Absorption of hemoglobin derivatives. *Source:* Van Assendelft, *Spectrocscopy of Hemoglobin Derivatives*

1064-nm neodymium:yttrium aluminum garnet (Nd:YAG) laser pulses, absorption at 1064 nm increases on the millisecond timescale by a factor of about 3, which can be explained by partial conversion of oxyhemoglobin to met-Hb.[40,41] Formation of a coagulum is also accompanied by loss of water from lumen blood, resulting in a higher concentration of chromophores. Optical scattering also increases in thermally coagulated blood. Black et al[42] reported that photocoagulation of human blood results in increased absorption by a factor of 2–10 and increased scattering by a factor of 2–4 in the wavelength range from 500 to 1100 nm.[42]

Water does not absorb light in the visible spectral range. However, at the wavelengths longer than 1100 nm, it becomes the major tissue chromophores. The light from resurfacing lasers, which include the erbium:YAG (Er:YAG) 2940 nm and carbon dioxide (CO_2) 10600 nm lasers, is mainly absorbed by water.

Lipids exhibit several sharp absorption bands around 915, 1205, 1715, and 2305 nm.[43] At these wavelengths, absorption of subcutaneous fat dominates that of the overlying skin layers, that is, epidermis and dermis. Therefore, selective and non-invasive fat removal by light should be possible.

1.3.1.3 Skin Fluorophores

The list and the emission spectral ranges of the major skin fluorophores are summarized in Fig. 1.17.[11,12,15,30-35] Native fluorophores in human skin include collagen, elastin, tryptophan, tyrosine, NADH, NAD, FAD, and porphyrins. Because emission spectra are sensitive to the changes in the fluorophore environment, fluorescence spectroscopy can be used for in vivo noninvasive evaluation of

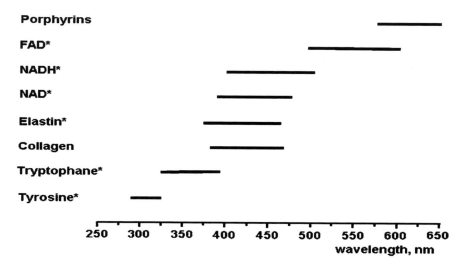

Fig. 1.17 The emission spectral ranges of the major skin fluorophores. For the fluorophores marked with the *asterisk*, the range is determined as half width at half the maximum

human skin structure, pathology, chronological, and sun-induced skin aging. In particular, the signals from tryptophan and collagen can be used for delineating nonmelanoma skin cancers.[11] It has also been demonstrated that quantification of the fluorescence spectra of collagen and tryptophan can serve as the markers for photoaging and natural aging.[44]

1.3.2 Photothermal Effects

As light is absorbed into the skin, it is absorbed and converted to energy, mostly in the form of heat. The temperature within the tissue influences the biological effect (Table 1.1). At temperature increases, cell injury, inflammation, and repair may occur.[45] When temperatures reach 60°C, protein denaturation is complete, while DNA denaturation occurs above 70°C.[46] Above 100°C, vaporization and ablation occur as intracellular water exceeds the boiling point. The rapid increase in pressure causes damage to the cells and blood vessels. Further heating over 100°C leads to charring and desiccation. At about 120°C, thrombosis of the blood vessels and necrotizing vasculitis have been demonstrated.[47-49] The Arrhenius model demonstrates that the rate of denaturation rises exponentially with temperature, thus the accumulation of denatured material also rises proportionally with time.[50] This accounts for the boundaries of dermal coagulation and laser-induced thermal injury. The influence of light energy heating a chromophore and the spread of heat to adjacent tissues by conduction constitutes the photothermal effect. This is influenced first by the height of temperature achieved, followed by the length of time the target is at that temperature. When light is absorbed, heat is lost by conduction to adjacent tissues in all directions, known as thermal relaxation. The thermal relaxation time (TRT) of the tissue is defined as the time it takes for a structure to cool to half the temperature to which it has been heated. Smaller objects have a shorter TRT than larger objects. For example, melanosomes measuring 0.5–1.0 μm have a TRT of approximately 1 μs, while capillaries measuring 10–100 μm have a TRT of approximately 1 ms.

1.3.2.1 Selective Photothermolysis

Introduced in the early 1980s, Anderson and Parrish developed a theory based on the preferential absorption by blood in the 577 nm, which led to the discovery of

Table 1.1 Thermal effects of light with human skin

Temperature (°C)	Effect
>60	Protein denaturation; melting of type 1 collagen (increased likelihood of scarring)
>70	DNA denaturation
>100	Vaporization, ablation
120	Blood vessel thrombosis, necrotizing vasculitis

Table 1.2 Thermal relaxation times (TRT) of target chromophores in the skin

Target chromophore	Diameter (μm)	TRT
Tattoo particle	0.1	10 ns
Melanosome	0.5	250 ns
Melanocyte	7	1 μs
Microvessel	50	1.4 ms
Blood vessel	150	12.8 ms
Terminal hair follicle	300	100 ms

selective laser treatment for vascular malformations. The *theory of selective photo-thermolysis* involves preferential absorption of a laser pulse shorter than the time associated with passive cooling of the target vessels by thermal conduction. Heat is produced in dermal microvessels at a rate faster than it is removed. For selective photothermolysis to occur, three components have to be taken into account: (1) wavelength, (2) fluence, and (3) pulse width (τ). The wavelength must be absorbed by the target chromophore more avidly than by other optically absorbing molecules. Using the optimal fluence to deliver enough energy to thermally alter the target tissue to achieve the desired tissue effects is important. τ must be less than TRT (i.e. $\tau <$ TRT) to spare the surrounding tissue. τ must be determined based on the working knowledge of the TRT of the target structures. For most tissues, TRT of a given target chromophore in seconds is approximately equal to the square of the diameter of the target in millimeters (Table 1.2). With longer laser exposure, most of the heat diffuses away from the target chromophore; hence, the absorbed energy is almost uniformly heating the target and its surrounding tissue. There is less spatial confinement and selectivity with longer τ, resulting in nonspecific thermal damage to adjacent structures. Conversely, shorter τ confine the energy to smaller targets with more spatial selectivity.

Altshuler et al[51] developed a new theory of selective thermal damage specifically for nonuniformly pigmented structures called the *extended theory of selective photothermolysis* (ESP). They demonstrated that primary targets can be used as subsurface heat sources to denature nearby tissue constituents. Thermal damage time (TDT) is the time required for irreversible target damage with sparing of the surrounding tissue. With ESP, the TDT can be longer than the TRT of the entire target. ESP is best illustrated with laser hair reduction. During LHR, the melanin in the hair shaft is the absorber. Although there is much controversy about the location of the follicular stem cells, data suggest that they are located either in the upper hair bulb or the bulge.[52–54] The authors assume that the bulge or vessels nearby the bulb should be destroyed for successful long-term laser hair removal. There is efficient heat transfer between absorber (hair shaft) and target (bulge, bulb) using longer pulses. TDT, in the case of the hair shaft, is defined as the minimum time that allows for simultaneous critical heating of the bulge without exceeding an absorber temperature that would result in fundamental changes in its optical thermal properties and loss of efficient heat transfer to surrounding tissue. The theory infers that the optimal τ should be between the TRT and the TDT. The authors infer that for nonuniformly pigmented targets, τ nearer the TDT will allow for maximal efficacy as well as optimized epidermal cooling. Another potential application of this theory is photosclerotherapy. The absorber for spider veins is hemoglobin. Controversy also exist as to how permanent vessel closure is achieved for optimal treatment effects, either denaturation of the endothelium or denaturation of the vessel wall structure.[55,56] The vessel structures do not contain any strong absorber and can be damaged by heat diffusion from blood. This theory provides new recommendation for hair removal and treatment of spider veins.

1.3.3 Photomechanical Effects

When the pulse duration is shorter than the TRT of the target chromophore, spatially localized heating occurs causing a sudden thermoelastic expansion. The sudden expansion generates acoustic or shock waves, damaging the surrounding structures. The rate of temperature increases can be notably remarkable with very short pulses, causing a steep temperature gradient between the target and the surrounding tissues. The mechanical damage can be illustrated in the treatment of pigmented lesions and tattoos using the Q-switched lasers.[57,58] Cavitation is another form of mechanical damage that is attributed to the dominant mechanism of vessel rupture. The precipitous rise in temperature may be responsible for initiating pressure waves which vaporizes water, developing a vapor bubble that expands and collapses violently. Cutaneous vessels treated with the pulsed dye laser at 1.5 μs pulse duration causes vessel rupture.[59]

1.3.4 Photochemical Effects

The vast majority of photobiological reactions that occur in dermatology are attributed to photochemical processes. Psoralen ultraviolet A (PUVA), extracorporeal photopheresis (ECP), and photodynamic therapy (PDT) are examples of treatments utilizing photochemical effects. PUVA and ECP are beyond the scope of this chapter, and will be discussed throughout this book. PDT utilizes a combination of a photosensitizer drug, light energy, and molecular oxygen to selectively destroy pathological cells. The photosensitizers in the cells, which are wavelength specific, act as the chromophore. The objective of PDT is selective destruction of abnormal cells, with preservation of normal adjacent structures. The excited photosensitizer transfers its energy with a molecular oxygen to produce highly reactive singlet oxygen to induce cytotoxicity (Box 1.1). The sequence of events occurs without the generation of heat. Although PDT can produce apoptosis, necrosis, or a combination, it is highly efficient in inducing apoptosis. The primary role of PDT is to kill unwanted cells in the vast majority of clinical applications (Box 1.2). Photosensitizers such as methylene blue derivative, Photofrin, and silicon phthalocyanine Pc 4, known to localize in mitochondria are reported to be more efficient in inducing apoptosis than those found at

---

Box 1.1 Sequence of Events in PDT

Photosensitization of neoplastic or pathological cells
Absorption of light energy
Transformation of the photosensitizer to a singlet state
Singlet state either returns to the ground state or to an excited triplet state
Photosensitizer at the excited triplet state interacts with molecular oxygen
Photo-oxidative reactions to induce cytotoxicity

Box 1.2 Key mechanisms of PDT on Tumor Destruction

Direct cell destruction
Vascular damage leading to tissue infarction
Immune activation against tumor cells

---

other cellular sites. With mitochondrial damage, the intrinsic pathway for apoptosis is activated, releasing cytochrome c, followed by activation of the caspase series, which play a central role in PDT apoptosis.[60,61]

1.4 Medical Light Sources

1.4.1 Spontaneous and Stimulated Emission

Light is emitted by atoms (molecules) from a light source material that can be either in the form of gas, liquid, or solid. The energy of an electron cannot change continuously. It changes in finite steps. The positions of the electrons with respect to the nucleus depend on their energy and are called energy levels and sublevels. Under normal conditions, most atoms and molecules exist in their ground states, that is, the lowest-energy states. Excitation of atoms (molecules) results by either heating, producing electrical discharge, or by optical pumping. Excitation is an elevation in energy of the system, such as an atom or molecule, above the ground state. An excited atom (molecule) returns to its ground state with time. In other words, the excited state has a lifetime that is defined by the time the atom (molecule) stays in its excited state before emitting a photon spontaneously. The schematic demonstrating spontaneous emission is shown in Fig. 1.18a. An atomic optical transition is typically an electronic transition, where energy is emitted as an electromagnetic radiation in the optical range. Direction of spontaneously emitted photons is random and frequency (wavelength) is random too in the limits of the bandwidth of luminescence of the excited transition. As a result, most spontaneous emitting light sources have an isotropic direction of emission and a wide range of frequencies (polychromatic).

approximately equal to the pulse duration of the pulsed light source or inversely proportional to the wavelength bandwidth $\Delta\lambda$ of a CW light source, $\tau_{c} \sim \lambda^{2}/(c\Delta\lambda)$. For example, a single-frequency CW gas-discharge He-Ne laser with a narrow bandwidth $\Delta\lambda = 10^{-6}$ nm and wavelength $\lambda = 632.8$ nm has a coherence length $l_{c} \approx$ 400 m; a multimode diode laser with $\Delta\lambda = 30$ nm and $\lambda = 830$ nm has $l_{c} \approx 23$ μm; for a titanium sapphire laser with $\lambda = 820$ nm, the bandwidth may be as big as 140 nm, therefore coherence length is very short $l_{c} \approx 2$ μm; the shortest $l_{c} \approx 0.9$ μm is for a white light source ($\Delta\lambda = 400$ nm).

Monochromatic light is light of one wavelength or frequency. Quasi-monochromatic light is the light that has a very narrow wavelength (frequency) bandwidth. Nonmonochromatic (polychromatic) light has a broad wavelength bandwidth.

1.4.5   Halogen Lamps

In halogen lamps, a tungsten filament is heated by electric current until it glows or emits light. A halogen lamp is an iodine-cycle tungsten incandescent lamp that emits the visible and NIR (360 nm to >1 μm) light. These lamps are widely used for spectrophotometry and phototherapy. Tungsten electrode can be heated up to 4000 K. The maximum of the emission spectrum for tungsten lamps is about $\lambda_{max} = 750$ nm. About 30% of the total power is emitted at the wavelengths shorter than λ_{max} and 70% of the total power is emitted at the wavelengths longer than λ_{max}.

1.4.6   Arc Lamps

An arc or flash lamp is a lamp that uses heat emission of plasma bridge formed in a gap between two conductors when they are separated. A mercury arc lamp is a discharge arc lamp filled with mercury vapor at high pressure. It emits UV, visible light, and NIR light. Another arc lamp that produces the IPL (intense pulsed light) is a xenon or krypton lamp that is filled with xenon or krypton. It is often used in tissue spectroscopy and dermatology. It emits UV, visible, and IR light in the range from 200 nm to >3.0 μm. The output spectrum of an arc lamp is a mix of plasma emission spectrum and spontaneous fluorescence of plasma ions. For a high energy short pulse, the temperature of arc lamp plasma should be very high (6000–10000 K). For CW or long pulse mode, the temperature of the arc lamp plasma is relatively low (3000–6000 K).

1.4.7   Light-Emitting Diodes

Light-emitting diode (LED) is a semiconductor device.[13] It consists of a chip of semiconducting material treated to create a structure called a *p–n* (positive–negative) junction. When connected to a power source, current flows from the *p*-side or anode to the *n*-side or cathode, but not in the reverse direction. Charge carriers (electrons and electron holes) flow into the junction from electrodes. When an electron meets a hole, it returns to a lower energy state and releases the energy in the form of a photon (light). The specific wavelength or color emitted by the LED depends on the semiconductor used. The LED light output power ranges from milliwatts to watts. Their typical light beam divergence is approximately ±120°. However, it can be as small as approximately ±5° for the special constructions. LEDs are very cheap and popular light sources. They are widely used in photomedicine. LEDs convert electrical energy to light with high efficiency and have a long lifetime (more than 10^5 h). They are the light sources that are available in a wide range of wavelengths from UV to IR, including multicolor and white light LEDs. To increase the output power, the LED arrays with 2–60 chips in one unit were designed.

1.4.8 Superluminescent Diodes

A superluminescent diode is a very bright diode light source with a broad bandwidth. It is usually manufactured using a laser diode technology, but without reflecting mirrors. Its main difference from an LED is that it has a uniform wave front of the output radiation, which allows to couple its radiation into a single mode fiber. Superluminescent diodes are used in medical optical coherence tomography (OCT) systems.

1.4.9 Lasers

Laser is an acronym for *light amplification by the stimulated emission of radiation*. Laser is a device that generates a beam of light that is collimated, monochromatic, and coherent. A laser is an active medium with inversed population that is placed between two paralleled mirrors. During lasing, the photon avalanche is propagating between two mirrors and is amplified each time it traverses the active medium. As a result, laser beam is forming with a very low divergence and single wavelength (monochromatic beam).

Laser radiation is characterized by its wavelength, power, and pulse- or CW-mode of generation. Normally, lasers are characterized by the output wavelength (nm or μm), spectral bandwidth (nm), energy characteristics, such as power (mW, W, kW) for CW laser, and energy per pulse (J), pulse width (ns, μs, ms, s), repetition rate (Hz), and average power (mW, W, kW) for pulse lasers. Important practical characteristic of a laser is its efficiency, which is the ratio of the output laser power to the input electrical power of laser pumping and expressed in percentage. In general, lasers with higher efficiency have the smallest size and low cost. There is a huge variety of lasers and laser systems available in the market. Lasers can be classified according to the active media. For example, a gas laser is a laser whose active medium is a gas or mixture of gases. There exist gas, solid, liquid, and semiconductor (diode) lasers. The most popular medical lasers are described below.[14,62,63] Most lasers emit at a particular wavelength (Fig. 1.19). In tunable lasers or laser systems with nonlinear conversion (Fig. 1.20), one can vary the wavelength over some spectral range.

CO_2 laser is a laser whose lasing medium is CO_2 gas with an IR emission from 9.2 to 11.1 μm with the maximal efficiency at 10.6 μm, and a power from a few watts to a few kilowatts. Both CW and pulsed regimes are available. Lasers are tunable in the limits of CO_2 molecules spectral range (from 9.2 to 11.1 μm). CO_2 laser has an efficiency of up to 40%. Because of a high water absorption in this wavelength range, CO_2 laser is mostly used for tissue ablation.

The lasing medium of an excimer laser is an excited molecular complex, an excimer (molecule dimer). Examples of excimer lasers are: ArF laser, 193 nm; KrF laser, 248 nm; XeCl laser, 308 nm; and XeF laser, 351 nm. These lasers are tunable within 10–20 nm. Because of a high tissue absorption and scattering in the UV range, excimer lasers are widely used for eye refractive surgery, psoriasis treatment, and ablation with high precision.

The lasing medium of a dye laser is a liquid dye. Dye lasers emit in a broad spectral range and are tunable. Its wavelengths range is from 340 to 960 nm, at optical frequency doubling from 217 to 380 nm, and at parametric conversion from 1060 to 3100 nm. Its emitted energy is from 1 mJ to 50 J in periodic pulse mode. The mean power is from 0.06 to 20 W. Pulse duration is from several nanoseconds to several microseconds, and pulse frequency from a single pulse to 1 kHz. A train of microsecond pulses can be used to generate millisecond pulses. These lasers are used for spectroscopy and photochemistry of biological molecules. This is one of the best lasers for targeting blood vessels. Therefore, pulsed dye lasers are widely used in dermatology for treating portwine stains (PWSs).

A solid-state laser has an active medium as a matrix of a crystal, glass, or ceramic doped by active ions. Crystal matrices such as sapphire, YAG, alexandrite, yttrium scandium gallium garnet (YSGG), and others are used in lasers. Active ions, such as Nd (neodymium), Cr (chromium), Er (erbium), Ho (holmium), Tm (thulium), in combination with different matrices provide a range of emission wavelengths. For example, Cr^{3+}-doped sapphire (ruby laser) emits at 694 nm, whereas Cr^{3+}-doped alexandrite crystal (alexandrite laser) emits at 755 nm. Solid-state lasers are pumped by optical radiation from a flash (arc) lamp or from the other laser. The efficiency of a flash lamp pumped laser is about 0.1–5%. Pumping with the diode laser increases the efficiency to 10–50%.

Nd:YAG laser is one of the most efficient solid-state lasers whose lasing medium is the crystal Nd:YAG with emission in the NIR at 1064 nm, other emission lines are at 946, 1319, 1335, 1338, 1356, and 1833 nm. The second harmonic (532 nm) and the third harmonic (355 nm) of this laser are also widely used in photomedicine. Both CW and pulsed regimes are available. Typical power of the main harmonic (1064 nm) is from a few watts to a few hundred watts in CW mode. Pulsed lasers are characterized by the high repetition rate of up to 300 Hz. Their pulse duration varies from few nanoseconds to hundred milliseconds, and the pulse energy is between

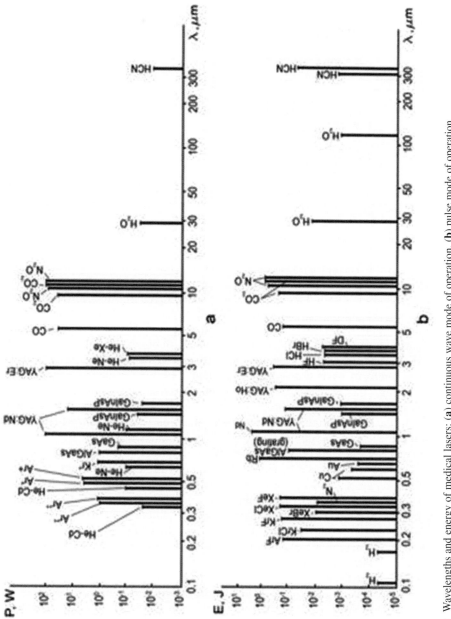

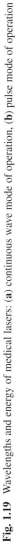

Fig. 1.19 Wavelengths and energy of medical lasers: (**a**) continuous wave mode of operation, (**b**) pulse mode of operation

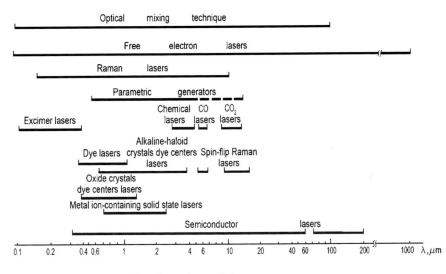

Fig. 1.20 Spectral ranges of tunable coherent light sources

0.05 and 100 J. The pulse power of such lasers can reach several megawatts (MW), and an average power up to 1000 W.

Er:YAG laser is a solid-state laser whose lasing medium is the Er:YAG crystal. Its emission is in MIR region, around 2.79–2.94 μm. It is one of the most effective lasers that are used for ablation of biotissue, including skin. It can be used for hard tissues as well, as its emission wavelength coincides with the strongest absorption band of water (2.94 μm). Typical power range of this laser is from watts to tenths of watts. For miniature systems (a crystal 4 mm in diameter and 75 mm long), the pulse duration is in the microsecond range with the pulse-repetition rate of 25 Hz, pulse energy of a few joules, and average power of a few watts. In the Q-switching regime, the pulse duration is in the nanosecond range with pulse energy of ~100 mJ.

Diode laser is a semiconductor laser. One of the widely used diode lasers is gallium arsenide (GaAs) laser. Its emission is in the NIR, at about 830 nm. To obtain the broad range of emission wavelengths, more complex compositions are available. For example, GaP_xAs_{1-x} lasers emit light from 640 ($x = 0.4$) to 830 nm ($x = 0$). The maximum output power of a single diode laser emitter is in the range from 0.5 to 10 W. High-power diode lasers (laser bars) usually comprise 10–90 single laser emitters. Maximum output power of a diode laser bar is in the range from twenty to several hundred watts. Diode lasers are the most efficient lasers with efficiency up to 70%. The divergence of most diode lasers is in the range from 50° to 90°. Diode laser can work in the CW mode or in the pulsed mode. Diode lasers are often used for pumping other lasers, such as a diode-pumped Nd:YAG, which is an integrated solid-state laser with an Nd:YAG crystal as a lasing medium and optical pumping provided by a single diode lasers or by a diode bars. Table 1.3 summarizes some wavelength related parameters of the lasers that are used in medicine.

Table 1.3 Wavelengths, wave numbers, and quantum energies of some lasers

Laser	λ (nm)	$\tilde{v} \times 10^3$ (cm^{-1})	$hv \times 10^{-19}$ (J)	hv (eV)	$N_A hv$ (kcal/mole)	$hv/k \times 10^3$ (κ)
He–Ne	543.3	18.4	3.65	2.28	52.5	26.3
	632.8	15.8	3.14	1.96	45.0	22.6
	1152.3	8.7	1.72	1.08	24.7	12.4
	3391.2	2.9	0.59	0.37	8.4	4.2
Ar$^+$	351.1	28.5	5.66	3.53	81.2	40.7
	363.8	27.5	5.46	3.41	78.3	39.3
	488.0	20.5	4.07	2.54	58.4	29.3
	514.5	19.4	3.86	2.41	55.4	27.8
Kr$^+$	647.1	15.5	3.07	1.92	44.0	22.1
He–Cd	325.0	30.8	6.11	3.82	87.7	44.0
	441.6	22.6	4.50	2.81	64.5	32.4
CO$_2$	9600	1.0	0.21	0.13	3.0	1.5
	10600	0.9	0.19	0.12	2.7	1.3
CO	5500	1.8	0.36	0.22	5.2	2.6
N$_2$	337.1	29.7	5.89	3.68	84.5	42.4
ArF	193	51.8	10.29	6.42	147.7	74.1
XeCl	308	32.5	6.45	4.03	92.5	46.4
XeF	350	28.6	5.67	3.54	81.4	40.8
Rodamin dye	600	16.7	3.31	2.07	47.5	23.8
Ruby	694.3	14.4	2.86	1.79	41.0	20.6
Nd:YAG	1064	9.4	1.87	1.17	26.8	13.4
Alexandrite	760	13.2	2.61	1.63	37.5	18.8
Ho:YAG	2088	4.8	0.95	0.59	13.6	6.8
Er:YAG	2940	3.4	0.68	0.42	9.7	4.9
LiF $-$ F$_2^+$	1000	10.0	1.99	1.24	28.5	14.3
GaAs	830	12.0	2.39	1.49	34.3	17.2
CH$_3$I	1.25×10^6	8×10^{-3}	1.6×10^{-3}	9.9×10^{-4}	0.2	1.1×10^{-2}

$v = 3 \times 10^{17}/\lambda$, Hz; $\tilde{v} = v/c = 10^7/\lambda$, cm^{-1} $hv = (1986/\lambda) \times 10^{-12}$, erg $= (1986/\lambda) \times 10^{-19}$, $J = 1240/\lambda$, eV; $N_A hv = (28.5/\lambda) \times 10^3$, kcal/mole; $hv/k = (14.3/\lambda) \times 10^6$, κ, where λ is the wavelength (nm), c is the light speed (cm/c), h is the Planck's constant, N_A is the Avogadro's number, and k is the Boltzmann's constant

1.5   Light Applications in Dermatology

1.5.1   Diagnostic

Skin biopsy remains to be the mainstay for diagnosis and occasionally is also used for monitoring treatment response in dermatology. There are currently available optical devices which are used clinically and in research to aid in the noninvasive diagnosis of dermatological diseases, following disease progression and/or treatment effects over time. Interest in skin optics is enhanced with available optical devices, which provide useful information about the physiology, morphology, composition, and perhaps mechanistic and therapeutic responses. Optical spectroscopy, confocal microscopy, polarization imaging (PLI), and OCT will be discussed here.

1.5.1.1   Optical Spectroscopy

Diffuse reflectance spectroscopy has been widely used in dermatology, particularly looking at the hemodynamics of the skin, skin pigmentation, and inflammation. Diffuse reflectance spectroscopy can be used as a tool to quantitatively measure melanin and hemoglobin content of the skin. Reflectance measurements can also be used to provide information about the light scattering properties of the skin. For example, scattering properties can reveal information about the morphology and architecture of the skin such as the arrangement and density of the collagen fibers. In vivo and ex vivo measurements can be done to gather useful information to aid in the assessment and diagnosis of a variety of dermatological conditions. Diffuse reflectance spectroscopy have been used to determine skin hyperpigmentation and hypopigmentation (pigmentation index),[64] inflammation, erythema (erythema index), occlusion, and hemodynamic response (i.e. reactive hyperemia) after occlusion by means of hemoglobin content and oxygen saturation level.[10,65,66] Pre- and post-treatment diagnostics for photochemical and photothermal procedures have also utilized spectroscopic measurements.

1.5.1.2   Confocal Microscopy

The confocal microscope was invented by Marwin Minsky in 1957. Initial experiments were performed in vitro using a bright mercury lamp light source. Following advances in light sources, scanning, and computer technologies, in vivo tissue imaging emerged in the 1980s. In vivo imaging of skin began in the early 1990s. In 1995, confocal laser scanning microscopy was introduced for rapid in vivo imaging of human skin.[67] The laser light utilizes the NIR wavelengths to provide high illumination power and deeper penetration. With this device, high-resolution images at the nuclear and cellular level in vivo with good correlation to conventional histology were achieved.[68] The optical section is oriented parallel to the skin surface. The optical section in confocal microscopy contrasts with the conventional orthogonal sections of histopathology, which are oriented perpendicular to the skin surface. The confocal microscope images a series of parallel planes tacked vertically in depth with a very thin section and high lateral resolution. Melanin is the strongest endogenous contrast source for confocal imaging. The present commercially available confocal laser microscope uses a deeper penetrating NIR wavelength of 830 nm (diode laser) with an illumination power of 1–5 mW. Confocal microscopy is superior to ultrasound scanners and conventional OCT with regard to the resolution. Reflectance mode confocal microscopy offers the highest resolution imaging down to 0.5 μm comparable to routine histology.[69] However, imaging is limited to the superficial dermis due to tissue-induced scattering and aberrations, its depth of penetration to at most 300–400 μm.[70] Imaging of benign and malignant skin conditions have been reported with good histopathological correlations which include psoriasis,[71] irritant contact dermatitis,[72] discoid lupus erythematosus,[73] sebaceous hyperplasia,[74] cherry angioma,[75] actinic keratosis,[76,77] basal cell carcinoma,[7,9] squamous cell carcinoma,[78,79] and melanoma.[80,81] Recently, multimodal reflectance fluorescence and fluorescence polarization confocal detection of skin cancers was reported by Al-Arashi et al.[4] Real-time in vivo imaging offers the advantage of viewing cellular details in human skin safely and rapidly, which aid in the diagnosis and management of several dermatological diseases.

1.5.1.3 Polarization Imaging

PLI is an optical technique that is capable of obtaining superficial images of thick tissue layers. When the light incident on the sample is linearly polarized, subtraction of two images acquired with the copolarized and cross-polarized light can be used to largely isolate the single-scattered component, which arises mainly from superficial skin layers. The advantages of the polarized light imaging include the ability to image comparatively thin tissue layers (~75–200 µm in the visible spectral range) and to retain a large field of view. It is relatively insensitive to small shifts in the position of the imaged object. Combination of the large field-of-view and sufficient lateral resolution enables rapid examination of large surfaces, thus facilitating tumor margin delineation.[5,6,82] It has been shown to successfully discriminate malignant and benign pigmented skin lesions[5,6,82] and to accurately delineate nonmelanoma and melanoma skin cancer margins.[5,6,83–85]

1.5.1.4 Optical Coherence Tomography

OCT was introduced in 1991 and was first demonstrated for cross-sectional retinal imaging. Since then, it has been used by different medical and surgical specialties including dermatology. OCT utilizes NIR light that maps depth-wise reflections from tissue to capture high-resolution, cross-sectional images at the micrometer scale.[86] OCT is an interferometric imaging technique that enables noninvasive, two- to three-dimensional cross-sectional imaging of microstructural morphology in biological tissue in situ. Conventional OCT has a lateral resolution of 10–15 µm, and a field of view covering several millimeters. Depending on the light source used, with emission centered at around 800–1310 nm, the penetration depth ranges from about 0.7 to 1.4 mm.[86–89] Epidermal and dermal layers can be delineated, and skin appendages which include hair follicles and eccrine ducts can be identified.[89–91] Doppler OCT has also emerged as a powerful skin imaging modality capable of demonstrating microvascular blood flow at flow rates as low as 20 µm/s, which is up to approximately 100 times more sensitive than Doppler ultrasound. Applications of this technique can be used to monitor changes in blood flow and vessel structure following laser treatment,[92] PDT, and pharmacological intervention.[70] Birefringence in the skin is attributed to the regular arrangements of collagen fibers in the dermis. Polarization-sensitive OCT is able to quantify and detect changes in the structural integrity of collagen scaffolding, which is demonstrated in thermally damaged skin.[88] New areas of investigation are spectroscopic OCT and OCT elastography. Spectroscopic OCT might serve as a type of "spectroscopic staining" analogous to staining in histology and elasticity imaging, while OCT elastography serves to detect alterations in the elastic modulus of the extracellular tissue matrix as seen in tissue edema, fibrosis, and calcification.

1.5.2   Therapeutic

1.5.2.1   Pigmented Lesions and Tattoos

Pigmented lesions include endogenous (melanin) and exogenous (tattoo particles, carbon, etc.) absorption band of melanin which stretches from UV to NIR region. Melanin is contained in melanosomes, 0.5–1.0 μm in size, with a τ between 70 and 250 ns. Tattoo particles usually range from 0.5 to 100 μm in size, with a τ between 10 and 50 ns. Black tattoo pigments are most responsive to laser treatment. Green, red, yellow, orange, purple, white, and flesh pigments are more resistant to laser treatment. Q-switched lasers in the green, red, and NIR wavelengths have been used to treat a wide variety of pigmented lesions which include lentigines, ephelides, nevus of Ota, and tattoos. Broadband light sources alone or combined treatment with Q-switched lasers have also demonstrated good results on lentigines, ephelides, and acquired bilateral nevus of Ota-like macules (also known as Hori's nevus). Disruption of melanosomes occurs during Q-switched laser treatment, producing a cavitation or shock wave due to the thermal expansion or the temperature gradient across pigmented cells. Tattoos, on the other hand, release fragmented ink particles, and are lost either in an epidermal crust, in the lymphatics, or phagocytosed by melanophages.[58]

1.5.2.2   Vascular Lesions

Hemoglobin, particularly oxyhemoglobin, is the main target for treating vascular lesions. PWS vessels range from 50 to 150 μm with a τ between 0.45 and 50 ms. Other vascular lesions that have shown good results with laser or light treatments include hemangiomas, spider angiomas, telangiectasias, venous lakes, poikiloderma of civatte, and a variety of dermatological conditions involving blood vessel formation. With hemoglobin's absorption peaks at 418, 542, and 577 nm, the light sources in the visible spectrum would be well absorbed at these wavelengths. Lasers and light sources in the blue, green, yellow, red, and NIR spectrum have been used successfully to treat vascular lesions. Pulsed dye lasers (yellow, 585–600 nm) remain to be the gold standard of treatment for PWS, hemangiomas, and telangiectasias. Since epidermal melanin is also absorbed during pulsed dye laser treatment, epidermal cooling is empiric to minimize epidermal damage. The use of long-pulsed alexandrite (755 nm), diode (800 nm), and Nd:YAG (1064 nm) lasers have been used with good results for deeply penetrating PWS lesions, venous lakes, leg veins, and other deeper vascular lesions. With deeper penetrating light sources, aggressive tissue cooling has to be done because of the risk of scarring.

1.5.2.3   Hair Removal

The chromophore for hair removal is the melanin-bearing structures, which include the hair shaft and the matrix cells. The other follicular tissues, which include the stem cells located in the bulb or bulge, around 1.5 mm and 2–7 mm in depth, respectively, do not contain an appreciable amount of any chromophore that absorbs in the red or NIR region. The target structures, which include the bulge and bulb, are damaged by heat diffusion from the hair shaft or matrix cells. Considering the depth of penetration required for hair removal, the most efficient light sources are long-pulsed light sources with optimized epidermal cooling in the red and NIR wavelengths which include the ruby, alexandrite, diode, and Nd:YAG lasers. Broadband light sources such as the IPLs have been used, but usually require more treatment visits.

1.5.2.4   Rejuvenation

Rejuvenation is achieved by both ablative and nonablative means. Carbon dioxide laser (FIR) and erbium laser (MIR) are used in ablative resurfacing. These are high-energy, short-pulsed lasers, which vaporize thin layers of tissue used to treat wrinkles, scars, and superficial lesions. In ablative resurfacing, water is the primary target chromophore. Light sources used for nonablative rejuvenation include the broadband light sources, fractional lasers in the visible and infrared (NIR to MIR) spectrum. Nonablative skin rejuvenation is a noninvasive approach to skin rejuvenation, eliminating the extended recovery period of traditional ablative resurfacing procedures. The nonablative approach primarily targets the subsurface, stimulating a wound healing response in the dermis. Fractional photothermolysis is a new concept in cutaneous remodeling where laser-induced microscopic zones of thermal injury, also known as *microscopic treatment zones*, are surrounded by normal, viable tissue. This unique thermal damage pattern allows tissue reepithelialization in less than 24 h without losing the epidermal barrier function.[93] Although effects are subtle and requires multiple treatments, nonablative rejuvenation has a high patient acceptability and satisfaction. Lasers and broadband light sources in the visible to MIR spectrum that are currently used for rejuvenation are listed in Table 1.4.

1.5.2.5   Acne Vulgaris

Light sources that are used to treat acne vulgaris act by destroying either (1) the sebaceous glands,[94] (2) the entire pilosebaceous unit, or (3) *Propionibacterium*

Table 1.4 Therapeutic applications in dermatology.

Application	Chromophore	Commonly used light devices
Pigmented lesions, tattoos	Melanin, tattoo ink particles	Q-switched Nd:YAG (532, 1064 nm) Q-switched alexandrite (755 nm) Q-switched ruby (694 nm)
Vascular lesions	Hemoglobin	Pulsed KTP (532 nm) Alexandrite (755 nm) Diode (800–980 nm) Nd:YAG (1064–1320 nm) Pulsed light (400–1400 nm)
Hair removal	Melanin (hair shaft)	Alexandrite (755 nm) Diode (800–980 nm) Nd:YAG (1064–1320 nm) Pulsed light (400–1400 nm)
Rejuvenation	Water	
Ablative		Er:YAG (2940 nm) CO_2 (10600 nm)
Nonablative		Pulsed KTP (532 nm) Pulsed dye (585–600 nm) Alexandrite (755 nm) Nd:YAG (1064–1320 nm) Pulsed light (400–1400 nm) Diode (532–1450 nm) Erbium glass (1540 nm) LED (417–880 nm) IR light (1100–1800 nm) Q-switched Nd:YAG (532, 1064 nm) Q-switched ruby (694 nm) RF, monopolar (RF current bipolar) RF, bipolar (RF current bipolar) RF, unipolar (RF EMR)

Ablative/Nonablative		Fractional
		  Diode (532 nm)
		  1320–2940 nm
		  IR light (850–1350 nm)
		  CO_2 (10600 nm)

Acne (*See also PDT*)		Pulsed dye (585–600 nm) Nd:YAG (1064–1320 nm) Diode (808–1450 nm) Erbium glass (1540 nm) Pulsed light (400–1400 nm) Q-switched Nd:YAG (532, 1064 nm) LED (414–880 nm) Blue light (405–420 nm) Red light (660 nm) Fractional CO_2 (10600 nm) RF, monopolar (RF current bipolar)
Psoriasis	Unknown Unknown Unknown Hemoglobin	UVB (280–320 nm); NB-UVB (311–313 nm) UVA (320–400 nm); PUVA Excimer (308 nm) Pulsed dye (585–600 nm)

(continued)

Table 1.4 (continued)

Application	Chromophore	Commonly used light devices
Vitiligo	Unknown	UVB (280–320 nm); NB-UVB (311–313 nm)
	Unknown	UVA (320–400 nm); PUVA
	Unknown	Excimer (308 nm)
	Hemoglobin	Pulsed dye (585–600 nm)
PDT	Photosensitizer	Blue light (417 nm)
		Red light (up to 740 nm)
		Pulsed dye (585–600 nm)
		Pulsed light (400–1400 nm)

Nd: YAG neodymium yttrium aluminum garnet, *KTP* potassium titanyl phosphate, *Er:YAG* erbium-doped yttrium aluminum garnet, CO_2 carbon dioxide, *LED* light-emitting diode, *IR* infrared, *RF* radiofrequency, *EMR* electromagnetic radiation, *NB-UVB* narrowband UVB, *PUVA* psoralen + UVA

acnes (*P. acnes*) through a PDT reaction with protoporphyrin IX (PpIX) and coproporphyrin and/or the addition of topical photosensitizers which include 5-aminolevulinic acid (ALA) and the methyl ester of ALA. As *P. acnes* proliferate, transforming noninflammatory to inflammatory lesions, PpIX and coproporphyrin III are produced. These porphyrins have an absorption in the near-UV and visible spectrum, with major absorption peaks at 415 (Soret band, blue light) and 630 nm (red light). Light devices that are used to treat inflammatory acne vulgaris by destroying the sebaceous glands include the NIR lasers and radiofrequency (RF) devices. Light devices that destroy *P. acnes* bacteria include blue, green, red, yellow, and RF sources. The addition of exogenous photosensitizers (ALA, methyl ester of ALA) with PDT has demonstrated a synergistic effect on the treatment of inflammatory acne vulgaris.[95,96]

1.5.2.6 Photodynamic Therapy

PDT involves a photosensitizer (chromophore), light (at wavelengths absorbed by the chromophore), and molecular oxygen to generate a photochemical reaction. The photosensitizers clinically approved by the US FDA for PDT of various indications are Photofrin, benzoporphyrin derivative (Verteporfin), and ALA. In Europe, methyl aminolevulinate (MAL), the methyl ester of ALA marketed as Metvix®, is currently the drug of choice for PDT. ALA and MAL are not photosensitizers, but are prodrugs that are transformed into a highly photoactive endogenous porphyrin derivative, PpIX via the heme biosynthetic pathway. PpIX can be activated by a blue or red light source for tissue destruction.[73] ALA-PDT has been studied and used successfully for the prevention and treatment of premalignant and non-melanoma skin cancers which include actinic keratosis,[97–100] Bowen's disease (squamous cell carcinoma in situ),[101–110] and superficial basal cell carcinoma.[97,99,100,109–116] PDT is also used for the treatment of cutaneous T-cell lymphoma,[117] acne,[96,118] and photorejuvenation.[119,120] For the treatment of nonmalignant skin conditions, PDT is used for the stimulation of immunomodulatory effects in contrast to the induction of necrosis and apoptosis as produced in the treatment of skin tumors. Other diseases where PDT has been reported to have some improvement were verruca vulgaris,[121,122] condyloma acuminata,[123] sebaceous hyperplasia,[124,125] nevus sebaceous,[126] psoriasis,[121,127–129] squamous cell carcinoma,[100,111,112,114,116] hidradenitis suppurativa,[125] and PWS.[130]

1.5.2.7   Others

Lasers and light sources have been used to treat other dermatological conditions which include psoriasis, vitiligo, precancerous lesions, and nonmelanoma skin cancers.

1.6   Summary

Rapid development and success of photomedicine is determined by the multifaceted variety and specificity of light-skin interactions. In particular, light provides more specific interactions with biological systems as compared to the short-wavelength X-ray and γ-radiation or longer wavelengths radiowaves. The wide variety of interactions of light with biological molecules include, but are not limited to, the dissociation, electronic excitation, vibrational, and rotational excitations. Low-energy photons (FIR, terahertz, and microwaves) may have some selective interaction with biological molecules due to the excitation of rotational levels, mechanical vibrations of molecules, or acoustic vibrations in the cell membranes. However, in general, their action is nonspecific and is related to thermal interaction. Photons of X-rays and shorter wavelengths have extremely high energy that can ionize any biological molecule with similar efficiency. Thus, their interaction with molecules of complex biological matter does not depend on the chemical structure of molecule. Therefore, skin optics is highly dynamic with a multitude of factors contributing to the skin's highly specialized functions. In the epidermis, melanin plays a major chromophore in light absorption, while in the dermis, hemoglobins are the major light absorbers except for the NIR wavelengths, where water and lipids are the major absorbers. The optics of the dermis is dominated by light scattering. In the red and NIR wavelength ranges, the scattering is reduced, enabling deeper light penetration. In the MIR, absorption by water becomes the dominant attenuation mechanism. The least penetrating wavelengths are in the far-UV and FIR regions. Research aimed at understanding skin optics has broadened the clinical applications of lasers and light sources. Real-time, noninvasive, in vivo optical imaging offers the unique advantage of viewing details of the human skin morphology and biochemistry on the subsurface safely and rapidly, which aids in the evaluation, diagnosis, and management of several dermatological diseases. Lasers and light sources for clinical applications are constantly being developed and upgraded to offer safe, efficacious, and innovative treatments. Spectacular advances in technology will improve the depth of penetration, portability, ease of use, and lower the cost of light treatments and devices in dermatology.

Appendix Optical properties of human skin measured ex vivo (standard error values are given in parentheses)

Tissue	λ (nm)	μa (mm^{-1})	$\mu s'$ (mm^{-1})	Effective penetration depth (mm)
Epidermis	370	1.35(0.16)	11.56(1.25)	0.14
	420	1.20(0.12)	9.82(0.99)	0.16
	470	0.84(0.06)	7.96(0.82)	0.21
	488	0.76(0.07)	7.41(0.74)	0.23
	514	0.63(0.07)	6.67(0.66)	0.27
	520	0.60(0.07)	6.51(0.64)	0.28
	570	0.39(0.08)	5.52(0.55)	0.38
	620	0.28(0.07)	4.90(0.47)	0.48
	633	0.26(0.07)	4.76(0.45)	0.51
	670	0.26(0.08)	4.48(0.43)	0.52
	720	0.24(0.07)	4.11(0.39)	0.56
	770	0.19(0.06)	3.79(0.37)	0.66
	820	0.15(0.06)	3.60(0.35)	0.77
	830	0.14(0.06)	3.56(0.35)	0.80
	870	0.10(0.05)	3.41(0.34)	0.97
	920	0.07(0.04)	3.32(0.34)	1.19
	970	0.06(0.03)	3.15(0.34)	1.32
	1020	0.04(0.03)	3.02(0.33)	1.64
	1064	0.02(0.02)	2.97(0.32)	2.38
	1070	0.02(0.02)	2.97(0.32)	2.38
	1120	0.02(0.02)	2.86(0.32)	2.38
	1170	0.06(0.04)	2.71(0.31)	1.41
	1220	0.07(0.04)	2.63(0.31)	1.33
	1270	0.06(0.04)	2.62(0.31)	1.45
	1320	0.11(0.05)	2.53(0.30)	1.08
	1370	0.56(0.14)	2.50(0.31)	0.44
	1420	2.36(0.35)	3.01(0.41)	0.16
	1470	2.96(0.42)	3.08(0.45)	0.14
	1520	1.89(0.29)	2.66(0.39)	0.20
	1570	1.01(0.20)	2.39(0.34)	0.31
Dermis	370	0.98(0.14)	8.76(1.36)	0.19
	420	0.85(0.11)	6.85(0.89)	0.23
	470	0.43(0.06)	5.36(0.60)	0.37
	488	0.36(0.05)	4.90(0.51)	0.42
	514	0.31(0.04)	4.32(0.41)	0.48
	520	0.30(0.04)	4.20(0.39)	0.50
	570	0.22(0.03)	3.50(0.31)	0.64
	620	0.15(0.02)	3.07(0.28)	0.83
	633	0.15(0.02)	2.99(0.27)	0.84
	670	0.15(0.02)	2.78(0.26)	0.87
	720	0.15(0.02)	2.54(0.24)	0.91
	770	0.13(0.02)	2.33(0.24)	1.02
	820	0.11(0.02)	2.18(0.23)	1.15
	830	0.11(0.02)	2.15(0.23)	1.16
	870	0.09(0.02)	2.05(0.22)	1.32
	920	0.08(0.02)	1.99(0.23)	1.43
	970	0.08(0.02)	1.90(0.22)	1.45
	1020	0.07(0.02)	1.84(0.22)	1.59

(continued)

Appendix (continued)

Tissue	λ (nm)	μa (mm^{-1})	$\mu s'$ (mm^{-1})	Effective penetration depth (mm)
	1064	0.05(0.02)	1.80(0.21)	1.89
	1070	0.05(0.02)	1.79(0.21)	1.89
	1120	0.06(0.02)	1.74(0.21)	1.75
	1170	0.12(0.02)	1.69(0.20)	1.23
	1220	0.13(0.02)	1.65(0.20)	1.20
	1270	0.10(0.02)	1.63(0.20)	1.39
	1320	0.15(0.03)	1.61(0.19)	1.12
	1370	0.48(0.04)	1.66(0.19)	0.57
	1420	1.76(0.18)	2.03(0.21)	0.22
	1470	2.19(0.20)	2.13(0.21)	0.19
	1520	1.41(0.11)	1.87(0.20)	0.27
	1570	0.85(0.07)	1.65(0.19)	0.40
	370	1.18(0.21)	5.27(0.69)	0.21
	420	1.65(0.33)	4.59(0.59)	0.18
	470	0.75(0.09)	3.92(0.50)	0.31
	488	0.63(0.08)	3.69(0.47)	0.35
	514	0.47(0.07)	3.37(0.43)	0.43
	520	0.44(0.07)	3.31(0.42)	0.45
	570	0.31(0.09)	2.89(0.36)	0.58
	620	0.15(0.03)	2.59(0.31)	0.90
	633	0.14(0.03)	2.54(0.30)	0.94
	670	0.13(0.03)	2.40(0.27)	1.01
	720	0.12(0.02)	2.22(0.24)	1.09
	770	0.11(0.02)	2.07(0.21)	1.18
	820	0.10(0.02)	1.98(0.20)	1.27
	830	0.10(0.02)	1.96(0.20)	1.27
	870	0.09(0.02)	1.89(0.19)	1.37
	920	0.09(0.02)	1.81(0.18)	1.39
	970	0.09(0.03)	1.76(0.18)	1.41
	1020	0.08(0.02)	1.72(0.16)	1.52
	1064	0.07(0.02)	1.69(0.15)	1.64
	1070	0.07(0.02)	1.68(0.15)	1.64
	1120	0.08(0.02)	1.65(0.15)	1.56
	1170	0.14(0.03)	1.63(0.15)	1.16
	1220	0.15(0.03)	1.61(0.15)	1.12
	1270	0.10(0.03)	1.59(0.14)	1.41
	1320	0.12(0.03)	1.58(0.14)	1.28
	1370	0.27(0.04)	1.60(0.15)	0.81
	1420	0.93(0.14)	1.77(0.18)	0.36
	1470	1.08(0.18)	1.81(0.19)	0.33
	1520	0.70(0.12)	1.70(0.17)	0.45
	1570	0.43(0.07)	1.60(0.16)	0.62
Infiltrative basal cell carcinoma	370	0.68(0.08)	6.52(0.92)	0.26
	420	0.67(0.11)	5.89(0.52)	0.28
	470	0.33(0.04)	4.88(0.36)	0.44
	488	0.29(0.05)	4.50(0.33)	0.49
	514	0.26(0.06)	4.04(0.30)	0.55
	520	0.25(0.06)	3.95(0.30)	0.56
	570	0.20(0.07)	3.33(0.28)	0.68

(continued)

Appendix (continued)

Tissue	λ (nm)	μa (mm^{-1})	$\mu s'$ (mm^{-1})	Effective penetration depth (mm)
	620	0.15(0.06)	2.90(0.28)	0.85
	633	0.15(0.05)	2.81(0.28)	0.87
	670	0.14(0.05)	2.59(0.28)	0.93
	720	0.13(0.05)	2.35(0.28)	1.02
	770	0.11(0.04)	2.12(0.26)	1.16
	820	0.09(0.04)	1.96(0.25)	1.35
	830	0.09(0.04)	1.92(0.25)	1.35
	870	0.07(0.03)	1.80(0.24)	1.59
	920	0.06(0.03)	1.66(0.20)	1.79
	970	0.08(0.03)	1.50(0.15)	1.61
	1020	0.07(0.03)	1.36(0.11)	1.82
	1064	0.08(0.04)	1.26(0.09)	1.75
	1070	0.08(0.04)	1.25(0.09)	1.75
	1120	0.10(0.06)	1.19(0.09)	1.61
	1170	0.16(0.07)	1.15(0.09)	1.27
	1220	0.17(0.09)	1.09(0.10)	1.25
	1270	0.18(0.12)	1.05(0.11)	1.22
	1320	0.27(0.15)	1.04(0.10)	0.97
	1370	0.69(0.27)	1.09(0.10)	0.52
	1420	2.21(0.46)	1.54(0.25)	0.20
	1470	2.75(0.54)	1.66(0.32)	0.17
	1520	1.90(0.47)	1.33(0.27)	0.23
	1570	1.12(0.31)	1.11(0.16)	0.36
Nodular basal cell carcinoma	370	0.87(0.29)	4.62(0.61)	0.26
	420	0.73(0.20)	4.36(0.38)	0.30
	470	0.40(0.12)	3.85(0.22)	0.44
	488	0.34(0.12)	3.60(0.20)	0.50
	514	0.28(0.11)	3.27(0.18)	0.58
	520	0.27(0.11)	3.20(0.18)	0.60
	570	0.18(0.09)	2.71(0.16)	0.80
	620	0.13(0.06)	2.34(0.13)	1.02
	633	0.12(0.06)	2.27(0.12)	1.08
	670	0.09(0.05)	2.07(0.11)	1.32
	720	0.07(0.04)	1.84(0.10)	1.59
	770	0.04(0.03)	1.66(0.09)	2.22
	820	0.02(0.02)	1.52(0.07)	3.33
	830	0.02(0.01)	1.49(0.07)	3.33
	870	0.01(0.01)	1.40(0.07)	4.76
	920	0.01(0.00)	1.31(0.06)	5.00
	970	0.01(0.01)	1.25(0.06)	5.26
	1020	0.00(0.00)	1.20(0.06)	–
	1064	0.00(0.00)	1.16(0.06)	–
	1070	0.00(0.00)	1.15(0.06)	–
	1120	0.00(0.00)	1.09(0.05)	–
	1170	0.01(0.01)	1.04(0.04)	5.56
	1220	0.02(0.01)	1.01(0.04)	4.00
	1270	0.01(0.01)	1.00(0.04)	5.88
	1320	0.05(0.01)	0.97(0.04)	2.56
	1370	0.32(0.03)	1.03(0.06)	0.88

(continued)

Appendix   (continued)

Tissue	λ (nm)	μa (mm^{-1})	$\mu s'$ (mm^{-1})	Effective penetration depth (mm)
	1420	1.46(0.20)	1.44(0.13)	0.28
	1470	1.86(0.16)	1.59(0.15)	0.23
	1520	1.19(0.07)	1.31(0.10)	0.33
	1570	0.67(0.04)	1.06(0.08)	0.54
Squamous cell carcinoma	370	0.94(0.20)	4.36(0.61)	0.26
	420	1.21(0.23)	4.21(0.50)	0.23
	470	0.41(0.06)	3.38(0.47)	0.46
	488	0.34(0.05)	3.13(0.43)	0.53
	514	0.32(0.04)	2.80(0.39)	0.58
	520	0.32(0.04)	2.74(0.38)	0.58
	570	0.29(0.04)	2.35(0.32)	0.66
	620	0.14(0.02)	1.95(0.26)	1.06
	633	0.13(0.02)	1.88(0.25)	1.12
	670	0.11(0.02)	1.71(0.23)	1.30
	720	0.09(0.02)	1.52(0.20)	1.52
	770	0.07(0.02)	1.35(0.18)	1.82
	820	0.05(0.02)	1.24(0.16)	2.27
	830	0.05(0.02)	1.22(0.15)	2.27
	870	0.04(0.01)	1.16(0.14)	2.63
	920	0.03(0.01)	1.09(0.13)	3.13
	970	0.04(0.02)	1.02(0.12)	2.78
	1020	0.04(0.02)	0.94(0.12)	2.94
	1064	0.04(0.02)	0.88(0.12)	3.03
	1070	0.04(0.02)	0.88(0.12)	3.03
	1120	0.04(0.02)	0.85(0.12)	3.03
	1170	0.10(0.03)	0.84(0.11)	1.89
	1220	0.11(0.03)	0.81(0.11)	1.82
	1270	0.11(0.03)	0.78(0.11)	1.85
	1320	0.17(0.04)	0.77(0.11)	1.45
	1370	0.43(0.05)	0.85(0.11)	0.78
	1420	1.70(0.12)	1.29(0.18)	0.26
	1470	2.35(0.21)	1.44(0.23)	0.19
	1520	1.50(0.15)	1.16(0.16)	0.29
	1570	0.92(0.12)	0.92(0.13)	0.44

References

1. Mueller GJ, Sliney DH, eds. *Dosimetry of Laser Radiation in Medicine and Biology*, SPIE Inst. Advanced Opt. Techn. IS5, Bellingham, WA: SPIE Press; 1989.
2. Anderson RR, Parrish JA. The optics of human skin. *J Invest Dermatol*. 1981;77:13–19.
3. Jobsis FF. Noninvasive, infrared monitoring of cerebral and myocardial oxygen sufficiency and circulatory parameters. *Science*. 1977;198:1264–1267.
4. Al-Arashi MY, Salomatina E, Yaroslavsky AN. Multimodal confocal microscopy for diagnosing nonmelanoma skin cancers. *Lasers Surg Med*. 2007;39:696–705.
5. Yaroslavsky AN, Neel V, Anderson RR. Demarcation of nonmelanoma skin cancer margins in thick excisions using multispectral polarized light imaging. *J Invest Dermatol*. 2003;121:259–266.

6. Yaroslavsky AN, Neel V, Anderson RR. Fluorescence polarization imaging for delineating nonmelanoma skin cancers. *Opt Lett.* 2004;29:2010–2012.
7. Gonzalez S, Tannous Z. Real-time, in vivo confocal reflectance microscopy of basal cell carcinoma. *J Am Acad Dermatol.* 2002;47:869–874.
8. Marghoob AA, Charles CA, Busam KJ, et al. In vivo confocal scanning laser microscopy of a series of congenital melanocytic nevi suggestive of having developed malignant melanoma. *Arch Dermatol.* 2005;141:1401–1412.
9. Nori S, Rius-Diaz F, Cuevas J, et al. Sensitivity and specificity of reflectance-mode confocal microscopy for in vivo diagnosis of basal cell carcinoma: a multicenter study. *J Am Acad Dermatol.* 2004;51:923–930.
10. Zonios G, Bykowski J, Kollias N. Skin melanin, hemoglobin, and light scattering properties can be quantitatively assessed in vivo using diffuse reflectance spectroscopy. *J Invest Dermatol.* 2001;117:1452–1457.
11. Brancaleon L, Durkin AJ, Tu JH, Menaker G, Fallon JD, Kollias N. In vivo fluorescence spectroscopy of nonmelanoma skin cancer. *Photochem Photobiol.* 2001;73:178–183.
12. Lakowic JR. *Principles of Fluorescence Spectroscopy.* New York: Plenum Press; 1983.
13. Schubert EF. *Light-Emitting Diodes.* Cambridge: Cambridge University Press; 2003.
14. Tuchin VV. Lasers and fiber optics in biomedicine. *Laser Physics.* 1993;3:767–820, 925-950.
15. Tuchin VV. *Tissue Optics: Light Scattering Methods and Instruments for Medical Diagnosis.* Vol. TT38, Tutorial texts in optical engineering. Bellingham, WA: SPIE Press; 2000:352 p.
16. Ishimaru A. *Wave Propagation and Scattering in Random Media.* New York: Academic Press; 1978;1:66.
17. Bashkatov AA, Genina EA, Kochubey VI, Tuchin VV. Optical properties of human skin, subcutaneous and mucous tissues in the wavelength range from 400 to 2000 nm. *J Phys D Appl Phys.* 2005;15:2543–2555.
18. Graaff R, Dassel ACM, Koelink MH, de Mul FFM, Aarnoudse JG, Zijistra WG. Optical properties of human dermis in vitro and in vivo. *Appl Opt.* 1993;32:435–447.
19. Jacques SL, Alter CA, Prahl SA. Angular dependence of HeNe laser light scattering by human dermis. *Lasers Life Sci.* 1987;1:309–334.
20. Marchesini R, Bertoni A, Andreola S, Melloni E, Sichirollo AE. Extinction and absorption coefficients and scattering phase functions of human tissues in vitro. *Appl Opt.* 1989;28:2318–2324
21. Muller G, Roggan A, eds. *Laser-Induced Interstitial Thermotherapy.* Bellingham, WA: SPIE Press; 1995.
22. Peters VG, Wyman DR, Patterson MS, Frank GL. Optical properties of normal and diseased human breast tissues in the visible and near infrared. *Phys Med Biol.* 1990;35:1317–1314.
23. Prahl S. Light transport in tissue, PhD dissertation. University of Texas at Austin; 1988.
24. Salomatina E, Jiang B, Novak J, Yaroslavsky AN. Optical properties of normal and cancerous human skin in the visible and near-infrared spectral range. *J Biomed Opt.* 2006;11:064026.
25. Simpson CR, Kohl M, Essenpreis M, Cope M. Near-infrared optical properties of ex vivo human skin and subcutaneous tissues measured using the Monte Carlo inversion technique. *Phys Med Biol.* 1998;43:2465–2478.
26. Troy TL, Thennadil SN. Optical properties of human skin in the near infrared wavelength range of 1000 to 2200 nm. *J Biomed Opt.* 2001;6:167–176.
27. van Gemert MJ, Jacques SL, Sterenborg HJ, Star WM. Skin optics. *IEEE Trans Biomed Eng.* 1989;36:1146–1154.
28. Wan S, Anderson RR, Parrish JA. Analytical modeling for the optical properties of the skin with in vitro and in vivo applications. *Photochem Photobiol.* 1981;34:493–499.
29. Bolin FP, Preuss LE, Taylor RC, Ference RJ. Refractive index of some mammalian tissues using a fiber optic cladding method. *Appl Opt.* 1989;28:2297–2303.
30. Kollias N, Baqer A. Spectroscopic characteristics of human melanin in vivo. *J Invest Dermatol.* 1985;85:38–42.
31. Kollias N, Baqer A. On the assessment of melanin in human skin in vivo. *Photochem Photobiol.* 1986;43:49–54.

32. Konig K, Ruck A, Scheckenburger H. Fluorescence detection and photodynamic activity of endogenous protoporphyrin in human skin. *Opt Eng*. 1997;31:1470–1474.

33. Prahl S. www.omlc.ogi.edu

34. Sinichkin YP, Utz SR, Mavliutov AH, Pilipenko HA. In vivo fluorescence spectroscopy of the human skin: experiments and models. *J Biomed Opt*. 1998;3:201–211.

35. Tuchin VV, ed. *Handbook of Optical Biomedical Diagnostics*. Vol PM107. Bellingham, WA: SPIE Press; 2002.

36. Hannemann RE, Dewitt DP, Hanley EJ, Schreiner RL, Bonderman P. Determination of serum bilirubin by skin reflectance: effect of pigmentation. *Pediatr Res*. 1979;13:1326–1329.

37. Vitkin IA, Woolsey J, Wilson BC, Anderson RR. Optical and thermal characterization of natural (Sepia officinalis) melanin. *Photochem Photobiol*. 1994;59:455–462.

38. Zijistra WG, Buursma A, Meeuwsen-van der Roest WP. Absorption spectra of human fetal and adult oxyhemoglobin, de-oxyhemoglobin, carboxyhemoglobin, and methemoglobin. *Clin Chem*. 1991;37:1633–1638.

39. Kuenstner JT, Norris KH. Spectrophotometry of human hemoglobin in the near infrared region from 1000 to 2500 nm. *J Near Infrared Spectroscopy*. 1994;2:59–65.

40. Barton JK, Frangineas G, Pummer H, Black JF. Cooperative phenomena in two-pulse, two-color laser photocoagulation of cutaneous blood vessels. *Photochem Photobiol*. 2001;73:642–650.

41. Yang MU, Yaroslavsky AN, Farinelli WA, et al. Long-pulsed neodymium:yttrium-aluminum-garnet laser treatment for port-wine stains. *J Am Acad Dermatol*. 2005;52:480–490.

42. Black JF, Barton JK. Chemical and structural changes in blood undergoing laser photocoagulation. *Photochem Photobiol*. 2004;80:89–97.

43. Anderson RR, Farinelli W, Laubach H, et al. Selective photothermolysis of lipid-rich tissues: a free electron laser study. *Lasers Surg Med*. 2006;38:913–919.

44. Kollias N, Gillies R, Moran M, Kochevar IE, Anderson RR. Endogenous skin fluorescence includes bands that may serve as quantitative markers of aging and photoaging. *J Invest Dermatol*. 1998;111:776–780.

45. Parrish JA, Deutsch TF. Laser photomedicine. *IEEE J Quant Electron*. 1984;QE-20:1386–1396.

46. Anderson RR, Parrish JA. Selective photothermolysis: precise microsurgery by selective absorption of pulsed radiation. *Science*. 1983;220:524–527.

47. Gay-Crosier F, Polla LL, Tschopp J, Schifferli JA. Complement activation by pulsed tunable dye laser in normal skin and hemangioma. *J Invest Dermatol*. 1990;94:426–431.

48. Greenwald J, Rosen S, Anderson RR, et al. Comparative histological studies of the tunable dye (at 577 nm) laser and argon laser: the specific vascular effects of the dye laser. *J Invest Dermatol*. 1981;77:305–310.

49. Paul BS, Anderson RR, Jarve J, Parrish JA. The effect of temperature and other factors on selective microvascular damage caused by pulsed dye laser. *J Invest Dermatol*. 1983;81:333–336.

50. Welch AJ. The thermal response to laser irradiated tissue. *IEEE J Quant Electron*. 1984;QE-20:1471–1481.

51. Altshuler GB, Anderson RR, Manstein D, Zenzie HH, Smirnov MZ. Extended theory of selective photothermolysis. *Lasers Surg Med*. 2001;29:416–432.

52. Akiyama M, Smith LT, Shimizu H. Changing patterns of localization of putative stem cells in developing human hair follicles. *J Invest Dermatol*. 2000;114:321–327.

53. Cotsarelis G, Sun TT, Lavker RM. Label-retaining cells reside in the bulge area of pilosebaceous unit: implications for follicular stem cells, hair cycle, and skin carcinogenesis. *Cell*. 1990;61:1329–1337.

54. Lyle S, Christofidou-Solomidou M, Liu Y, Elder DE, Albelda S, Cotsarelis G. Human hair follicle bulge cells are biochemically distinct and possess an epithelial stem cell phenotype. *J Investig Dermatol Symp Proc*. 1999;4:296–301.

55. Neumann RA, Knobler RM, Leonhartsberger H, Gebhart W. Comparative histochemistry of port-wine stains after copper vapor laser (578 nm) and argon laser treatment. *J Invest Dermatol*. 1992;99:160–167.

56. van Gemert MJ, Welch AJ, Amin AP Is there an optimal laser treatment for port wine stains. *Lasers Surg Med.* 1986;6:76–83.

57. Anderson RR, Margolis RJ, Watenabe S, Flotte T, Hruza GJ, Dover JS. Selective photothermolysis of cutaneous pigmentation by Q-switched Nd:YAG laser pulses at 1064, 532, and 355 nm. *J Invest Dermatol.* 1989;93:28–32.

58. Taylor CR, Anderson RR, Gange RW, Michaud NA, Flotte TJ. Light and electron microscopic analysis of tattoos treated by Q-switched ruby laser. *J Invest Dermatol.* 1991;97:131–136.

59. Garden JM, Tan OT, Kerschmann R, et al. Effect of dye laser pulse duration on selective cutaneous vascular injury. *J Invest Dermatol.* 1986;87:653–657.

60. Oleinick NL, Morris RL, Belichenko I. The role of apoptosis in response to photodynamic therapy: what, where, why, and how. *Photochem Photobiol Sci.* 2002;1:1–21.

61. Yang MF, Baron ED. Update on the immunology of UV and visible radiation therapy: phototherapy, photochemotherapy and photodynamic therapy. *Expert Rev Dermatol.* 2008;3:85–98.

62. Altshuler GB, Tuchin VV. Physics behind the light-based technology: skin and hair follicle interactions with light in light-based systems for cosmetic application, ed. Gurpreet Ahluwalia, William Andrew, Inc., Norwich, NY, USA, 2008.

63. Splinter R, Hooper BA. *An Introduction to Biomedical Optics.* New York, London: Taylor & Francis; 2007.

64. Gniadecka M, Wulf HC, Mortensen NN, Poulsen T. Photoprotection in vitiligo and normal skin. A quantitative assessment of the role of stratum corneum, viable epidermis and pigmentation. *Acta Derm Venereol.* 1996;76:429–432.

65. Merschbrock U, Hoffmann J, Caspary L, Huber J, Schmickaly U, Lubbers DW. Fast wavelength scanning reflectance spectrophotometer for noninvasive determination of hemoglobin oxygenation in human skin. *Int J Microcirc Clin Exp.* 1994;14:274–281.

66. Svaasand LO, Norvang LT, Fiskerstrand EJ, Stopps EKS, Berns MW, Nelson JS. Tissue parameters determining the visual appearance of normal skin and port-wine stains. *Lasers Med Sci.* 1995;10:55–65.

67. Rajadhyaksha M, Anderson RR, Webb RH. Video-rate confocal scanning laser microscope for imaging human tissues in vivo. *Appl Opt.* 1999;38:2105–2115.

68. Rajadhyaksha M, Grossman M, Esterowitz D, Webb RH, Anderson RR. In vivo confocal scanning laser microscopy of human skin: melanin provides strong contrast. *J Invest Dermatol.* 1995;104:946–952.

69. Neerken S, Lucassen GW, Bisschop MA, Lenderink E, Nuijs TA. Characterization of age-related effects in human skin: a comparative study that applies confocal laser scanning microscopy and optical coherence tomography. *J Biomed Opt.* 2004;9:274–281.

70. Gambichler T, Moussa G, Sand M, Sand D, Altmeyer P, Hoffmann K. Applications of optical coherence tomography in dermatology. *J Dermatol Sci.* 2005;40:85–94.

71. Gonzalez S, Rajadhyaksha M, Rubinstein G, Anderson RR. Characterization of psoriasis in vivo by reflectance confocal microscopy. *J Med.* 1999;30:337–356.

72. Astner S, Burnett N, Rius-Diaz F, Doukas AG, Gonzalez S, Gonzalez E. Irritant contact dermatitis induced by a common household irritant: a noninvasive evaluation of ethnic variability in skin response. *J Am Acad Dermatol.* 2006;54:458–465.

73. Ardigo M, Maliszewski I, Cota C, et al. Preliminary evaluation of in vivo reflectance confocal microscopy features of Discoid lupus erythematosus. *Br J Dermatol.* 2007;156:1196–1203.

74. Aghassi D, Gonzalez E, Anderson RR, Rajadhyaksha M, Gonzalez S. Elucidating the pulsed-dye laser treatment of sebaceous hyperplasia in vivo with real-time confocal scanning laser microscopy. *J Am Acad Dermatol.* 2000;43:49–53.

75. Aghassi D, Anderson RR, Gonzalez S. Time-sequence histologic imaging of laser-treated cherry angiomas with in vivo confocal microscopy. *J Am Acad Dermatol.* 2000;43:37–41.

76. Aghassi D, Anderson RR, Gonzalez S. Confocal laser microscopic imaging of actinic keratoses in vivo: a preliminary report. *J Am Acad Dermatol.* 2000;43:42–48.

77. Ulrich C, Busch JO, Meyer T, et al. Successful treatment of multiple actinic keratoses in organ transplant patients with topical 5% imiquimod: a report of six cases. *Br J Dermatol.* 2006;155:451–454.

122. Stender IM, Na R, Fogh H, Gluud C, Wulf HC. Photodynamic therapy with 5-aminolae-vulinic acid or placebo for recalcitrant foot and hand warts: randomised double-blind trial. *Lancet.* 2000;355:963–966.
123. Frank RG, Bos JD. Photodynamic therapy for condylomata acuminata with local application of 5-aminolevulinic acid. *Genitourin Med.* 1996;72:70–71.
124. Gold MH, Bradshaw VL, Boring MM, Bridges TM, Biron JA, Lewis TL. Treatment of seba-ceous gland hyperplasia by photodynamic therapy with 5-aminolevulinic acid and a blue light source or intense pulsed light source. *J Drugs Dermatol.* 2004;3:S6–S9.
125. Rivard J, Ozog D. Henry Ford Hospital dermatology experience with Levulan Kerastick and blue light photodynamic therapy. *J Drugs Dermatol.* 2006;5:556–561.
126. Dierickx CC, Goldenhersh M, Dwyer P, Stratigos A, Mihm M, Anderson RR. Photodynamic therapy for nevus sebaceus with topical delta-aminolevulinic acid. *Arch Dermatol.* 1999;135:637–640.
127. Boehncke WH, Konig K, Kaufmann R, Scheffold W, Prummer O, Sterry W. Photodynamic therapy in psoriasis: suppression of cytokine production in vitro and recording of fluores-cence modification during treatment in vivo. *Arch Dermatol Res.* 1994;286:300–303.
128. Boehncke WH, Sterry W, Kaufmann R. Treatment of psoriasis by topical photodynamic therapy with polychromatic light. *Lancet.* 1994;343:801.
129. Tandon YK, Yang MF, Baron ED. Role of photodynamic therapy in psoriasis: a brief review. *Photodermatol Photoimmunol Photomed.* 2008;24:222–230.
130. Nelson JS, McCullough JL, Berns MW. Principles and applications of photodynamic therapy in dermatology. In: Arndt KA, Dover JS, Olbricht SM, eds. *Lasers in Cutaneous and Aesthetic Surgery.* Philadelphia, PA: Lippincott-Raven Publishers; 1997:349–382.

Chapter 2
Photoaging in Skin of Color

Mary F. Bennett and Kevin D. Cooper

2.1 Introduction

Chronological (intrinsic) aging is that associated with the passage of time and a consequent decline in biological functions. This form of aging has a signature in the skin, evident clinically as fine wrinkling and/or skin laxity. Photoaging occurs concurrently with chronological aging but only on sun-exposed sites, and is induced by repeated exposure to ultraviolet (UV) radiation. Chronically, sun-exposed skin has distinctive changes including coarse wrinkles, dyspigmentation, telangiectasias, and a propensity to develop precancerous lesions and subsequent skin cancer. Anecdotally, people of skin of color tend to "age better" than their white counterparts. At the same age, people with black skin are thought to have fewer wrinkles compared to those with lighter skin.[1] Differences in the structure and physiology of skin of color may account for observed differences in incidence and presentation of photoaging in people of color. In darker skin, the melanosomes are larger, more oval, and nonaggregated and along with a higher total melanin content, may confer an increased natural photoprotection from UV radiation.[2]

Studies exist to support the observation of decreased signs of aging in skin of color; however, evidence is hampered by the multitude of confounding factors that play a role in aging of the skin, including dietary intake and exposure to environmental toxins, such as smoking. Indeed, the primary environmental insult to the skin, UV radiation, is extremely difficult to match when studying different populations, confounded by differing latitude and sun exposure habits.

Demographic changes in westernized countries, including increasing life span and ethnic diversity, mean that photoaging in skin of color will become of greater relevance to a larger segment of the population than ever before. The age of the population is increasing rapidly. It is estimated that by the year 2040, over 30% of the US population will be older than 55 years old, over twice the current level.[3] The American population

M.F. Bennett (✉) and K.D. Cooper
Department of Dermatology, Veterans Affairs Medical Center, University Hospitals Case Medical Center and Case Western Reserve University, Cleveland, OH, USA
e-mail: marybennett@physicians.ie

E.D. Baron (ed.), *Light-Based Therapies for Skin of Color,*
DOI: 10.1007/978-1-84882-328-0_2, © Springer-Verlag London Limited 2009

classified as white will decrease from 75% to less than 50% by the year 2050, Hispanics and Latinos will constitute 25%, African-Americans 14%, and Asians 8% of the population.[4] This is likely to include a growing number of cosmetic concerns associated with photoaging in people with darker skin, whose complaints will differ from those of white patients. In general, white patients seek cosmetic procedures most frequently to reduce the signs of aging, that is, wrinkles, whereas African-Americans are more frequently concerned with dyschromic pigmentation.[5]

Habits such as sun-protective behavior may be culturally determined. What constitutes beauty is influenced by ethnic and cultural patterns. In the 1920s, a tanned complexion became desirable for white Caucasians but this trend did not follow in all cultures. In fact, attempts to lighten the skin tone in Asia and Africa has led to several cases of excessive use of inappropriate agents.[6] Asian women often avoid sun exposure to achieve a pale complexion.[7] With diversification of the American standard of beauty to include ethnic features comes a proliferation of products and services marketed toward the ethnic population wishing to enhance, not mask, these distinctive features.[8] Also differential skin care needs dictate preferences for different vehicles across skin types among other parameters.[9]

Our knowledge of the process of photoaging in the skin has greatly expanded with an intense interest in the area of prevention and treatment, not only for the purposes of cosmesis but also in the development of skin cancer. In white skin, wrinkling and telangiectasia are associated with increased risk of actinic keratosis and nonmelanoma skin cancers (age adjusted odd ratio, 2–9) (Fig. 2.1).[10-12] The presence of actinic keratoses is strongly associated with an increased risk of squamous cell carcinoma (SCC).[13] Skin cancer, although traditionally felt to be uncommon in people of skin of color, has a distinctive pattern of expression in certain ethnic groups. Risk factors associated with skin cancer are different in darker-skinned individuals, and although UV radiation is not always implicated, it still plays a role in many skin cancers seen, particularly in those with lighter complexions. The dermatologist needs to be cognizant of these patterns, and study of the risk factors associated with cancer development may lead to greater insights into the process of carcinogenesis. Skin cancer, in particular melanoma, presents late in African-Americans and Hispanics, who are less likely to perform self-skin examinations.[14-17]

Once melanoma is diagnosed in a patient or their family member, African-Americans do not adopt significant sunscreen use, whereas Mexican Americans adopt sunscreen habits similar to that of Caucasians (Summers and Cooper, in preparation). Thus, a concerted and ethnically tailored effort needs to be made to educate people with skin of color on the prevention and detection of skin cancer.

2.2   Pathophysiology of Photoaging

Aging of the skin is a function of the combined effects of genetics and the environment. The most important environmental inducer of skin aging is UV radiation. The main clinically relevant components, UVA and UVB, exert distinct effects on the skin. The contribution of each to aging is the cause of much debate. Traditionally,

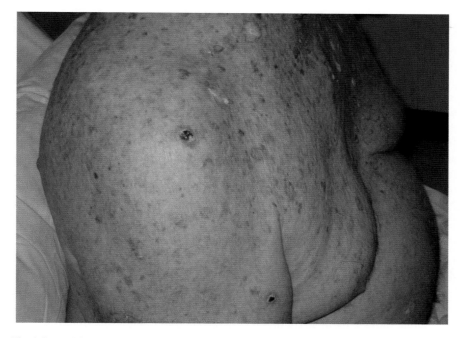

Fig. 2.1 Actinic keratoses and nonmelanoma skin cancers on a Caucasian male who had significant sun exposure in the past

UVA is felt to induce pigmentation and UVB causes sunburn predominantly but both are involved in the production of reactive oxygen species (ROS) and cellular damage. UVB absorption by DNA causes cross-linking of adjacent pyrimidines, whereas UVA chromophores transfer energy to oxygen to generate ROS, which oxidize cellular components including DNA, proteins, and lipids. UVB (290–320 nm) penetrates the epidermis and induces in DNA damaging both the keratinocytes and the melanocytes, leading to the release of soluble products into the dermis. UVA (320–400 nm) penetrates more deeply and has direct effects on both the epidermis and the dermis. Given the known association between UVA and pigmentation, it may be theorized that UVA is an important factor in the dyschromia associated with photoaging in skin of color.

Although chronological and photoaging produce a distinct clinical picture, the two processes share many fundamental molecular pathways.[18] Cellular changes occur that alter the balance between synthesis and degradation of structural proteins in the skin, reducing its strength and resiliency. UV radiation leads to a broad activation of cell surface growth factor and cytokine receptors, inducing many downstream signaling pathways, which converge on the transcription factor AP-1. AP-1 regulates the expression of many matrix metalloproteinases (MMPs) and type I procollagen. Chronological aging is also associated with increased AP-1 activity, increased MMP expression, impaired TGF-β signaling, enhanced collagen degradation, and decreased collagen synthesis. In chronological aging, ROS are thought to cause an accumulation of cellular damage. The production of ROS following UV irradiation of the skin has been well documented and again intrinsic and photoaging converge to alter gene and protein expression and function leading to the photoaged phenotype.

In skin of color, larger melanin granules are present throughout the epidermis and thus impede the penetration of UV photons through to the nuclei of basal layer keratinocytes and beyond. Only a small fraction of photons penetrates into the dermis leading to connective tissue damage and vascular ectasia. It is perhaps this responsive, labile nature of protective melanin production that can lead to dyschromia in these skin types and indeed, pigmentary change is a documented feature of photoaged skin in people of color. Increased levels of melanogenesis genes [e.g. tyrosinase (TYR), dopachrome tautomerase] and alterations in the epidermal–melanin axis and Factor XIIIa melanophages have been shown to be present in UV-induced solar lentigines ("age" or "liver spots").[19–22]

2.2.1 UV-Induced Damage to Cellular Genetic Components

DNA may directly absorb UVB, resulting in DNA photoproducts, cyclobutane pyrimidine dimers, particularly thymine dimers and pyrimidine (4–6) pyrimidone photoproducts. UVA can also generate thymine dimers.[23,24] These DNA changes are constantly repaired by nucleotide excision repair.[25] Signature C to T and CC to TT mutations occur in UV photodamage when repair is incomplete. ROS generated by UV (*see* Sect. 2.2.5) also induce characteristic mutations through 8-hydroxyguanine, during replication G:C to T:A transversions, by pairing of adenine, instead of cytosine.[26] These are primarily repaired by the base excision repair system. Dermal fibroblasts in elderly subjects have been shown to have decreased transcripts of DNA repair synthesis-related genes.[27] This reduced capacity of DNA repair seen in aging may be associated with accumulation of UV-induced abnormalities leading to the photodamage phenotype.

If genomic damage is extensive, p53 acting as "the guardian of the genome," and its associated proteins induce apoptosis of keratinocytes. p53 mutations may occur following UV irradiation, thus this genome checkpoint is lost and clonal expansion of irradiated, mutated keratinocytes may give rise to actinic keratoses.[28] If a second p53 allele is mutated, SCC will arise. DNA photodamage is undoubtedly implicated in skin carinogenesis, but it also triggers many molecular responses such as release of cytokines, activation of inflammatory responses, apoptosis, and pigmentation which contribute to clinically evident photoaging.

2.2.1.1 Telomeres

Telomeres are tandem repeats of a short sequence, accounting for several thousand base pairs at the end of chromosomes.[29] They serve to protect regulatory sequences and proximal genes. They have been termed the cell's "biological clock" preventing indefinite serial divisions of cells and thus are likely to have an anticancer effect.[30] Research over the last decade has established a central role for the telomere in maintaining genomic integrity. Telomere disruption, whether due to acute DNA damage or progressive telomere shortening, is the initial event that triggers multiple DNA damage responses. Telomeres are normally in a loop configuration with the double-stranded chromosome folded back on itself[31] and the loop secured by insertion of the 3' overhang into the proximal double-stranded DNA where it is held in place by binding proteins, notably telomere repeat factor 2.[32] Acute DNA damage, such as UV irradiation with production of photoproducts, distorts the telomere loop and exposes the TTAGGG repeat sequence. Tandem repeats of TTAGGG can be provided as a signal in the absence of DNA damage by exogenously provided telomere homologue oligonucleotides, "T-oligos."[33] Both cultured human melanocytes and intact guinea pig skin have been shown to respond to thymidine dinucleotide pTT (the thymine dimers that account for approximately 75% of all UV-induced DNA damage) treatment with dramatic increases in melanin production, precisely mimicking UV-induced tanning clinically and histologically.[34] pTT is able to induce photoprotective tanning and increase DNA repair capacity at least in part via the p53 signaling pathway.[35] Treatment of mammalian cells with T-oligos also initiates signaling through the ATM (ataxia telangiectasia-mutated), ATR (ATM-related, Sickle cell), and/or DNA-PK kinases, which in turn activates p53 and other effector proteins.[36] T-oligo treatment at low dose and/or short duration results in reversible cell cycle arrest, often with evidence of adaptive differentiation, such as enhanced melanogenesis in pigment cells, whereas higher doses or longer duration of therapy may push cells to the same cell-type-specific biological endpoints of apoptosis or senescence as observed after serial cell passage, acute DNA damage, or experimental telomere loop disruption.[37]

A Japanese study showed that telomere lengths in the epidermis and in the dermis was reduced with age, and average telomere shortening rates in the epidermis and in the dermis were 9 and 11 base pairs pear year, respectively. Unexpectedly, telomere length was not significantly different between epidermis from sun-exposed sites and from sun-protected sites, and hence, they were unable to show that telomere shortening is associated with photoaging of the skin.[38]

2.2.1.2 Mitochondrial DNA

Mitochondria are the main energy source that generates ATP through oxidative phosphorylation in mammalian cells.[39] The mitochondrial respiratory chain is the major source of intracellular ROS and free radicals. Each mitochondrion contains multiple copies of mitochondrial DNA (mtDNA), which codes for 13 polypeptides which form the respiratory enzyme complexes required for normal functioning of the oxidative phosphorylation system.[39] A wide spectrum of alterations in the mito-chondria and mtDNA is associated with chronological aging, including increased production of ROS, accumulation of point mutations in mtDNA, decline in mitochondrial respiratory function, and so on. Photoaged skin has been shown to exhibit mutations in mtDNA.[40-42] A common 4977 bp deletion has been shown to be increased by tenfold in photoaged skin.[43] Repeated sublethal doses of UVA to cultured primary human dermal fibroblasts have also been shown to induce mutations in mtDNA.[44] In vivo studies have shown that 2 weeks of repeated UVA exposure leads to an increase in the level of this common mutation by approximately 40% and that these changes persisted for at least 16 months postirradiation.[45] ROS induce further mtDNA mutations exacerbating ROS production. This chronic cellular damage due to mitochondrial dysfunction has been termed as the "defective powerhouse model" with the formation of a vicious cycle of inadequate energy production and chronic oxidative stress.[46]

2.2.2   Connective Tissue Remodeling

The hallmark changes that occur in photoaged skin are found in the connective tissue. In photoaged skin, collagen fibrils are abnormal and elastotic material accumulates.[47] The dermis becomes strikingly filled with an amorphous mass of deranged elastic tissue with a grenz zone in the superficial papillary dermis due to decreased volume of collagen bundles. Collagen type I and III are reduced and elastin is increased.[48,49] Oxidative stress results in a dose-related increase (up to 1.8-fold) in the level of elastin mRNA in cultured human dermal fibroblasts, accounting for elastotic changes seen in the photo-aged dermis.[50] In chronically photodamaged skin, collagen synthesis is downregulated compared with photoprotected skin.[51] This may be related to the fact that fibroblasts from photoaged skin show less interaction with intact collagen.[52] The induction of MMPs has been shown to follow UV irradiation and is an important factor in the observed connective tissue changes. MMPs are a group of zinc-dependent endopepti-dases capable of degrading the extracellular framework of the skin. MMP-1 initiates the cleavage of fibrillar collagen types I and III in the dermis, which is then further degraded by MMP-2 and -9.[53] UVB has been shown to induce the production of MMP-1, -3, -9 in normal human epidermis and UVA induces MMP-1 expression in dermal fibroblasts.[53-55] Solar irradiation may exacerbate chronological aging by further increasing elevated levels of MMPs in aged skin, confounded further by decreased levels of tissue inhibitors of metalloproteases.[56] In vivo comparison between lightly pigmented subjects and darkly pigmented subjects revealed that twice the UV expo-sure in lightly skinned individuals produced only modest MMP-1 mRNA expression induction and DNA photoproducts in the darkly pigmented group.[57] Not unexpectedly, DNA photoproducts in the lightly pigmented group were observed in cells throughout the layers of the epidermis and in the upper dermis. Whereas, in the darkly pigmented group, the modest level of increase in photoproducts was seen in the postmitotic cells of the upper epidermis, owing to the attenuation of UV penetration by melanin.

2.2.3 Vascular Changes

Clinically photoaged skin shows vascular changes in the form of telangiectasias, whereas chronologically aged skin does not. Comparison of the photoaged, dermal vasculature in different skin colors does not exist to date. A diminution of the cutaneous microvasculature occurs with age with a consequent decline in nutritional support for older skin.[58-60] Altered architecture of the dermal vascular plexus occurs due to vascular obliteration in photoaged skin in contrast to intrinsically aged skin.[58,61] In mildly photodamaged skin, there is thickening of the venule walls. In the severe form, there is thinning of the vessel walls and perivascular veil cells are reduced in number.[62] In a study of Korean adults, it was shown that in photoaged skin, there is a progressive loss of dermal blood vessels associated with a reduction in vessel size, especially in the upper dermis, features that do not occur in sun-protected skin.[63] Intrinsically aged skin did show significantly reduced average vessel size, possibly accounting for the pallor, decreased temperature, and reduced UV-induced erythema seen in aged skin.[63]

UVB radiation causes an acute upregulation of proangiogenic and proinflammatory mediators, including vascular endothelial growth factor (VEGF), with increased vascular permeability, activation of proteases, degradation of extracellular matrix molecules, vascular proliferation, and influx of inflammatory cells. Several angiogenic factors including VEGF, basic fibroblast growth factor (b-FGF), and interleukin-8 (IL-8) are upregulated after acute UVB irradiation of the skin.[64-66] The expression of the angiogenesis inhibitor, thrombospondin-1, is downregulated by UVB irradiation, contributing to the angiogenic switch and the creation of a proangiogenic environment.[67] Hence, it is felt that pro-angiogenic factors are involved in acute and subacute UV damage and the absence of normally present angiogenesis inhibitors results in enhanced dermal photodamage.[68,69]

In transgenic mice that overexpress VEGF, a 10-week course of irradiation with a subthreshold dose of UVB, resulted in the formation of cutaneous wrinkles and in the classical features of chronically UVB-damaged skin.[70] These features included epidermal hyperplasia, degradation of collagen and elastic fibers within the dermis, and inflammatory cell infiltration. Transgenic overexpression of thrombospondin 1 in the mouse epidermis reduced dermal damage, wrinkle formation, and angiogenesis after chronic UVB irradiation.[68]

2.2.4 Chronic Inflammation

UV radiation is a potent inducer of the inflammatory response designed to protect the skin from damage. Local defenses are brought into play, with the infiltration and activation of myeloid monocytic cells and macrophages (Mphs), for the "cleanup" of UV-induced apoptotic cells and cells displaying photooxidation. However, the immune system, the protector of the skin, may in actuality be promoting aging through the generation of ROS and UV-induced immunosuppression.[71] Chronic solar damage may result in chronic infiltrates that derive from repeated cycles of leukocytic infiltration after each acute exposure. Chronically sun-exposed skin contains more infiltrating mononuclear cells than sun-protected skin.[72] In contrast to the infiltrate present in the skin shortly after acute UV, chronically sun-exposed dermis shows an increased number of mast cells, Mphs, and CD4+ CD45RO+ T cells and in sun-exposed epidermis, higher numbers of CD1a+ dendritic cells.[72] The population of cells that influx into skin 6–72 h post-UV irradiation of human skin are myeloid monocytic cells, many of which undergo differentiation into activated Mphs.[73,74] These cells are a major source of IL-10 but fail to secrete IL-12, and play a critical role in the UV-induced immune suppression and tolerance,[75] including migration to regional lymph nodes, where they modify the T-cell sensitization environment by altering the cytokine milieu.[76] Activated Mph may be needed to phagocytose UV-induced apoptotic cells, and their production of IL-10 may help to modulate inflammation and prevent autoimmunity. These cells likely represent a blood-derived population of newly infiltrating monocytic cells that undergo transient arrest from dendritic cell differentiation with concomitant promotion of differentiation toward phagocytic, activated Mph.[75-79] When complement C3 is converted into iC3b, it induces ligation of the monocytes' β2-integrin receptors, thus, transforming CD11b+ monocytic cells into activated Mph with the consequent generation of MMPs and ROS.[80] Langerhan's cells (LCs) move to the draining lymph nodes immediately following UV damage, but within a few hours, the main antigen presenting cell that carries antigen to the draining lymph node is the tolerance-inducing, IL-10 high, IL-12 low, monocytic/macrophagic population that was activated through CD11b and other UV-induced skin cytokines critical for immunosuppression, such as IL-6.[76,81] Although the immune system is poised to defend our skin from environmental insults, cumulative damage occurs not only due the oxidative effects of UV but also due to the oxidative milieu generated by inflammatory cells. Resultant immunosuppression may also contribute to the increased propensity of photoaged skin to developed skin cancers due to decreased tumor surveillance.

2.2.5 *Reactive Oxygen Species*

ROS are implicated in the aging process and this fact has been utilized by the cosmetic industry with the marketing of an array of antioxidant products aimed at countering the effects of aging. ROS are highly reactive molecules that include singlet oxygen (O_2), superoxide (O_2^-), hydrogen peroxide (H_2O_2), and hydroxyl radical ($HO^•$). They strongly attract electrons from DNA, cell membranes, and proteins, which leads to damage of those components. Protein, carbohydrate, lipid, and DNA oxidation occur. Lipid peroxidation causes loss of integrity of the cellular membrane with leakage of cellular components and ultimately cell death. The skin is particularly vulnerable to lipid damage, being rich in unsaturated fatty acids. The damage done by free radicals contributes to aging. Both chronological and photo-aging generate free radicals either through the process of oxidative metabolism or through UV radiation.[82] Additionally, the respiratory burst of infiltrating polymor-phonuclear leucocytes and Mphs, following UV exposure, contributes to ROS production. DNA damage can be incurred indirectly through the generation of ROS, following either UVB or UVA, and this includes mtDNA mutations, generat-ing a vicious cycle.[44,83]

Repeated doses of UV radiation (UVA and UVB) to fibroblasts in culture causes an increase in oxidized proteins, which has been shown to occur in vivo also. ROS can modify proteins in tissue to form carbonyl derivatives.[84] These carbonyls accu-mulate in the papillary dermis of photodamaged skin as demonstrated by increase in oxidatively modified proteins in the skin, particularly the upper dermis, in skin biopsies demonstrating solar elastosis.[85] The proteosome is responsible for the deg-radation of oxidized proteins in the cell and its function declines with age, resulting in the accumulation of these oxidized proteins.

Proteomic profiles of immortalized kerationcytes in response to UV alone, dini-trobenzenesulfonic acid (DNBS) alone, and combined exposures showed a marked upregulation of memberane NOX5 (a potent producer of ROS), redox proteins, and cytosolic calmodulin (which functions as a switch in response to oxidative stress) when cells were treated with the immunosuppressive sequence of UV followed by an antigen (DNBS), but not with either agent alone.[86] These data are indicative of overwhelmed oxidative defenses. Thus, further evidence that there are at least two sources of ROS following exposure to UV irradiation: direct photon-induced ROS from lipid and other macromolecule photophysical interactions, and keratinocyte or fibroblast production of ROS.

2.2.6 UV-Induced Melanogenesis

Aging results in a decline in functional melanocytes in both the skin and the hair. The number to dopa-positive melanoctyes decreases with age by approximately 10–20% per decade.[87,88] The decrease in melanocytes occurs in both sun-exposed and sun-protected areas. Paradoxically, pigmentation is a feature of chronically sun-exposed skin, possibly explained by the greater functional activity in older melano-cytes after years of cumulative sun exposure.[89] With long-term sun exposure, the density of melanocytes increases and is about twice as high as sun-protected sites.[89]

UV induces pigmentation in the skin through a myriad of intracellular signals. UV increases the transcription of the TYR gene and the function of MC1-R on melanocytes. Keratinocyte and melanocyte proopiomelanocortin expression and its derivative peptides are increased. A range of UV-induced cytokines are produced by keratinocytes, including b-FGF, nerve growth factor, endothelin-1 (ET-1), and the proopiomelanocortin-derived peptides, MSH, ACTD, β-LPH, and β-endorphin. These act to stimulate melanocyte mitosis, increase melanogenesis, enhance melanocyte dendricity, and prevent apoptosis.[90] UV also induces nitric oxide production and increases cGMP. Inflammatory mediators formed during UV exposure such as leukotriene C1 stimulate growth of melanocytes and modifications in the normal melanocyte phenotype.[91] Telomere changes, as discussed in Sect. 2.2.1.1, including selective excision of thymidine oligonucleotides during the repair of UV-induced DNA photoproducts, have been shown to stimulate melanogenesis in mammalian pigment cells and intact skin, mimicking the direct effect of UV.[92] This mechanism may be through the activation of p53 and protein kinase cascades.[93,94]

Interesting studies, documenting the expression profiles of solar lentigines, have increased our insight into the changes in melanogenesis associated with photoaging.[95] There is a twofold increase in TYR-positive cells per length of dermoepidermal interface in solar lentigos compared to unaffected skin.[19] ET-1 and stem cell factor (SCF) are key regulators in the development of hyperpigmentation in solar lentigos.[96,97] Exposure to UV results in an increased secretion of ET-1 from keratinocytes, which stimulates melanin production by melanocytes, via signaling through PKC and MAPK. SCF, which is also produced by keratinocytes, binds to c-kit receptors on melanocytes and thus activates intrinsic tyrosine kinase activity.[98,99] Keratinocytes in solar lentigos are able to produce significantly more ET-1 than those in perilesional unaffected skin and ET receptor mRNA is increased in the lentigo.[19,100] The ET-1-inducible cytokine, tumor necrosis factor-α, is also consistently upregulated in lesional solar lentigo epidermis.[19] Solar lentigos have increased transcript and protein levels of SCF in the epidermis, as the membrane-bound form.[20] The number of melanophages in the dermis of solar lentigos has been shown to be increased compared to unaffected skin.[21]

Although UV increases expression of melanogenic genes similarly in skin of different racial/ethnic groups,[101] there are significant differences including melanin redistribution, protection against DNA damage, and induction of apoptosis in melanin-containing keratinocytes.[102-104]

2.3 Histological Features of Photoaged Skin

Distinct histological characteristics are evident in photoaged skin compared to skin subject to chronological aging only.[60] Most studies that have catalogued these differences were done in white skin, where differences are most dramatic. In intrinsic aging, there is both epidermal and dermal atrophy, with flattening (loss of undulation) of the dermoepidermal junction. Epidermal atrophy occurs due to the reduction of keratinocytes in the rete ridges, as well as melanocytes and LCs. Dermal atrophy is attributed to loss of fibroblasts, elastic fibers, vasculature, and appendages. In adults, the amount of collagen decreases by 1% per year due to decreased collagen synthesis and increased collagenase mRNA.[104,105] A loss of elastic fibers occurs with fragmentation of elastin fibers. The loss of skin appendages is due to a decrease in the number of hair follicles and in eccrine and apocrine gland size. There is also a decrease in the number of melanocytes in the hair bulb.

In contrast to sun-protected epidermis, epidermal thickness is increased in sun-exposed skin.[106] The stratum corneum of photodamaged skin is compact and laminated.[107] The transition between the stratum lucidum and the stratum corneum is often indistinct.[107] The stratum lucidum is thicker compared with normal epidermis, with two or more cell layers. In the epidermis, there is increased cell heterogeneity, vacuolization, dysplasia, and necrosis.[107] The epidermis contains intercellular and intracellular vacuoles in the basal and spinous layers. Fewer LCs are present in severely photodamaged skin compared with normal skin.[107]

Increased collagen fragments are also a prominent feature in photodamaged skin. Procollagen gene and protein expression are significantly reduced in the upper one-third of the dermis, reflecting UV penetrance.[49] In photoaged dermis, large quantities of abnormal, thickened, tangled, and nonfunctional elastic fibers are seen, which eventually degenerate into a nonfibrous, amorphous mass, a finding known histologically as solar elastosis.[108] In areas with enlarged, knotted, elastic fibers and rounded elastotic masses, fragmentation of fibers is found. The lower papillary and upper intermediate dermis of sun-exposed skin have numerous reticulin fibers accompanying the fibers of the elastotic masses.

In regard to pigmentary changes, in both photoaged and normal skin, basal and suprabasal keratinocytes contain more melanosomes.[107] In darkly pigmented areas of the skin, melanosomes are present through all the cellular layers of the epidermis, including corneocytes.[107]

Several investigators have evaluated the histological changes associated with photodamaged skin in diverse racial groups, utilizing various techniques.[107,109-112] A number of features that are found on skin biopsies of photodamaged white skin are not present in black skin, reflecting the clinical phenotype. Asian skin with actinic damage has more features in common with white skin, and in one study of Asians from Thailand, similarities were noted between white and Asian skin.[110] In a small study of sun-exposed skin of 19 African-American and 19 white women, it was reported that, after long-term sun exposure, striking racial differences are present in the skin of whites and African-Americans.[112] The epidermis of African-American skin showed only minor changes compared with the profound alterations that occurred in white skin. The epidermis was entirely normal histologically in most of the African-American women, with a limited few containing vacuoles and with dyskeratosis in the malpighian layer. In contrast, white epidermis was substantially altered, with many focal areas of atrophy and/or necrosis present. Only one of the 19 African-American women had mild epidermal atrophy. In unexposed skin, white and black, the stratum lucidum consisted of one or two thin layers. In photodamaged white skin, the stratum lucidum had increased cell layers. However, the stratum lucidum in African-American skin remained unaltered and compact.

In this study, the entire epidermis of photoaged African-Americans contained melanosomes in both the younger and older age groups. In white photodamaged skin, only a few melanosomes were seen in the basal layer. Melanophages in African-American photoaged dermis were more numerous and larger than that in white dermis.

African-American photoaged dermis contained close stacking of the small collagen bundles, running parallel to the surface of the epidermis. In white skin, collagen fibers were diffuse and many fragments were present in the dermal interstices.

Solar elastosis was not observed in the specimens of any of the African-American subjects. In white skin, variable amounts of moderate-to-extensive elastosis were observed with more elastic fibers in the dermis compared with African-American skin. In the reticular dermis of older African-American subjects, there was an increase in the number and thickness of elastic fibers. Thicker braid-like configurations of elastin were seen in African-Americans over 50 years of age.

A study of photodamage in 61 Asian women of Thai descent, with skin type IV, revealed epidermal atrophy, atypia, and dysplasia.[110] Basal layer keratinocytes contained dense clusters of highly melanized melanosomes. There was an overall increase in melanin in the keratinocytes. Numerous large, melanophages were identified in the dermis in most women. Moreover, marked elastosis presenting as twisted fibers in various stages of amorphous degeneration were noted.

Although this data is useful, few large-scale studies have been done to assess these histological differences and additionally, there is a complete lack of data in other ethnic groups, that is those of Hispanic, Native American, Asian-Indian origin, etc, reflecting the paucity of clinical data on the features of photoaging in other skin colors.

2.4   Clinical Features of Photoaged Skin

The changes that occur at a molecular and histological level, following chronic UV exposure, are evidenced clinically by wrinkles and solar lentigines; these are accentuated in the habitually exposed skin of the face and backs of the hands. The clinical characteristics of photoaged skin are more pronounced compared with those observed in intrinsic aging and as a result, the actinic changes are often of cosmetic concern to many individuals. In intrinsic aging, the skin has a pale appearance with fine wrinkling. This is due to the fact that the dermis thins by 20% with intrinsic aging, with greatest thinning occurring after 70 years of age. [60,113] Melanocytes also decrease during adulthood, with an estimated decrease of 10% per decade.[89]

All skin, including skin of color, is subject to the effects of intrinsic aging such as thinning of the epidermis, flattening of the dermoepidermal junction, and reduction of extracellular matrix components.[114,115] The impact of chronic sun exposure leading to photoaging, although attenuated in skin of color, undoubtedly contributes to the signs of aging, not only in subjects with white skin but also in Asian and African-American subjects.[1,5,110,116-119]

Natural pigmentation of the skin influences the manifestations of photoaging. The protective nature of melanin retards the photoaging process, with signs occurring at a later age in African-American subjects than in white subjects.[5] But it is this responsive nature of the pigmentary system in people with skin of color that leads to the manifestation of increased pigment irregularities in both black and Asian subjects compared to white subjects.[1,117,118] In intrinsically aged skin, pigmentary changes are not prominent, compared with photoaged skin. UV is the classic environmental agent that produces pigmentary abnormalities, whereas although pollution and smoking contribute to aging; resulting in wrinkling, pigmentation is not a feature. There are several different manifestations of pigmentary alterations associated with photoaged skin. These include mottled hyperpigmentation, solar lentigines, diffuse hyperpigmentation, pigmented seborrheic keratoses, and guttate hypopigmentation (idiopathic guttate hypomelanosis).[120] There are differences in the presentation of photodamage between and within racial groups, forming a spectrum of findings with most changes seen in lighter-skinned individuals.

Coarse wrinkling occurs in photoexposed areas in skin of color. Matrix degradation triggered by solar radiation causes the wrinkled phenotype, including facial wrinkles, and loss of volume with cheek sagging.[55,121] Well-defined furrows occur around the neck due to solar elastosis, a condition termed cutis rhomboidalis nuchae.

Although skin cancer is less common in people of skin of color than in whites, there is now a trend toward increased skin cancer rates in most ethnic groups. UV radiation is often not implicated in patients of color presenting with SCC and melanomas, as they tend to occur on nonexposed sites. However, UV is a definite etiological factor in basal cell carcinomas (BCCs) in all ethnic groups and UV becomes of increasing relevance, particularly in fair-skinned Asians and Hispanics with actinic damage.[14] Increased skin cancer rates can be attributed to childhood sun exposure, increased outdoor recreational activities, and destruction of the ozone layer. It is important to remember that people of color usually have higher morbidity and mortality rates for several types of skin cancer as compared with their white counterparts. This is probably secondary to late presentation and treatment and clinicians should focus on preventative measures, screening, and earlier diagnosis in these patients.

2.4.1 African-American Skin

Given the photoprotective effect of melanin, African-Americans display fewer changes associated with photoaging than white individuals. On the average, five times as much UV light (UVB and UVA) reaches the upper dermis of Caucasians as reaches that of blacks.[122] Melanin acts as a neutral density filter, reducing all wavelengths of light equally. The superior photoprotection of black epidermis is due not only to increased melanin content but also to other factors related to packaging and distribution of melanosomes. As a result of these qualities, the onset of photoaging occurs at a later age in African-Americans compared to whites and may not appear until the fifth or sixth decade.[1,5] Nonetheless, photoaging is still seen, especially in lighter-skinned individuals.[1]

The most frequently encountered manifestation of photoaging in African-Americans includes fine wrinkling, skin textural changes, benign cutaneous growths, and pigmentary abnormalities.[123]

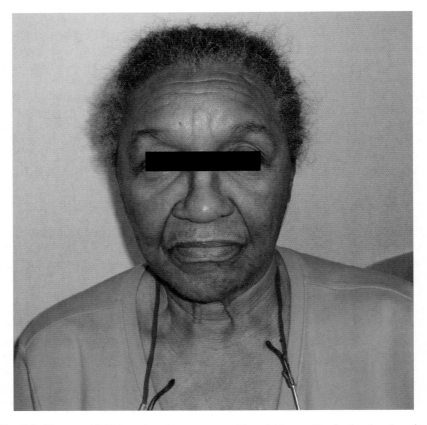

Fig. 2.2 82 year old African-American women with wrinkles on the forehead and neck and prominence of the nasolabial folds, but lateral canthal wrinkles and fine wrinkling are not a feature. Some generalized hyperpigmentation of the face and neck is present with lighter pigmentation on the anterior chest secondary to photoprotection

Patterns of wrinkling have been shown to be somewhat different in African-Americans, with wrinkling beside the lateral canthi of the eyes and at the corners of the mouth occurring less often when compared to whites of a similar age (Fig. 2.2).[112] There is a slower loss of dermal volume in the facial skin of young and middle-aged African-American women than in white women at that age, who tend to have more prominent facial sagging (Fig. 2.3).[112]

Pigment dyschromia is the most common reason for African-Americans to seek cosmetic procedures.[5] Pigment abnormalities due to actinic damage may present as focal areas of hyperpigmentation, either mottled or more confluent, resulting in an uneven skin tone, which is a common concern for African-American women. Solar lentigines are not a feature of African-American photoaging in general but a diffuse darkening of the facial skin can occur, compared with sun-protected areas.

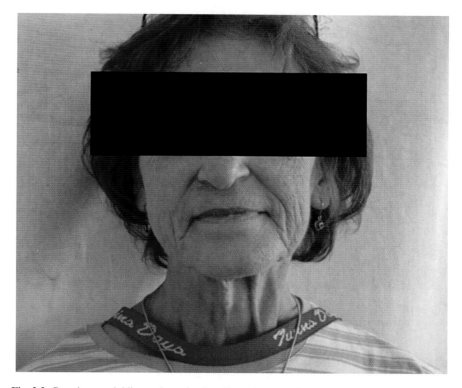

Fig. 2.3 Prominent wrinkling and sagging in a Caucasian woman who had significant sun exposure

Guttate hypomelanosis (also known as disseminate lenticular leukoderma) is another clinical entity seen in photoaging in African-Americans, and is characterized by multiple, small, depigmented macules on the anterior surface of the legs, lower abdomen, and arms (Fig. 2.4).[124,125] The macules are circular with well-defined borders. The differential diagnosis in this group would include vitiligo. Histologically, there is a decrease in pigment granules. Ultrastructural studies have shown a loss of melanocytes lacking mature melanosomes.[126]

Benign pigmented lesions are commonly found in skin of color patients, with 61% having ten or more seborrheic keratoses in one study.[127] Seborrheic keratoses can occur on sun-exposed as well as sun-protected areas and the reticulated seborrheic keratosis is the form most often found on sun-exposed skin. These lesions are papillomatous epithelial proliferations containing horn cysts without any tendency toward malignancy. Seborrheic keratoses are less common in populations with dark skin compared to those having white skin; however, black individuals develop a variant of seborrheic keratoses termed dermatosis papulosa nigra. These lesions affect the face, especially the upper cheeks and lateral orbital areas (malar regions), as well as the neck (Fig. 2.5). They are small, pedunculated, and heavily pigmented papules with a minimal keratotic element. The onset of these lesions generally is

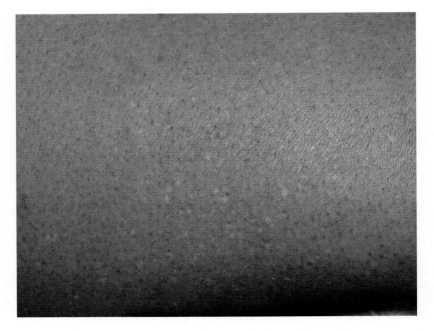

Fig. 2.4 Idiopathic guttate hypomelanosis (depigmented macules) on the upper arm of an African-American patient

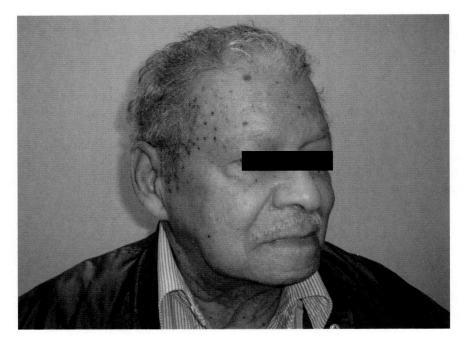

Fig. 2.5 80 year old African American male with multiple seborrheic keratoses on photoexposed areas, forming a pattern consistent with dermatitis papulosa nigra on the malar areas

earlier than that of ordinary seborrheic keratoses, being present in about 5% of black people in the tenth decade, rising to over 40% by the third.[128] These lesions appear to be caused by a nevoid developmental defect of the pilosebaceous follicles. Histologically, they show irregular acanthosis and hyperkeratosis.[128]

The average natural sun-protective factor of African-American skin is approximately 13.4,[122] making sun-induced skin cancers less prevalent. SCC is the most common cutaneous malignancy in African-Americans at 30% of total skin cancers in this group.[14,129-131] SCC mostly occurs on sun-protected sites, anogenital areas, legs, and feet suggesting distinct causative factors other than UV radiation, for instance scarring or chronic inflammation often precedes SCC formation.[116,129,132-136]

The prevalence of BCC in African-Americans averages 1–2% per year.[129,132] BCC is primarily related to long-term intensive UV exposure and this is the case for all skin colors.[14] Other risk factors in African-Americans include albinism, scars, ulcers, chronic infections, sebaceous nevus, arsenic ingestion, immunosuppression, previous radiation, xeroderma pigmentosum, and trauma.[14] Some studies have shown an association with BCC in African-Americans with other malignancies. Transurocanic acid, which is a photoreceptor in the skin, involved in UV immunosuppression, has been found to be at higher concentrations in African-Americans and may, in part, explain the observed phenomenon of increased frequency of second malignancies seen in patients with BCCs.[137] A subset of African Americans demonstrate immunosuppression from UV exposure; these subjects correlate with those in whom redness can be induced in the skin by UV exposure.[138] (Selgrade et al); whether this trait correlates with cancer risk or photoaging risk is unknown.

Over 90% of melanomas occur in sun-exposed skin in the white population.[139] About 67% of melanomas in people of color arise in non-sun-exposed areas (i.e. palmar, plantar, subungal, and mucosal) without exhibiting usual risk factors associated in white people;[140] therefore, UV radiation is felt to be less important as an etiological agent in theses cases.[130] African-Americans have an incidence of malignant melanoma 5–18 times less than whites.[139] The acral lentiginous form of melanoma was once thought to be found more commonly in African-Americans than whites, but in more recent studies, there was no significant difference found.[141] Lenitigo maligna melanoma is very rare in African-Americans, although it has been described on the face.[142] Early detection and recognition are key steps in the improvement of prognosis of African-Americans with melanoma.

2.4.2   Asian Skin

The population of Asia is more than half the total population of the Earth. The people of Asia are primarily of Mongolian extraction, this includes the people of China, Japan, and Korea. These three countries account for one-fourth of the world's population.[143] For the purpose of clarity, the people of Central Asia and India (who are Caucasian but with brown skin) and Pacific Islanders are excluded from this discussion.

In contrast to other skin colors, there is substantial data on photoaging in Asians. Many authors define pigmentary change as the primary manifestation of photodamage in Asians, rather than wrinkles but more and more studies are also documenting the presence and patterns of wrinkle formation.[144-146] Relative pigmentation between subjects may be an important variable in the study of aging Asian skin. In a study of 404 Chinese females, skin phototyping showed the predominant skin type to be type III (71.4%), followed by type II and then type IV, but some studies in Asian patients have shown that constitutive skin color does not always correlate with skin response to UV radiation.[147,148]

In a study of 1,500 people from China, Indonesia, and Malaysia of skin types III and IV, hyperpigmentation was found to be an early and prominent feature of photoaging.[145] Coarse and fine wrinkling came later and was more inconspicuous. Wrinkling and dyspigmentation were the primary characteristics of photodamage in 407 Koreans between the ages of 30 and 92 years.[118] Dyspigmentation was of two types: hyperpigmented macules on sun-exposed skin and pigmented seborrheic keratoses. In those over 60 years of age, seborrheic keratoses were more common in men than women. Pigmented macules were more common in women at 50 years and older. A direct correlation with UV irradiation was shown, with wrinkling present in 19.2% of Koreans with a daily exposure of 1–2 h per day, compared with 64.6% of those that had more than 5 h per day. Smoking was also shown to multiply this risk. In another study of Koreans (40–70 years of age), men were found to have seborrheic keratoses on sun-exposed skin, with the majority on the face and dorsa of hands and the prevalence increased with age. Both chronological aging and cumulative sun exposure were independent variables for the development of seborrheic keratoses.[149] Figure 2.6 is an example of seborrheic keratoses on the neck of an elderly Asian woman.

Comparing Japanese ($n = 258$) versus French ($n = 280$) women, pigment spots were found to occur at higher grades and earlier in life in Japanese women than French. However, wrinkles including expression lines on the forehead, frown lines, crow's feet, wrinkles under the eyes, and wrinkles on the upper lip were more pronounced at an earlier age in French women than in Japanese women.[150] Figure 2.7 shows some pigmentation and mild fine wrinkling on the cheek of an elderly Asian woman.

Nonmelanoma skin cancer is relatively uncommon in Asians. The incidence of BCC, SCC, and Bowen's disease in the Japanese population in Kauai, Hawaii is 12, 4, and 11 times lower, respectively. than whites in the area.[151] But those rates are at least 45 times higher than for Japanese in Japan.[151] More intense UV radiation and greater outdoor activities may account for this. The incidence of actinic keratoses, a premalignant form of SCC, in Japan is approximately 414 per 100,000, with a sharp increase from 1987 to 1996.[152-154] This may reflect a more westernized lifestyle with vacations to sunny climates.[151] Suzuki et al found that the presence of seborrheic keratoses may be a risk factor for actinic keratoses among Japanese.[153]

The incidences of BCCs in Asians per 100,000 population have been reported as follows: Chinese men (6.4), Chinese women (5.8), Japanese (15–16.5), Japanese residents of Kauai, Hawaii (29.7), Japanese residents of Okinawa (26.1).[151,154-157]

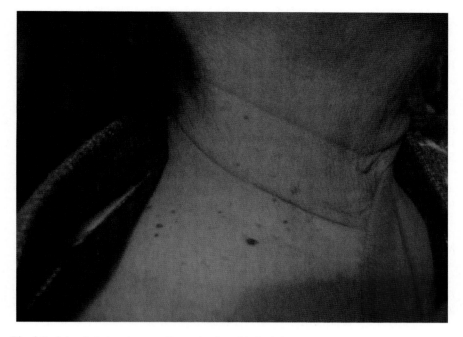

Fig. 2.6 Seborrheic keratoses on the neck of an elderly Asian woman

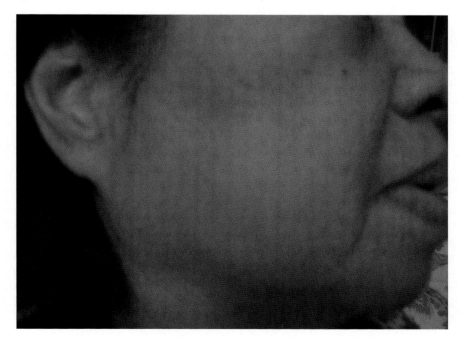

Fig. 2.7 Pigmentation and fine wrinkling on the cheek of an elderly Asian woman

In Japan and Singapore, data suggest that there is an increasing trend in the incidence of BCCs.[156,158,159] An analysis in Singapore showed that fairer-skinned Chinese had a twofold increased incidence of BCC compared with darker-skinned Malays and Indian.[160,161] BCC occurs most often in persons after the fifth decade on sun-exposed areas of the head and neck, regardless of the degree of pigmentation of the skin.[161,162] BCCs in Asians have been reported clinically to appear brown to glossy black and have the so-called "black pearly" appearance, a characteristic clinical feature of BCC in Asian races.[160,161] Pigmentation is present in more than 50% of BCCs in Japanese.[14] In contrast, only 6% of BCCs in Caucasians are pigmented.[14] In Asians, nodular BCC is the most common histopathological type of BCC.[160,161]

SCC is the second most common skin cancer in Chinese Asians and Japanese.[154,156] The incidence of SCC among Chinese Asians, which is reported to range from 2.6 to 2.9 per 100,000, has decreased 0.9% annually from 1968 to 1997.[156]

In Asians, the incidence of melanoma, is similar to those in African-Americans, ranging form 0.5 to 1.5 per 100,000.[162] Acral-lentiginous melanoma (ALM) is the most common histological subtype in Asians.[14] ALM represented 50% of melanomas in a study form Japan between 1987 and 1996.[154] However, there has been an increase in superficial spreading melanoma in Japan, again in keeping with the increased incidence of actinic keratoses and perhaps associated with vacationing abroad and a tanning culture.[154,157]

2.4.3 Hispanic Skin

The Hispanic population is the fastest growing minority in the USA. The nation's Hispanic population increased by 1.4 million to reach 45.5 million on July 1, 2007, totaling 15.1% of the estimated US population of 301.6 million.[163] With a 3.3% increase between in the preceding 12-month period, Hispanics were the fastest-growing minority group. Hispanics and Latinos have a wide range of skin phototypes and pigmentation due to their ancestral diversity. The term Hispanic is considered as an ethnicity by the US Census Bureau, to identify people who indicate that their origin is from a Spanish-speaking country. Their countries of origin range from Mexico to South and Central America to Spain and the Caribbean Islands of Peurto Rico, Dominican Republic, and Cuba. In some of these countries, mestizos, persons of Native American and European ancestry predominate, whereas mulattos, persons of African and European descant predominate in others. Given the ancestral diversity and wide range of skin types in these patients, the study of photoaging is difficult in this group. As a result, there is little published information regarding photoaging in Hispanics. Halder and Ara observed that those who have had many years of exposure during outdoor occupations can exhibit marked deep wrinkling.[117] Anecdotally, Hispanic people can develop seborrheic keratoses and solar lentigines in sun-exposed sites, with lighter-skinned individuals at greatest risk for the latter (Figures 2.8, 2.9).

The rising incidence of skin neoplasms in the Hispanic population has been identified as an emerging concern. BCC is the most common skin cancer in

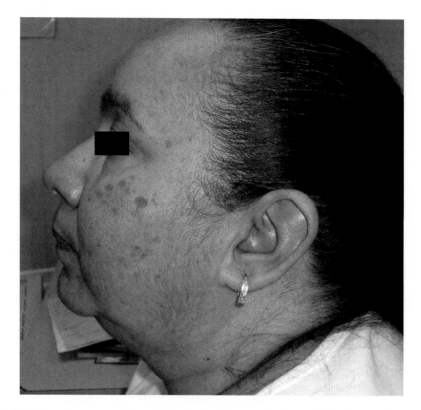

Fig. 2.8 Hispanic woman with multiple solar lentigines on the face and dyspigmentation

Hispanics with an incidence of 113–171 per 100,000 in New Mexican Hispanics.[164] Pigmented BCCs are more common in Hispanics than non-Hispanics, which is probably related to their darker skin color or possibly some genetic predisposition.[165] SCC has a reported incidence of 21 per 100,000 in New Mexican Hispanics and 13.8–32.9 per 100,000 in Hispanic residents of southeastern Arizona.[166] In some provinces in Argentina, Chile, Mexico, Bolivia, and Peru, BCCs and SCCs are seen in association with chronic arsenic exposure.[167]

The incidence of melanoma in Hispanics is three to seven times less than whites.[14] Malignant melanoma has been reported in both the Southeastern and Southwestern Hispanic populations.[168,169] Data from the California Cancer Registry reported that rates of invasive melanoma have increased markedly among Hispanics since 1988.[170] The incidence of melanoma in Puerto Ricans increased from 0.92 to 1.59 per 100,000 from 1977 to 1987.[171] Light-skinned Hispanics do have a lower incidence of melanoma, 4.3 compared with 20.8 per 100,000 white Caucasians. However, sun protection advice is still imperative in the prevention of melanoma in these individuals. Especially given the findings that Hispanic high school students

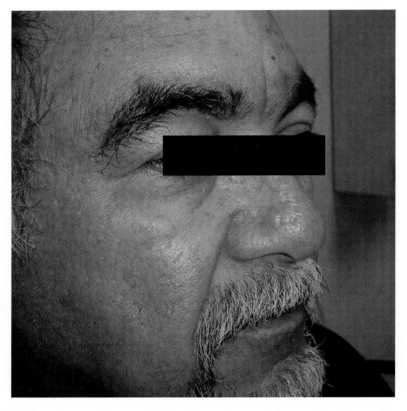

Fig. 2.9 Hispanic man with some solar lentigines and textural changes. There is a small scar on the right side of nose from a previous excision of a pigmented basal cell carcinoma

are 2.5 times more likely to use tanning beds, less likely to use sunscreen, and unaware of skin self-examination compared to their white Caucasian peers.[172,173]

2.5 Prevention of Photoaging

2.5.1 Photoprotection

Protection from the sun at any age reduces the risk of actinic keratoses and SCC and the progression of photoaging.[174-178] However, BCC risk reduction is dependent on reducing sun exposure during childhood.[179] Prevention of photoaging involves sun avoidance when possible, wearing protective clothing and daily use of sunscreens. Patients should not only avoid excessive intermittent sun exposure, as in intentional sunbathing, but also minimize the cumulative daily UV exposure.

2.5.2 Sunscreens

There is evidence to suggest that, apart from a preventative role, sunscreens may permit photodamaged skin to repair itself.[178] In animal studies, the use of sunscreen led to the improvement of preexisting damage and prevention of further changes induced by UV radiation.[175,178] Histological features were stabilized in patients following a 2-year application of sun protection factor (SPF) 29, contrasted with progressive changes in the placebo group.[176] The use of broad-spectrum sunscreens for up to 4.5 years has been shown to reduce the incidence of actinic keratoses by approximately 40% and SCC by 25%.[180,181] The internationally recognized standard of measuring the efficacy of sunscreen, the SPF, may be a poor indicator of a sunscreen's effectiveness in preventing photodamage. SPF is defined as the minimal erythema dose ratio between sun-protected and -unprotected skin, that is SPF 2 equals a 50% block, SPF 15 equals a 93% block, and SPF 45 equals a 98% block. As UVB is 1,000 times more capable of inducing erythema than UVA, SPF really reflects protection against UVB only. In vivo testing methods for UVA exist but are cumbersome or impractical compared to UVB testing. Immediate pigment darkening, persistent pigment darkening (PPD), and the protection factor in the UVA (PFA). IPD describes the immediate brown pigmentation of the skin caused by oxidation of preformed melanosomes in the skin.[182] It can only be tested in skin types III–V. PPD measures melanin photooxidation between 2 and 24 h postexposure and can be tested in skin types II–IV but exposure times need to be prolonged (up to 1 h).[183] PFA measures either erythema or tanning following UVA 24 h after exposure in skin types I–IV.[184] None of these tests indicate the level of UV-induced immunosuppression.

Sunscreens can be classified as either chemical blockers, which absorb UV radiation, or physical blockers, which reflect and scatter UV. Physical blockers such as titanium dioxide and zinc oxide are effective against both UVB and UVA. These sunscreens provide good protection but they are opaque and cosmetically unacceptable to patients, especially those with skin of color. Most sunscreens are designed to prevent UVB-induced sunburn. Sunscreen ingredients effective against UVB include cinnamtes, PABA and esters, salicylates, and octocrylene. UVA chemical absorbers include avobenzone, ecamsule, and oxybenzone. The use of sunscreens is not as prevalent in those with skin of color compared to individuals with white skin, who are used to the practice of sunscreen application often from early childhood. Reluctance to apply sunscreen may be overcome by education on the merits of the prevention of photoaging and with improved formulations for ease of use, and in those with lighter skin color, an emphasis on skin cancer prevention becomes pertinent.

2.5.3 Antioxidants

Antioxidants have become very popular ingredients of cosmetic products that claim anti-aging properties. The role of oxidative stress in aging and photodamage is well documented. The skin has intrinsic antioxidants to protect it from environmental stressors including glutathione and ubiquinol and from the diet, vitamin C and E.[185] Vitamin C has been shown to protect the skin against sunburn, delay the onset of tumors in animals, and reduce photoaging.[186-189] Vitamin E acts to prevent lipid peroxidation, through scavenging by its constituent tocopherols and tocotrienols. Several studies have documented the photoprotective effects of vitamin E in animals.[190-193] Plant antioxidants have also been studied including silymarin (milk thistle extract), soy isoflavones (genistein, daidzein, etc.), and tea polyphenols. The epicatechin derivatives, commonly called polyphenols, present in green tea possess antioxidant, anti-inflammatory, and anticarcinogenic properties, specifically epigallocatechin-3-gallate. Topical treatment or oral consumption of green tea polyphenols inhibits chemical carcinogen- or UV radiation-induced skin carcinogenesis in different laboratory animal models.[185] Treatment of epigallocatechin-3-gallate to human skin results in the inhibition of UVB-induced erythema, oxidative stress, and infiltration of inflammatory leukocytes.[194] In animal models of photocarcinogenesis, and in some in vivo human studies, antioxidants show photoprotection when given either systemically or topically, but their potential is yet to be fully evaluated in human clinical trials.

2.6 Treatment of Photoaging

2.6.1 Hydroxy Acids

The alpha- and polyhydoroxy acids (AHAs, PHAs) are organic carboxylic acids that cause exfoliation of the stratum corneum, as well as dermal changes. Many nonprescription creams, that claim to reverse the signs of aging, contain hydroxyl acids in low concentration (4–12%). In high concentrations, these agents are used as chemical peels. Skin treated with hydroxyl acids is much more likely to burn with exposure to UVB and concomitant sunscreen application is essential. Five percent glycolic acid and 8% lactic acid cream for 5 months improved mottling and roughness compared to placebo and sunscreen but did not improve wrinkles or actinic keratoses.[195,196] PHAs provide similar results to AHAs but cause less skin irritation, and hence are better tolerated in treating patients with skin of color.[197]

2.6.2 Retinoids

A large number of controlled clinical studies have been published demonstrating that topical application of all-trans retinoic acid improves the appearance of photoaged skin.[198-200] Retinoids (i.e. tretinoin, taxarotene, and adapalene) mediate cellular responses primarily through the activation of nuclear retinoid receptors.[198] Tretinoin and tazarotene are approved by the US Food and Drug Administration for the use of "palliation" of fine wrinkles and irregular pigmentation of photoaging. Tretinoin has been extensively studied for the treatment of photodamage.[176] Photoaging amelioration was assessed in Asian patients ($n = 45$), treated with tretinoin 0.1% or vehicle for 40 weeks.[201] At the end of the treatment period, hyperpigmented lesions on the face and hands were lighter or much lighter in 90% of the tretinoin group, compared with 33% of the vehicle group. In a largely African-American group, 0.1% topical tretinoin improved postinflammatory hyperpigmentation.[202]

Tazarotene is a synthetic retinoid that mediates cell differentiation and proliferation and it has been shown effective as a treatment for photodamage.[203] The penetration of UVB radiation in skin treated with topical retinoids is over 30% higher than untreated skin, so care needs to be taken in photoprotecting these patients while on treatment.[204]

In general, retinoids are well tolerated in darker skin types; however, retinoid dermatitis may cause postinflammatory hyperpigmentation. In addition, progressive hyperpigmentation can occur with retinoids without any clinical evidence of irritation.

Vitamin A derivatives, such as retinol and retinaldehyde, are often found in over-the-counter antiaging creams but little evidence exists for their efficacy in photoaging.[176]

2.6.3 Skin-Lightening Agents

Skin-lightening (bleaching) agent use in people of skin of color is commonplace in many patients, and is used for a variety of skin conditions including the hyperpigmentation associated with photodamage. Skin-lightening agents target several points of melanogenesis at either inhibition of melanocyte stimulation (e.g. antioxidants, anti-inflammatory agents), cell receptor antagonism (e.g. α-melanocyte-stimulating hormone antagonists), inhibition of melanin synthesis enzymes [e.g. TYR, TRP (tyrosinase-related protein)-1, TRP-2], inhibition of melanosome transport within the melanocyte and transfer to the keratinocyte (e.g. PAR-2 antagonists), and activation of melanin degradation within the keratinocyte (Table 1).[205] Agents such as hydroquinone,

Table 1 Molecular Targets of Skin-lightening Agents. Adapted from Ortonne at al, 2008 [203]

Molecular Targets	Agents Used
Tyrosinase inhibition	Hydroquinone, kojic acid, arbutin, ascorbic acid (vitamin C), deoxyarbutin
Tyrosinase copper chelation	Ellagic acid
Inhibition of tyrosinase glycosylation	Glucosamine, N-acetyl glucosamine, tunicamycin
Melanosome transfer	Niacinamide, protease inhibitors
Downregulation of tyrosinase	Retinoid (trans-retinoic acid, retinol and its esters, retinaldehyde)
Antioxidant	Vitamin C compounds, vitamin E, sulfhydryl compounds
Anti-inflammatory agent	Hydrocortisone, phytosterol, glycyrrhetinic acid
Increase epidermal turnover	Retinoids, salicylic acid

kojic acid, arbutin, ascorbic acid, ellagic acid, sulfhydryl compounds, and resorcinols are effective in interfering with TYR, the first enzyme in the conversion of tyrosine to melanin. Hydroquinone is the most commonly employed topical agent for the treatment of hyperpigmentation. A number of side effects are associated with its use, including local irritation, contact dermatitis, and in particular in dark-skinned people, exogenous ochronosis. This disorder is characterized by progressive sooty darkening of the skin area in patients who have used high concentrations of hydroquinone for many years. Often for better efficacy, hydroquinone is compounded into various mixtures for the treatment of hyperpigmentation, for example the "Kligman formula" contains 5% hydroquinone with 0.1% retinoic acid and 0.1% dexamethasone.

Many plant extracts are used for skin-lightening, as a "natural" alternative to hydroquinone. These include arbutin, kojic acid, aloesin, flavonoids, hesperiden, niacinamide, licorice extract, mulberry, polyphenols to name but a few.[206] Azelaic acid, derived from *Pityrosporum ovale*, is a weak inhibitor of TYR in vitro and when it is prescribed topically as a 20% cream with glycolic acid (15% and 20%), its efficacy has been compared with 4% hydroquinone in the treatment of facial hyperpigmentation in dark-skinned patients. Kojic acid, a fungal metabolite, inhibits the catecholase activity of TYR, and is used in concentrations ranging from 1% to 4%. It has been reported to have high sensitizing potential and may cause irritant contact dermatitis.

2.6.4 Lasers

The treatment of hyperpigmentation with laser (light amplification by stimulated emission of radiation) techniques is a fast-growing field. Many lasers have the capability to treat pigmentation of photoaging but not in all skin types. Inappropriate destruction of melanocytes and postinflammatory hyperpigmentation remain an important problem for darker skin types. Therefore, laser is used infrequently in darker skin types. The superficially located melanin pigment in solar lentigines lends them to treatment with the rapid-firing Q-switched lasers, ruby, alexandrite and Nd:YAG. Lentigines when treated with Q-switched Alexandrite laser in patients with skin types IV resulted in no hypo- or hyperpigmentation in one study.[207] In 34 Asian patients, solar lentigines were treated with Versapulse Q-switched Nd-YAG 532 versus Versapulse long-pulse versus conventional Q-switched Nd:YAG. A range of adverse events occurred including hyperpigmentation, hypopigmentation, erythema, which tended to be more pronounced with Versapulse Q-switched Nd:YAG 532.[208] CO_2 and Er:YAG will treat both wrinkles and pigmentary changes but are not appropriate for darker skin types with risk of postinflammatory hyperpigmentation. When treating patients with laser, a test spot should always be performed before a full treatment.

Intense pulsed light (IPL) uses high-intensity pulses of a broad wavelength (515–1200 nm) of light to deliver energy to the skin. IPL has been employed for lentigines and vascular lesions associated with photoaging. Photorejuventation was conducted with IPL in Asian skin types IV–V, with 97 patients receiving 3–6 treatments using 550 and 570 nm filters.[209] Treatment results were evaluated and rated by both patients and physicians at the end of the third treatment based on improvement in pigmentation, telangiectasia, and skin texture. A combined rating of "good" or "excellent" was given to more than 90% of the patients for pigmentation, more than 83% for telangiectasia, and more than 65% for skin texture.[209] Some inflammation did occur but resolved without any postinflammatory hyperpigmentation.

In another study on Asian patients, IPL treatment of solar lentigines and ephelides on the face, 48% of patients had more than 50% improvement and 20% had more than 75% improvement, with small plaques of solar lentigines responded best.[210] Adverse effects of IPL treatment include pain, local irritation, and postinflammatory hyperpigmentation. Further comparison studies of the laser treatments and depigmenting agents will determine the optimal treatment for patients of varying skin colors with hyperpigmentation.

2.6.5 Chemical Peels

Chemical peeling is used extensively in fair-skinned individuals for the treatment of photoaging. The potential to cause postinflammatory hyperpigmentation and scarring is a real risk in patients with skin of color. Deep peels are not suitable for skin types IV–VI as they may lead to pigmentary changes and scarring. Patient selection and counseling is important prior to utilizing a chemical peel. Solar lentigines may be spot-peeled.

Superficial peeling agents (epidermis to upper papillary dermis) include trichloroacetic acid 10–35%, glycolic acid solution 30–50% or glycolic gel 70%, salicylic acid 20–30% in ethanol, Jessner's solution. Medium depth peeling agents (epidermis to upper reticular dermis) include TCA 50%, glycolic acid solution 70%, TCA 25% and glycolic gel 70%, and Jessner's solution with TCA.[211] Little data exists to support the use of chemical peels for photoaging in skin of color and risks associated with treatment may outweigh the benefits.

2.7 Conclusion

UV radiation is a potent inducer of multiple signaling cascades. Differences in the pigmentary system associated with differing skin color can alter the impact of UV on the skin. In skin of color, less wrinkling and laxity occur due to the protective nature of melanin. However, the ability of dark skin to pigment is a double-edged sword, with the development of significant dyschromia following chronic sun damage in this population. Dyschromia in skin of color will be an increasing problem presented to dermatologists, with the rapidly expansion of minority populations. Our current armamentarium is insufficient to treat these conditions, often inducing postinflammatory hyperpigmentation in darker skin types. Evolving technology and understanding of the pathophysiology of photoaging in skin of color will undoubtedly expand our therapeutic and preventative options in these patients.

For migrant populations, the interaction of varying skin types with foreign environments will be an increasing important phenomenon in the presentation of skin diseases, with UV exposure at new latitudes altering their skin cancer risk. The emerging increase in skin cancer in ethnic populations may reflect new cultural habits and cumulative UV exposure. Photoaging, as part of the process of skin carcinogenesis, is becoming increasingly relevant in patients with skin of color.

References

1. Halder RM. The role of retinoids in the management of cutaneous conditions in blacks. *J Am Acad Dermatol.* 1998;39(2 Pt 3):S98–S103.
2. Sturm RA, Box NF, Ramsay M. Human pigmentation genetics: the difference is only skin deep. *Bioessays.* 1998;20(9):712–721.
3. Smith ES, Fleischer Jr. AB, Feldman SR. Demographics of aging and skin disease. *Clin Geriatr Med.* 2001;17(4):631–641, v.
4. US census data 2000 [cited 2008; Available from: http://censtats.census.gov/pub
5. Halder RM, Grimes PE, McLaurin CI, Kress MA, Kenney Jr. JA. Incidence of common dermatoses in a predominantly black dermatologic practice. *Cutis.* 1983;32(4):388, 390.
6. Petit A, Cohen-Ludmann C, Clevenbergh P, Bergmann JF, Dubertret L. Skin lightening and its complications among African people living in Paris. *J Am Acad Dermatol.* 2006;55(5):873–878.
7. Kimball AB. Skin differences, needs, and disorders across global populations. *J Investig Dermatol Symp Proc.* 2008;13(1):2–5.
8. Jackson BA. Cosmetic considerations and nonlaser cosmetic procedures in ethnic skin. *Dermatol Clin.* 2003;21(4):703–712, ix.
9. Maibach HI, Berardesca E. Racial and skin color differences in skin sensitivity: implications for skin care products. *Cosmetics and Toiletries.* 1990;105:35–36.
10. Holman CD, Armstrong BK, Evans PR, et al. Relationship of solar keratosis and history of skin cancer to objective measures of actinic skin damage. *Br J Dermatol.* 1984;110(2):129–138.
11. Memon AA, Tomenson JA, Bothwell J, Friedmann PS. Prevalence of solar damage and actinic keratosis in a Merseyside population. *Br J Dermatol.* 2000;142(6):1154–1159.
12. Brooke RC, Newbold SA, Telfer NR, Griffiths CE. Discordance between facial wrinkling and the presence of basal cell carcinoma. *Arch Dermatol.* 2001;137(6):751–754.
13. Foote JA, Harris RB, Giuliano AR, et al. Predictors for cutaneous basal- and squamous-cell carcinoma among actinically damaged adults. *Int J Cancer.* 2001;95(1):7–11.
14. Gloster HMJr., Neal K. Skin cancer in skin of color. *J Am Acad Dermatol.* 2006;55(5):741–760; quiz 761-764.
15. Byrd-Miles K, Toombs EL, Peck GL. Skin cancer in individuals of African, Asian, Latin-American, and American-Indian descent: differences in incidence, clinical presentation, and survival compared to Caucasians. *J Drugs Dermatol.* 2007;6(1):10–16.
16. Friedman LC, Bruce S, Weinberg AD, Cooper HP, Yen AH, Hill M. Early detection of skin cancer: racial/ethnic differences in behaviors and attitudes. *J Cancer Educ.* 1994;9(2):105–110.
17. Pipitone M, Robinson JK, Camara C, Chittineni B, Fisher SG. Skin cancer awareness in suburban employees: a Hispanic perspective. *J Am Acad Dermatol.* 2002;47(1):118–123.
18. Rittie L, Fisher GJ. UV-light-induced signal cascades and skin aging. *Ageing Res Rev.* 2002;1(4):705–720.
19. Kadono S, Manaka I, Kawashima M, Kobayashi T, Imokawa G. The role of the epidermal endothelin cascade in the hyperpigmentation mechanism of lentigo senilis. *J Invest Dermatol.* 2001;116(4):571–577.

20. Imokawa G. Autocrine and paracrine regulation of melanocytes in human skin and in pigmentary disorders. *Pigment Cell Res.* 2004;17(2):96–110.
21. Unver N, Freyschmidt-Paul P, Horster S, et al. Alterations in the epidermal-dermal melanin axis and factor XIIIa melanophages in senile lentigo and ageing skin. *Br J Dermatol.* 2006;155(1):119–128.
22. Motokawa T, Kato T, Katagiri T, et al. Messenger RNA levels of melanogenesis-associated genes in lentigo senilis lesions. *J Dermatol Sci.* 2005;37(2):120–123.
23. Young AR, Potten CS, Nikaido O, et al. Human melanocytes and keratinocytes exposed to UVB or UVA in vivo show comparable levels of thymine dimers. *J Invest Dermatol.* 1998;111(6):936–940.
24. Kielbassa C, Epe B. DNA damage induced by ultraviolet and visible light and its wavelength dependence. *Methods Enzymol.* 2000;319:436–445.
25. Goukassian D, Gad F, Yaar M, Eller MS, Nehal US, Gilchrest BA. Mechanisms and implications of the age-associated decrease in DNA repair capacity. *FASEB J.* 2000;14(10):1325–1334.
26. Kielbassa C, Roza L, Epe B. Wavelength dependence of oxidative DNA damage induced by UV and visible light. *Carcinogenesis.* 1997;18(4):811–816.
27. Moriwaki S, Takahashi Y. Photoaging and DNA repair. *J Dermatol Sci.* 2008;50(3):169–176.
28. Ziegler A, Jonason AS, Leffell DJ, et al. Sunburn and p53 in the onset of skin cancer. *Nature.* 1994;372(6508):773–776.
29. Greider CW. Telomere length regulation. *Annu Rev Biochem.* 1996;65:337–365.
30. Campisi J. Cellular senescence as a tumor-suppressor mechanism. *Trends Cell Biol.* 2001;11(11):S27–S31.
31. Griffith JD, Comeau L, Rosenfield S, et al. Mammalian telomeres end in a large duplex loop. *Cell.* 1999;97(4):503–514.
32. van Steensel B, Smogorzewska A, de Lange T. TRF2 protects human telomeres from end-to-end fusions. *Cell.* 1998;92(3):401–413.
33. Eller MS, Li GZ, Firoozabadi R, Puri N, Gilchrest BA. Induction of a p95/Nbs1-mediated S phase checkpoint by telomere 3' overhang specific DNA. *FASEB J.* 2003;17(2):152–162.
34. Eller MS, Yaar M, Gilchrest BA. DNA damage and melanogenesis. *Nature.* 1994;372(6505):413–414.
35. Gilchrest BA, Eller MS. The tale of the telomere: implications for prevention and treatment of skin cancers. *J Investig Dermatol Symp Proc.* 2005;10(2):124–130.
36. Yang J, Yu Y, Hamrick HE, Duerksen-Hughes PJ. ATM, ATR and DNA-PK: initiators of the cellular genotoxic stress responses. *Carcinogenesis.* 2003;24(10):1571–1580.
37. Gilchrest BA. Using DNA damage responses to prevent and treat skin cancers. *J Dermatol.* 2004;31(11):862–877.
38. Sugimoto M, Yamashita R, Ueda M. Telomere length of the skin in association with chronological aging and photoaging. *J Dermatol Sci.* 2006;43(1):43–47.
39. Lee HC, Wei YH. Oxidative stress, mitochondrial DNA mutation, and apoptosis in aging. *Exp Biol Med (Maywood).* 2007;232(5):592–606.
40. Birch-Machin MA, Tindall M, Turner R, Haldane F, Rees JL. Mitochondrial DNA deletions in human skin reflect photo- rather than chronologic aging. *J Invest Dermatol.* 1998;110(2):149–152.
41. Berneburg M, Gattermann N, Stege H, et al. Chronically ultraviolet-exposed human skin shows a higher mutation frequency of mitochondrial DNA as compared to unexposed skin and the hematopoietic system. *Photochem Photobiol.* 1997;66(2):271–275.
42. Yang JH, Lee HC, Wei YH. Photoageing-associated mitochondrial DNA length mutations in human skin. *Arch Dermatol Res.* 1995;287(7):641–648.
43. Koch H, Wittern KP, Bergemann J. In human keratinocytes the Common Deletion reflects donor variabilities rather than chronologic aging and can be induced by ultraviolet A irradiation. *J Invest Dermatol.* 2001;117(4):892–897.
44. Berneburg M, Grether-Beck S, Kurten V, et al. Singlet oxygen mediates the UVA-induced generation of the photoaging-associated mitochondrial common deletion. *J Biol Chem.* 1999;274(22):15345–15349.

45. Berneburg M, Plettenberg H, Medve-Konig K, et al. Induction of the photoaging-associated mitochondrial common deletion in vivo in normal human skin. *J Invest Dermatol.* 2004;122(5):1277–1283.
46. Krutmann J, Gilchrest BA. Photoaging of skin. In: Gilchrest BA, Krutmann J, eds. Skin Aging. Berlin Heideleberg: Springer Verlag; 2006:33–43.
47. Smith Jr. JG, Davidson EA, Sams Jr. WM, Clark RD. Alterations in human dermal connective tissue with age and chronic sun damage. *J Invest Dermatol.* 1962;39:347–350.
48. Braverman IM, Fonferko E. Studies in cutaneous aging: I. The elastic fiber network. *J Invest Dermatol.* 1982;78(5):434–443.
49. Talwar HS, Griffiths CE, Fisher GJ, Hamilton TA, Voorhees JJ. Reduced type I and type III procollagens in photodamaged adult human skin. *J Invest Dermatol.* 1995;105(2):285–290.
50. Kawaguchi Y, Tanaka H, Okada T, et al. Effect of reactive oxygen species on the elastin mRNA expression in cultured human dermal fibroblasts. *Free Radic Biol Med.* 1997;23(1):162–165.
51. Fisher GJ, Datta S, Wang Z, et al. c-Jun-dependent inhibition of cutaneous procollagen transcription following ultraviolet irradiation is reversed by all-trans retinoic acid. *J Clin Invest.* 2000;106(5):663–670.
52. Varani J, Schuger L, Dame MK, et al. Reduced fibroblast interaction with intact collagen as a mechanism for depressed collagen synthesis in photodamaged skin. *J Invest Dermatol.* 2004;122(6):1471–1479.
53. Kahari VM, Saarialho-Kere U. Matrix metalloproteinases in skin. *Exp Dermatol.* 1997;6(5):199–213.
54. Fisher GJ, Choi HC, Bata-Csorgo Z, et al. Ultraviolet irradiation increases matrix metalloproteinase-8 protein in human skin in vivo. *J Invest Dermatol.* 2001;117(2):219–226.
55. Fisher GJ, Datta SC, Talwar HS, et al. Molecular basis of sun-induced premature skin ageing and retinoid antagonism. *Nature.* 1996;379(6563):335–339.
56. Pillai S, Oresajo C, Hayward J. Ultraviolet radiation and skin aging: roles of reactive oxygen species, inflammation and protease activation, and strategies for prevention of inflammation-induced matrix degradation - a review. *Int J Cosmet Sci.* 2005;27(1):17–34.
57. Fisher GJ, Kang S, Varani J, et al. Mechanisms of photoaging and chronological skin aging. *Arch Dermatol.* 2002;138(11):1462–1470.
58. Kligman AM. Perspectives and problems in cutaneous gerontology. *J Invest Dermatol.* 1979;73(1):39–46.
59. Kelly RI, Pearse R, Bull RH, Leveque JL, de Rigal J, Mortimer PS. The effects of aging on the cutaneous microvasculature. *J Am Acad Dermatol.* 1995;33(5 Pt 1):749–756.
60. Yaar M, Gilchrest BA. Aging of skin. In: Freedberg IM, Eisen AZ, Wolff K, Austen KF, Goldsmith LA, Katz SI, Fitzpatrick TB, eds. Dermatology in General Medicine. New York: McGraw-Hill; 1999:1697–1706.
61. Gilchrest BA, Stoff JS, Soter NA. Chronologic aging alters the response to ultraviolet-induced inflammation in human skin. *J Invest Dermatol.* 1982;79(1):11–15.
62. Braverman IM, Fonferko E. Studies in cutaneous aging: II The microvasculature. *J Invest Dermatol.* 1982;78(5):444–448.
63. Chung JH, Yano K, Lee MK, et al. Differential effects of photoaging vs intrinsic aging on the vascularization of human skin. *Arch Dermatol.* 2002;138(11):1437–1442.
64. Kramer M, Sachsenmaier C, Herrlich P, Rahmsdorf HJ. UV irradiation-induced interleukin-1 and basic fibroblast growth factor synthesis and release mediate part of the UV response. *J Biol Chem.* 1993;268(9):6734–6741.
65. Strickland I, Rhodes LE, Flanagan BF, Friedmann PS. TNF-alpha and IL-8 are upregulated in the epidermis of normal human skin after UVB exposure: correlation with neutrophil accumulation and E-selectin expression. *J Invest Dermatol.* 1997;108(5):763–768.
66. Bielenberg DR, Bucana CD, Sanchez R, Donawho CK, Kripke ML, Fidler IJ. Molecular regulation of UVB-induced cutaneous angiogenesis. *J Invest Dermatol.* 1998;111(5):864–872.
67. Yano K, Kajiya K, Ishiwata M, Hong YK, Miyakawa T, Detmar M. Ultraviolet B-induced skin angiogenesis is associated with a switch in the balance of vascular endothelial growth factor and thrombospondin-1 expression. *J Invest Dermatol.* 2004;122(1):201–208.

68. Yano K, Oura H, Detmar M. Targeted overexpression of the angiogenesis inhibitor thrombospondin-1 in the epidermis of transgenic mice prevents ultraviolet-B-induced angiogenesis and cutaneous photo-damage. *J Invest Dermatol.* 2002;118(5):800–805.

69. Brauchle M, Funk JO, Kind P, Werner S. Ultraviolet B and H2O2 are potent inducers of vascular endothelial growth factor expression in cultured keratinocytes. *J Biol Chem.* 1996;271(36):21793–21797.

70. Hirakawa S, Fujii S, Kajiya K, Yano K, Detmar M. Vascular endothelial growth factor promotes sensitivity to ultraviolet B-induced cutaneous photodamage. *Blood.* 2005;105(6):2392–2399.

71. Bennett MF, Robinson MK, Baron ED, Cooper KD. Skin immune systems and inflammation: protector of the skin or promoter of aging. *J Investig Dermatol Symp Proc.* 2008;13(1):15–19.

72. Bosset S, Bonnet-Duquennoy M, Barre P, et al. Photoageing shows histological features of chronic skin inflammation without clinical and molecular abnormalities. *Br J Dermatol.* 2003;149(4):826–835.

73. Hammerberg C, Duraiswamy N, Cooper KD. Active induction of unresponsiveness (tolerance) to DNFB by in vivo ultraviolet-exposed epidermal cells is dependent upon infiltrating class II MHC+ CD11bbright monocytic/macrophagic cells. *J Immunol.* 1994;153(11):4915–4924.

74. Meunier L, Bata-Csorgo Z, Cooper KD. In human dermis, ultraviolet radiation induces expansion of a CD36+ CD11b+ CD1− macrophage subset by infiltration and proliferation; CD1+ Langerhans-like dendritic antigen-presenting cells are concomitantly depleted. *J Invest Dermatol.* 1995;105(6):782–788.

75. Kang K, Gilliam AC, Chen G, Tootell E, Cooper KD. In human skin, UVB initiates early induction of IL-10 over IL-12 preferentially in the expanding dermal monocytic/macrophagic population. *J Invest Dermatol.* 1998;111(1):31–38.

76. Toichi E, Lu KQ, Swick AR, McCormick TS, Cooper KD. Skin-infiltrating monocytes/macrophages migrate to draining lymph nodes and produce IL-10 after contact sensitizer exposure to UV-irradiated skin. *J Invest Dermatol.* 2008.

77. Yoshida Y, Kang K, Berger M, et al. Monocyte induction of IL-10 and down-regulation of IL-12 by iC3b deposited in ultraviolet-exposed human skin. *J Immunol.* 1998;161(11):5873–5879.

78. Hammerberg C, Katiyar SK, Carroll MC, Cooper KD. Activated complement component 3 (C3) is required for ultraviolet induction of immunosuppression and antigenic tolerance. *J Exp Med.* 1998;187(7):1133–1138.

79. Takahara M, Kang K, Liu L, Yoshida Y, McCormick TS, Cooper KD. iC3b arrests monocytic cell differentiation into CD1c-expressing dendritic cell precursors: a mechanism for transiently decreased dendritic cells in vivo after human skin injury by ultraviolet B. *J Invest Dermatol.* 2003;120(5):802–809.

80. Takahara M, Kang K, Liu L, Yoshida Y, McCormick TS, Cooper KD. CD11b-dependent iC3b transient arrest of dermal and blood monocytic dendritic cell precursor differentiation. *J Invest Dermatol.* 2002;119:328.

81. Toichi E, McCormick TS, Cooper KD. Cell surface and cytokine phenotypes of skin immunocompetent cells involved in ultraviolet-induced immunosuppression. *Methods.* 2002;28(1):104–110.

82. Fridovich I, Superoxide dismutases. An adaptation to a paramagnetic gas. *J Biol Chem.* 1989;264(14):7761–7764.

83. Cadet J, Douki T, Pouget JP, Ravanat JL. Singlet oxygen DNA damage products: formation and measurement. *Methods Enzymol.* 2000;319:143–153.

84. Stadtman ER. Protein oxidation and aging. *Science.* 1992;257(5074):1220–1224.

85. Sander CS, Chang H, Salzmann S, et al. Photoaging is associated with protein oxidation in human skin in vivo. *J Invest Dermatol.* 2002;118(4):618–625.

86. Bennett M, Liu L, Liu S, Biljanovska NC, McCormick TS, Chance MR, Cooper KD, Karnik P. Combined exposure to UV and Di-nitro benzene sulfonic acid (DNBS) profoundly modulates Ca++-binding proteins and alters redox signaling. *J Invest Dermatol.* 2007;127:S143.

87. Quevedo WC, Szabo G, Verks J. Influence of age and UV on the population of dopa-positive melanocytes in human skin. *J Invest Dermatol.* 1969;52:287–290.

88. Snell RS, Bischitz PG. The melanocytes and melanin in human abdominal wall skin: a survey made at different ages in both sexes and during pregnancy. *J Anat.* 1963;97:361–376.

89. Gilchrest BA, Blog FB, Szabo G. Effects of aging and chronic sun exposure on melanocytes in human skin. J Invest Dermatol. 1979;73(2):141–143.

90. Gilchrest BA, Park HY, Eller MS, Yaar M. Mechanisms of ultraviolet light-induced pigmentation. Photochem Photobiol. 1996;63(1):1–10.

91. Medrano EE, Farooqui JZ, Boissy RE, Boissy YL, Akadiri B, Nordlund JJ. Chronic growth stimulation of human adult melanocytes by inflammatory mediators in vitro: implications for nevus formation and initial steps in melanocyte oncogenesis. Proc Natl Acad Sci U S A. 1993;90(5):1790–1794.

92. Gilchrest BA, Eller MS. DNA photodamage stimulates melanogenesis and other photoprotective responses. J Investig Dermatol Symp Proc. 1999;4(1):35–40.

93. Eller MS, Maeda T, Magnoni C, Atwal D, Gilchrest BA. Enhancement of DNA repair in human skin cells by thymidine dinucleotides: evidence for a p53-mediated mammalian SOS response. Proc Natl Acad Sci U S A. 1997;94(23):12627–12632.

94. Wu C, Marks S, Park H-Y, Howard C, Gilchrest BA. T-Oligos induce mitf, tyrosinase and pkc-beta in cultured human melanocytes. Pigment Cell Res. 2004;17(4):452–452(1).

95. Ortonne JP, Bissett DL. Latest insights into skin hyperpigmentation. J Investig Dermatol Symp Proc. 2008;13(1):10–14.

96. Imokawa G, Kobayasi T, Miyagishi M. Intracellular signaling mechanisms leading to synergistic effects of endothelin-1 and stem cell factor on proliferation of cultured human melanocytes. Cross-talk via trans-activation of the tyrosine kinase c-kit receptor. J Biol Chem. 2000; 275(43):33321–33328.

97. Hattori H, Kawashima M, Ichikawa Y, Imokawa G. The epidermal stem cell factor is overexpressed in lentigo senilis: implication for the mechanism of hyperpigmentation. J Invest Dermatol. 2004;122(5):1256–1265.

98. Blume-Jensen P, Claesson-Welsh L, Siegbahn A, Zsebo KM, Westermark B, Heldin CH. Activation of the human c-kit product by ligand-induced dimerization mediates circular actin reorganization and chemotaxis. EMBO J. 1991;10(13):4121–4128.

99. Costin GE, Hearing VJ. Human skin pigmentation: melanocytes modulate skin color in response to stress. FASEB J. 2007;21(4):976–994.

100. Imokawa G, Yada Y, Miyagishi M. Endothelins secreted from human keratinocytes are intrinsic mitogens for human melanocytes. *J Biol Chem.* 1992;267(34):24675–24680.

101. Tadokoro T, Yamaguchi Y, Batzer J, et al. Mechanisms of skin tanning in different racial/ ethnic groups in response to ultraviolet radiation. *J Investig Dermatol.* 2005;124:1326–1332.

102. Tadokoro T, Kobayashi N, Zmudzka BZ, et al. UV-induced DNA damage and melanin content in human skin differing in racial/ethnic origin. *FASEB J.* 2003;17:1177–1179.

103. Yamaguchi Y, Brenner M, Hearing VJ. The Regulation of skin pigmentation. *J Biol Chem.* 2007;282(38):27557–27561.

104. Shuster S, Black MM, McVitie E. The influence of age and sex on skin thickness, skin collagen and density. *Br J Dermatol.* 1975;93(6):639–643.

105. Burke EM, Horton WE, Pearson JD, Crow MT, Martin GR. Altered transcriptional regulation of human interstitial collagenase in cultured skin fibroblasts from older donors. *Exp Gerontol.* 1994;29(1):37–53.

106. El-Domyati M, Attia S, Saleh F, et al. Intrinsic aging vs. photoaging: a comparative histopathological, immunohistochemical, and ultrastructural study of skin. *Exp Dermatol.* 2002;11(5):398–405.

107. Montagna W, Kirchner S, Carlisle K. Histology of sun-damaged human skin. *J Am Acad Dermatol.* 1989;21(5 Pt 1):907–918.

108. Kligman LH, Kligman AM. The nature of photoaging: its prevention and repair. *Photodermatol.* 1986;3(4):215–227.

109. Toyoda M, Nakamura M, Luo Y, Morohashi M. Ultrastructural characterization of microvasculature in photoaging. *J Dermatol Sci.* 2001;27(Suppl 1):S32–S41.

110. Kotrajaras R, Kligman AM. The effect of topical tretinoin on photodamaged facial skin: the Thai experience. *Br J Dermatol.* 1993;129(3):302–309.

111. Warren R, Gartstein V, Kligman AM, Montagna W, Allendorf RA, Ridder GM. Age, sunlight, and facial skin: a histologic and quantitative study. *J Am Acad Dermatol*. 1991;25(5 Pt 1):751–760.

112. Montagna W, Carlisle K. The architecture of black and white facial skin. *J Am Acad Dermatol*. 1991;24(6 Pt 1):929–937.

113. de Rigal J, Escoffier C, Querlex B, Faivre B, Agache P, Leveque, JL. Assessment of aging of human skin by in vivo ultrasonic imaging. *J Invest Dermatol*. 1989;93(5):621–625.

114. Jenkins G. Molecular mechanisms of skin ageing. *Mech Ageing Dev*. 2002; 123(7):801–810.

115. Lavker R. Cutaneous aging: chronological versus photoaging. In: Gilchrest BA, ed. Photodamage. Carlton; 1995:123-135.

116. Halder RM, CJ Ara. Skin cancer and photoaging in ethnic skin. *Dermatol Clin*. 2003;21(4):725–732, x.

117. Hillebrand GG, Miyamoto K, Schnell B, Ichihashi M, Shinkura R, Akiba S. Quantitative evaluation of skin condition in an epidemiological survey of females living in northern versus southern Japan. *J Dermatol Sci*. 2001;27(Suppl 1):S42–S52.

118. Chung JH, Lee SH, Youn CS, et al. Cutaneous photodamage in Koreans: influence of sex, sun exposure, smoking, and skin color. *Arch Dermatol*. 2001;137(8):1043–1051.

119. Yaar M, Eller MS, Gilchrest BA. Fifty years of skin aging. *J Investig Dermatol Symp Proc*. 2002;7(1):51–58.

120. Taylor SC. Photoaging and pigmentary changes of the skin. In: Burgess CM, ed. Cosmetic Dermatology. Berlin Heidelberg: Springer; 2005:29–51.

121. Fisher GJ, Wang ZQ, Datta SC, Varani J, Kang S, Voorhees JJ. Pathophysiology of premature skin aging induced by ultraviolet light. *N Engl J Med*. 1997;337(20):1419–1428.

122. Kaidbey KH, Agin PP, Sayre RM, Kligman AM. Photoprotection by melanin-a comparison of black and Caucasian skin. *J Am Acad Dermatol*. 1979;1(3):249–260.

123. Taylor S, DeYampert NM. Treatment of photoaging in African American and Hispanic patients. In: Rigel DS, Weiss RA, Lim HW, Dover JS, eds. Photoaging. New York: Marcel Dekker; 2004:365–377.

124. Argüelles-Casals D, González D. [Disseminated lenticular leukodermia]. *Ann Dermatol Syphiligr (Paris)*. 1969;96(3):283–286.

125. Cummings KI, Cottel WI. Idiopathic guttate hypomelanosis. *Arch Dermatol*. 1966;93(2): 184–186.

126. Ortonne JP, Perrot H. Idiopathic guttate hypomelanosis. Ultrastructural study. *Arch Dermatol*. 1980;116(6):664–668.

127. Tindall JP, Smith JG. Skin lesions of the aged and their association with internal changes. *JAMA*. 1963;186:1039–1042.

128. Hairston MA, Reed RJ, Derbes VJ. Dermatosis Papulosa Nigra. *Arch Dermatol*. 1964;89:655–658.

129. Halder RM, Bang KM. Skin cancer in blacks in the United States. *Dermatol Clin*. 1988;6(3):397–405.

130. Halder RM, Bridgeman-Shah S. Skin cancer in African Americans. *Cancer*. 1995;75(2 Suppl):667–673.

131. Mora RG, Perniciaro C. Cancer of the skin in blacks. I. A review of 163 black patients with cutaneous squamous cell carcinoma. *J Am Acad Dermatol*. 1981;5(5):535–543.

132. Fleming ID, Barnawell JR, Burlison PE, Rankin JS. Skin cancer in black patients. *Cancer*. 1975;35(3):600–605.

133. Singh B, Bhaya M, Shaha A, Har-El G, Lucente FE. Presentation, course, and outcome of head and neck skin cancer in African Americans: a case-control study. *Laryngoscope*. 1998;108(8 Pt 1):1159–1163.

134. Gray DT, Suman VJ, Su WP, Clay RP, Harmsen WS, Roenigk RK. Trends in the population-based incidence of squamous cell carcinoma of the skin first diagnosed between 1984 and 1992. *Arch Dermatol*. 1997;133(6):735–740.

135. McCall CO, Chen SC. Squamous cell carcinoma of the legs in African Americans. *J Am Acad Dermatol*. 2002;47(4):524–529.

185. Pinnell SR. Cutaneous photodamage, oxidative stress, and topical antioxidant protection. *J Am Acad Dermatol.* 2003;48(1):1–19; quiz 20-22.
186. Bissett DL, Chatterjee R, Hannon DP. Photoprotective effect of topical anti-inflammatory agents against ultraviolet radiation-induced chronic skin damage in the hairless mouse. *Photodermatol Photoimmunol Photomed.* 1990;7(4):15.
187. Darr D, Combs S, Dunston S, Manning T, Pinnell S. Topical vitamin C protects porcine skin from ultraviolet radiation-induced damage. *Br J Dermatol.* 1992;127(3):247–253.
188. Black HS. Potential involvement of free radical reactions in ultraviolet light-mediated cutaneous damage. *Photochem Photobiol.* 1987;46(2):213–221.
189. Eberlein-Konig B, Placzek M, Przybilla B. Protective effect against sunburn of combined systemic ascorbic acid (vitamin C) and d-alpha-tocopherol (vitamin E). *J Am Acad Dermatol.* 1998;38(1):45–48.
190. Lopez-Torres M, Thiele JJ, Shindo Y, Han D, Packer L. Topical application of alpha-tocopherol modulates the antioxidant network and diminishes ultraviolet-induced oxidative damage in murine skin. *Br J Dermatol.* 1998;138(2):207–215.
191. Jurkiewicz BA, Bissett DL, Buettner GR. Effect of topically applied tocopherol on ultraviolet radiation-mediated free radical damage in skin. *J Invest Dermatol.* 1995;104(4):484–488.
192. Steenvoorden DP, Beijersbergen van Henegouwen G. Protection against UV-induced systemic immunosuppression in mice by a single topical application of the antioxidant vitamins C and E. *Int J Radiat Biol.* 1999;75(6):747–755.
193. Burke KE, Clive J, Combs Jr. GF, Commisso J, Keen CL, Nakamura RM. Effects of topical and oral vitamin E on pigmentation and skin cancer induced by ultraviolet irradiation in Skh:2 hairless mice. *Nutr Cancer.* 2000;38(1):87–97.
194. Katiyar SK. Skin photoprotection by green tea: antioxidant and immunomodulatory effects. *Curr Drug Targets Immune Endocr Metabol Disord.* 2003;3(3):234–242.
195. Stiller MJ, Bartolone J, Stern R, et al. Topical 8% glycolic acid and 8% L-lactic acid creams for the treatment of photodamaged skin. A double-blind vehicle-controlled clinical trial. *Arch Dermatol.* 1996;132(6):631–636.
196. Thibault PK, Wlodarczyk J, Wenck A. A double-blind randomized clinical trial on the effectiveness of a daily glycolic acid 5% formulation in the treatment of photoaging. *Dermatol Surg.* 1998;24(5):573–577; discussion 577-578.
197. Grimes PE. Photoaging. In: Tosti A, Grimes PA, DePadova MP, eds. Color Atlas of Chemical Peels. New York: Springer; 2006;15:151–175.
198. Kang S, Voorhees JJ. Photoaging therapy with topical tretinoin: an evidence-based analysis. *J Am Acad Dermatol.* 1998;39(2 Pt 3):S55–S61.
199. Weinstein GD, Nigra TP, Pochi PE, et al. Topical tretinoin for treatment of photodamaged skin. A multicenter study. *Arch Dermatol.* 1991;127(5):659–665.
200. Griffiths CE, Kang S, Ellis CN, et al. Two concentrations of topical tretinoin (retinoic acid) cause similar improvement of photoaging but different degrees of irritation. A double-blind, vehicle-controlled comparison of 0.1% and 0.025% tretinoin creams. *Arch Dermatol.* 1995;131(9):1037–1044.
201. Griffiths CE, Goldfarb MT, Finkel LJ, et al. Topical tretinoin (retinoic acid) treatment of hyperpigmented lesions associated with photoaging in Chinese and Japanese patients: a vehicle-controlled trial. *J Am Acad Dermatol.* 1994;30(1):76–84.
202. Bulengo-Ransby SM, Griffiths CE, Kimbrough-Green CK, et al. Topical tretinoin (retinoic acid) therapy for hyperpigmented lesions caused by inflammation of the skin in black patients. *N Engl J Med.* 1993;328(20):1438–1443.
203. Phillips TJ, Gottlieb AB, Leyden JJ, Lowe NJ, Lew-Kaya DA, Sefton J, Walker PS, Gibson JR; Tazarotene Cream Photodamage Clinical Study Group. Efficacy of 0.1% tazarotene cream for the treatment of photodamage: a 12-month multicenter, randomized trial. *Arch Dermatol.* 2002;138(11):1486–1493.
204. Hecker D, Worsley J, Yueh G, Kuroda K, Lebwohl M. Interactions between tazarotene and ultraviolet light. *J Am Acad Dermatol.* 1999;41(6):927–930.

205. Ortonne JP, Bissett DL. Latest insights into skin hyperpigmentation. *J Investig Dermatol Symp Proc.* 2008;13(1):10–14.
206. Zhu W, Gao J. The use of botanical extracts as topical skin-lightening agents for the improvement of skin pigmentation disorders. *J Investig Dermatol Symp Proc.* 2008;13(1):20–24.
207. Rosenbach A, Lee SJ, Johr RH. Treatment of medium-brown solar lentigines using an alexandrite laser designed for hair reduction. *Arch Dermatol.* 2002;138(4):547–548.
208. Chan H. Treatment of photoaging in Asian skin. In: Rigel D, Weiss RA, Lim HW, Dover JS, eds. Photoaging. New York: Marcel Dekker; 2004:343–364.
209. Negishi K, Tezuka Y, Kushikata N, Wakamatsu S. Photorejuvenation for Asian skin by intense pulsed light. *Dermatol Surg.* 2001;27(7):627–631; discussion 632.
210. Kawada A, Shiraishi H, Asai M, et al. Clinical improvement of solar lentigines and ephelides with an intense pulsed light source. *Dermatol Surg.* 2002;28(6):504–508.
211. Roberts WE. Chemical peeling in ethnic/dark skin. *Dermatol Therapy.* 2004;17:196–205.

Chapter 3
Endogenous Protection by Melanin

Bernhard Ortel, Mark Racz, Deborah Lang, and Pier G. Calzavara-Pinton

Melanin is the dominant skin pigment, and the intensity of pigmentation is a conspicuous component of distinction between racially different human populations. Humans evolved in sub tropical Africa and constitutive pigmentation was likely dark to protect from damage by intense sun exposure, a persistent feature of highly melanized skin.[1,2] When descendants of these early humans moved north, dark skinned people were at a disadvantage for vitamin D (ViD) conversion and thus paler skinned descendants had a selective advantage in moderate climates and far northern latitudes. At the same time, the loss of dark pigment made these fair skinned people more prone to acute and chronic adverse effects of sun exposure, such as sunburn and skin cancer.[3] This chapter discusses the endogenous protection that epidermal pigment provides to humans. The sole source of cutaneous melanin are melanocytes that reside in the epidermis. They provide the surrounding keratinocytes with melanosomes, specialized organelles that contain melanins. Darkness and hue of constitutive pigmentation are not due to different densities of melanocytes but rather caused by differences in size and distribution of melanosomes, the overall melanin content of the epidermis and the relative amounts of eumelanin and pheomelanin. Although there is no doubt that melanin is protective from environmental ultraviolet (UV) exposure, the mechanisms by which this happens are not completely clarified. In addition to constitutive differences, multiple exogenous and endogenous agents modulate melanin pigmentation. This chapter will focus primarily on those changes that are induced by UV radiation (UVR). However, as will become evident, this approach does not lead to exclusion but rather to the inclusion of other factors that regulate epidermal melanization.

B. Ortel (✉), M. Racz, D. Lang, and P.G. Calzavara-Pinton
Dermatology, University of Chicago, Chicago, IL, USA
e-mail: bernhard.ortel@uchospitals.edu

E.D. Baron (ed.), *Light-Based Therapies for Skin of Color*,
DOI: 10.1007/ 978-1-84882-328-0_3, © Springer-Verlag London Limited 2009

83

3.1   Melanocytes

The physiological activity of pigment production and distribution by the melanocyte is readily noticed by simple inspection. Therefore, aberrations in melanocyte
development and function have been noticed and documented since many years.[4]
The advent of modern biomolecular analysis has helped identify many mechanisms
that underlie ethnic and racial differences in pigmentation, as well as genetic and
acquired diseases that affect melanocytes.[1,5] Conversely, the understanding of the
disease-associated defects has furthered our knowledge about the complex process
of melanization.[6] Well over a hundred genes have been identified that affect pigmentation. Half of them have been cloned and most have relevance for specific
human pigmentary disorders. All the functionally relevant mutations that are analogous to those in human disorders have been described in inbred mice, which
received descriptive names matching the colors of their coats (e.g. *silver*, *cappuc-
cino*, *mocha*, *sandy*, *leaden*, and *cocoa*). This chapter will concentrate on melanin
pigmentation in human skin; however, recent reviews of the murine melanocytic
system are available for reference.[7,8]

3.1.1   Development and Homeostasis

Melanocytes are derived from an embryonic tissue called the neural crest. The
neural crest consist of a highly plastic and migratory population of cells that arises
after the formation of the other dominant embryonic cell layers (ecto-, endo-, and
mesoderm). As embryogenesis progresses, the neural crest cells migrate to other
regions of the embryo where the primitive organs are developing (Fig. 3.1). The
melanocyte precursor cells migrate to populate numerous locations in the skin,
including the epidermis, dermis, and hair follicles. Immunohistochemistry and
electron microscopy have demonstrated melanocytes in fetal skin as early as in the
eighth week.[9] Once melanoblasts reach the epidermis and hair follicles, they establish a stem cell compartment from which the epidermal melanocytes are regener-
ated. The melanocyte stem cells reside in the lower bulge of the hair follicle, where
they have been identified by immunostaining for markers of early melanocyte
development, such as dopachrome tautomerase and PAX3. When melanocytes die,
cells from the stem cell population migrate from the bulge and replace them. In
vitiligo, where epidermal melanocytes are lost due to an autoimmune disease, repigmentation in response to therapy occurs typically as centrifugal spread from follicular openings, supporting the concept of repopulation from the follicular stem
cell compartment.
Melanocytes are also found in the eye, the inner ear, and the leptomeninges (Fig. 3.2).
This explains why disturbances of melanocytes and their precursors are not always
confined to the skin and its appendages. There are several transcription factors that
are essential for melanocyte development in the embryo. These include PAX3,
SOX10, and microphthalmia transcription factor (MITF).[10–13] PAX3 is a transcription

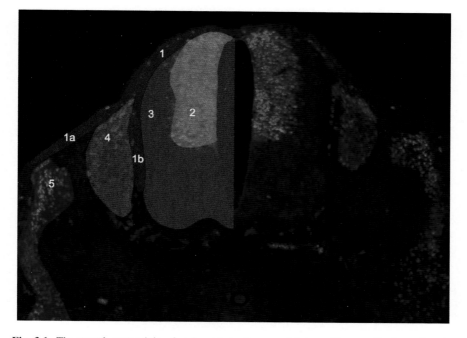

Fig. 3.1 The neural crest origin of melanoblasts. Immunostaining with an antibody against the transcription factor Pax3 highlights multiple populations of cells in a cross section of a 12.5-day-old mouse embryo. Neural crest (area 1) forms between the neural tube and the nonneural ectoderm. Neural crest cells migrate both mediolaterally dorsal to the somites (area 1a) and dorsoventrally (area 1b). The former population (area 1a) is generally restricted to the melanoblasts. Pax3 is also expressed in nonneural crest populations, such as the dorsomedial neuronal cells (area 2) in the neural tube (areas 3), the dorsal root ganglia (area 4), and the somite (area 5)

factor instrumental in the development of several cell types including melano-cytes.[10] The importance of PAX3 to the melanocyte population during development is evident by the loss of hair and skin pigmentation in mice and humans with *PAX3* gene mutations. PAX3 functions as a transcription factor in these melanoblasts by regulating the expression of melanocyte-specific genes including *MITF*.[11] The basic helix-loop-helix leucine zipper transcription factor MITF is often referred to as a "master regulator of melanocyte development" due to its function in regulating several genes involved in melanocyte development, differentiation, and survival.[14] MITF directly activates several melanocyte-specific differentiation genes, includ-ing *TRP-1*, *TRP-2*, and *tyrosinase*. Mutations in *MITF* lead to pigmentation defects in the skin, as well as hearing defects due to a loss of pigment cells in the ear.[14,15] The promotion, survival, and migration of the neural crest-derived cells are sup-ported by the expression of several receptors and the presence of their complemen-tary ligands. These include components of the WNT signaling pathway, the KIT tyrosine kinase receptor and its ligand SCF (stem cell factor, also known as steel factor), and endothelin (ET) receptors and ligands. KIT and SCF play a role in

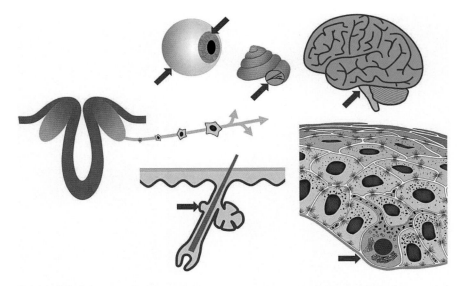

Fig. 3.2 Melanoblast migration. Originating from the neural crest, melanoblasts migrate to their target destination in the eye, the inner ear, brain, and skin. Mutation in one of multiple molecules that are important for melanoblast migration and melanocyte survival can lead to deficiencies in each of the target structures. Clinically, the epidermal pigment deficiency is most conspicuous

melanogenesis, proliferation, migration, and survival.[16] Humans with mutations in *KIT* present with unpigmented patches of skin (Fig. 3.3). Similarly, the interaction between the ET-3 and the ET receptor B results in maintenance of melanoblasts as well as precursors of ganglion cells. Mutations in either of these molecules lead to severe pigmentation defects in mice, and in humans they result in Waardenburg syndrome IV, which is associated with megacolon.[17] The four known subsets of Waardenburg syndrome are associated with mutations in transcription factor genes including *PAX3*, *MITF*, *SOX10*, and *SLUG*.[18] Depending on the ontogenetic role of the defective molecule and its tissue specificity, a variety of associations are seen that go beyond depigmented areas of skin, including deafness, heterochromia iridum (Fig. 3.4), dystopia canthorum, upper limb hypoplasia, and megacolon.[18]

3.1.2 Melanization

The melanocyte is the only source of melanin in human epidermis and its primary role is to produce and distribute melanin. Melanization is the process of melanin synthesis within the melanocytes and transfer to the keratinocytes of each epidermal melanin unit. This functional unit consists of 1 melanocyte and 36 basal keratinocytes that receive melanosomes through the dendrites of the melanocyte (Fig. 3.5).[19] The synthetic process is highly specialized and sequestered to melanosomes within the

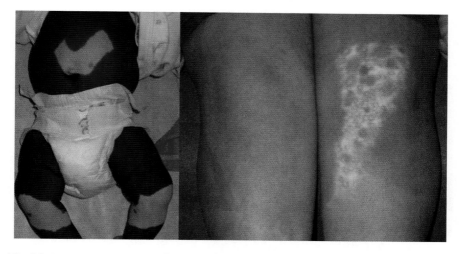

Fig. 3.3 Localized melanocyte deficiency. These children were born with piebaldism, an autosomal dominant disorder due to *KIT* tyrosine kinase gene mutations resulting in defective melanocyte migration and development. (Images reproduced with permission by Dr. S. Stein, University of Chicago, from the website http://dermatlas.bsd.uchicago.edu)

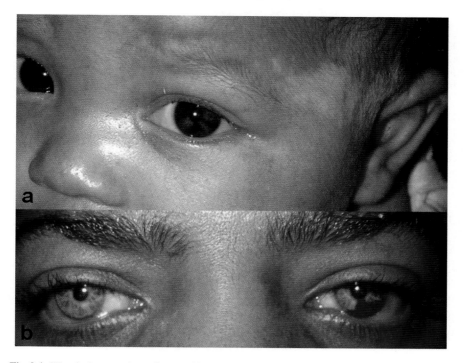

Fig. 3.4 Waardenburg syndrome is caused by genetic defects of one of several proteins (MITF, PAX-3, SOX10, and others) that are involved in melanocyte development, resulting in patchy lack of pigmentation of skin and eyes as shown in two subjects. (**a**) Leukoderma on the face and heterochromia of the left iris of an infant (Image reproduced with permission by Dr. S. Stein, University of Chicago, from the website http://dermatlas.bsd.uchicago.edu); (**b**) Heterochromia iridum in an adult African-American (Image courtesy of Dr. Reshma Haugen, Rush University). In Waardenburg syndrome, multiple developmental defects of the nervous system may be associated with melanocyte defects

a   b

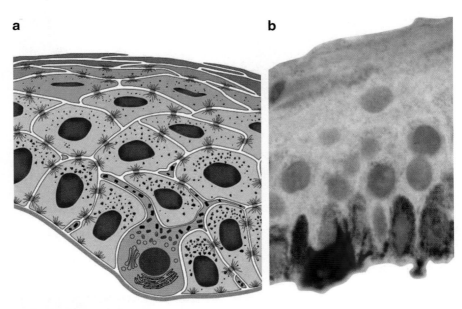

Fig. 3.5 (**a**) The epidermal melanin unit is a functional grouping of one melanocyte and about 36 basal keratinocytes that are recipients of melanosome transfer from the melanocyte. (**b**) Matching histological section stained with *Mart-1* (melanocyte antigen recognized by T lymphocytes-1) highlighting the melanocyte and its dendrites

melanocyte. This subcelluar compartmentalization prevents toxic intermediates of melanin synthesis from causing unwanted toxicity to the melanocyte and provides neatly packaged units of pigment for transfer to the keratinocytes.

3.1.2.1 Melanosome Formation

Melanocytes maintain a highly dynamic endosomal system to create cell-specific lysosome-related organelles (LROs), the melanosomes. The melanization process depends on the sequential delivery of structural proteins and melanogenic enzymes to the melanosomes (Fig. 3.6). Melanosomes are recognized in four stages by their ultrastructural features.[20,21] Stage I melanosomes are spherical and contain intraluminal vesicles. Stage II melanosomes are oval and contain a fibrillary protein structure. Stage III and IV show gradually increasing melanin deposition. Stage IV melanosomes are opaque on electron microscopy and show minimal tyrosinase activity, which is highest in stage III melanosomes.[22] Pheomelanosomes retain a spherical structure through all stages and are smaller than eumelanosomes.[23] Melanosome maturation is regulated by timed targeting of proteins to this developing organelle. The first component, PMEL (PMEL17, HMB45, silver, GP100) forms

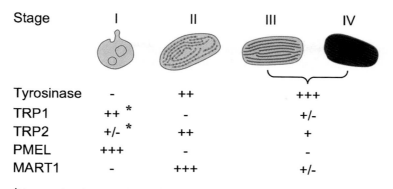

Stage	I	II	III	IV
Tyrosinase	-	++		+++
TRP1	++ *	-		+/-
TRP2	+/- *	++		+
PMEL	+++	-		-
MART1	-	+++		+/-

* Low molecular weight cleavage products

Fig. 3.6 Melanosome maturation. Four stages of melanosomes differ in their ultrastructural morphology and biochemistry. For details, see text. Figure adapted from Kushimoto et al[22]

the internal structure where the melanin polymers get deposited once tyrosinase and related proteins have been imported.[24] In early endosomes, a proteolytic milieu seems to dominate. This is important for PMEL processing in order to form the internal fibrillar component of the melanosome. For the same reason, tyrosinase-related proteins TRP-1 and TRP-2 (dopachrome tautomerase) are found in early melanosomes in cleaved low molecular weight forms that are inactive.[22] Once the melanosomes transition to stage II, proteolysis subsides and full-length enzymes initiate melanin synthesis.[22]

The sequential delivery of melanosomal proteins is critical to the melanization process. The analysis of genetic defects in Hermansky Pudlak syndrome (HPS) has elucidated many of the steps involved in early melanosome formation.[25] HPS is inherited in an autosomal recessive manner and features pigment dilution in hair, skin, and eyes. All eight currently known HPS subtypes have mutations in genes encoding proteins involved in the function of LROs, including melanosomes. HPS-2 has a defective adapter protein-3 that sorts tyrosinase and possibly other melanogenic proteins to the melanosomes.[6] In the other HPS variants, components of the biogenesis of lysosome-related organelles complex (BLOC-1, -2, -3) are affected.[6] Depending on the specific gene product, additional features are associated with the reduced pigmentation in HPS, such as excessive bleeding due to platelet dysfunction, immunodeficiency, and compromise of the lungs, the GI tract, and the kidneys.[25] Another defect in lysosomal transport presenting with silvery hair and reduced pigmentation is Chédiak-Higashi syndrome, where a gene defect in LYST results in compromised fission and fusion of LROs. The molecular defect results in giant melanosomes and enlarged granulocytic granules. Hypopigmentation, immune dysfunction, bleeding diathesis, and neurological degeneration all result from LRO compromise.[26]

3.1.2.2 Melanin Synthesis

Melanin synthesis is initiated from L-phenylalanine or from L-tyrosine by hydroxylation that results in the formation of L-dihydroxyphenylalanine (L-DOPA), a precursor for both catecholamines and melanins.[21] After oxidation to dopaquinone and dopachrome, the synthetic pathways leading to eumelanin and pheomelanin diverge. Eumelanins result from the formation of dihydroxyindole (DHI) and DHI carbolic acid (DHICA), while pheomelanin is a polymer of L-DOPA condensation products with cysteine (Fig. 3.7).[21,27] Three structurally closely related enzymes, tyrosinase, TRP-1 and TRP-2, are involved in melanin synthesis.[22] These molecules contain cysteine-rich regions and metal-binding domains.[28] The catalytic domain of tyrosinase contains six histidine residues that bind two copper atoms. An N-terminal peptide signal mediates import into the endoplasmic reticulum where the proteins are glycosylated. A C-terminal transmembrane fragment localizes tyrosinase to the melanosomal membrane. Most of these features are shared by TRP-1 and TRP-2 including metal binding, with TRP-1 binding iron and TRP-2 containing zinc. Both TRP-1 and TRP-2 modify, stabilize, and regulate the eumelanogenic process but their exact roles are still being evaluated. There are additional proteins involved in melanization, including peroxidase, PMEL, and catechol-*O*-methyltransferase.[29] PMEL is rich in cysteine and histidine and catalyzes DHICA polymerization.[30] It forms a scaffold for melanin deposition and stabilization.[24] Melanogenesis is

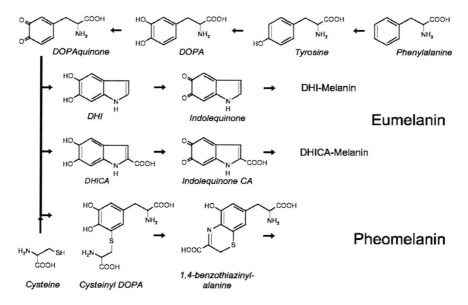

Fig. 3.7 Biosynthesis of melanin. The two major forms of melanin are brown-black eumelanin and orange pheomelanin. *DOPA* dihydroxyphenylalanine, *DHI* 5,6-dihydroxyindole, *DHICA* 5,6-dihydroxyindole-2-carboxylic acid

affected by levels of glutathione oxidase and glutathione reductase that balance glutathione levels, as well as catalase that controls H_2O_2 levels, the latter a potent inhibitor of tyrosinase.[31]

Eumelanins contain variable proportions of DHI and DHICA depending on its source. Synthetic, enzymatically prepared melanins contain about 10% carboxylated molecules, while natural melanins consist of up to 50% DHICA.[32] There is no general agreement on the secondary structure and higher organization of melanins that *in vivo* are tightly associated with proteins, forming melanoproteins. One of the reasons is that only harsh solubilization methods can be used for melanosome extraction, but these break up the very structure that is the object of the study. Even for synthetic melanins, the arrangement within the oligomers and larger aggregates has not been resolved at this time. Moreover, synthetic melanins are in many ways not a good substitute for the study of the naturally occurring polymer aggregates. The planar structure of the primary molecules has led to the proposal of aggregates of stacked oligomers that assemble in fibrillary structures.[33] Aggregates of the fibrillary polymers form the melanin granules in the melanosomes (Fig. 3.8).[34] Melanin remains an analytical challenge and an object of creative modeling.[35]

While eumelanins are dark brown (DHICA) or black (DHI), pheomelanin confers an orange-red pigmentation that is dominant in Celtic skin types (phototype I). The naturally occurring shades and variations of skin pigmentation are due in part to variable contributions of eumelanins and pheomelanin.[36] As mentioned above, pheomelanin synthesis requires cysteine; however, it is not clear how cysteine availability in melanosomes is regulated. The transformation of oxidized glutathione (GSSG) to reduced glutathione (GSH) is crucial for the formation of glutathionyldopa, a source of cysteinyldopa, and thus a starting point for pheomelanogenesis. Glutathione oxidase and reductase regulate the GSH levels. At low concentrations of sulfhydryl compounds, the synthesis gets rerouted from pheomelanin to eumelanin formation.[37]

The importance of the critical melanogenic proteins is highlighted by genetic disorders. In different forms of albinism, pigmentation is absent or greatly reduced because melaninogenesis is compromised by loss-of-function mutations in one of the proteins involved in the melanization process. In oculocutaneus albinism (OCA) types 1 and 3, tyrosinase and TRP-1 are defective, respectively, while in

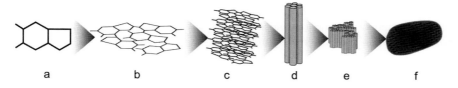

    a   b   c   d   e   f

Fig. 3.8 Current concepts of the macromolecular structure of melanin. DHI and DHICA (**a**, *see* Fig. 3.7) form planar oligomers (**b**) that are stacked (**c**) and form filaments (**d**). These are condensed into aggregates (**e**), which represent the granular subunits of melanosomes (**f**). Figure adapted from Clancy and Simon[34]

OCA2 and OCA4, two putative transmembrane transporter proteins, OCA2 and MATP, are mutated.[38] It is unknown, by which mechanism the defective gene product OA1 affects melanogenesis in ocular albinism 1.

3.1.2.3 Melanosome Transfer

Once melanosomes have formed and are melanized, they are transported peripherally through the branching extensions of the melanocyte known as dendrites. The intradendrite movement requires actin filaments and microtubules and is mediated through the interaction of three proteins, myosin Va, RAB27A, and melanophilin, that bridge the melanosomes with the actin filaments.[39] The importance of the close interaction of these three proteins is supported by the fact that mutations in any one of these genes lead to Griscelli syndrome, presenting with pigmentary dilution and silvery hair.[39,40] Depending on which protein is affected, neurological and hematological abnormalities may be associated with the pigmentation defect.[40]

When the melanosomes have reached the tips of the dendrites, they need to be transferred to keratinocytes, a continuous and dynamic process. The ability of keratinocytes to uptake the melanosomes is critical for successful particle transfer as demonstrated by phagocytosis of latex particles by keratinocytes.[41] Keratinocyte growth factor (KGF) has been shown to activate the phagocytic activity of keratinocytes and also to enhance melanosome transfer.[42] In addition to the KGF receptor, other signaling mechanisms, such as through the protease-activated receptor-2 (Par-2), have been identified that regulate constitutive and UVR-stimulated transfer of melanosomes from melanocytes to keratinocytes.[43] Par-2 is thought to modify the phagocytotic process involved in melanosome transfer.[44] Increased phagocytic activity by keratinocytes has also been reported after their treatment with α-MSH.[45] Melanosomes are distributed within the keratinocytes by intracellular trafficking mechanisms in a predominantly supranuclear distribution (Fig. 3.11). During terminal keratinocyte differentiation from basal cell to corneocyte, the melanosomes are gradually lost. The process of melanosome degradation within the keratinocytes has not been clarified but is most likely a phagolysosomal process.[46,47] In view of the technical difficulties involved in the analysis of the macromolecular structure of melanin, an understanding of its degradation would be helpful in developing novel analytical approaches. Some authors suggest that melanosomes are gradually eliminated by enzymatic degradation.[48] Acid hydrolases have been proposed to act on the protein component of melanosomes.[49] The degradation of the aromatic hydrocarbons constituting melanin may be mediated by NAPDH oxidase.[49]

3.2 Protection by Melanin

Melanin protects from acute and chronic effects of UVR. Skin phototyping itself uses sun sensitivity and protective properties of melanin pigmentation as defining criteria.[50] Constitutively darker skin of phototypes IV to VI is less likely to burn after solar UV exposure, indicating an inherent protective effect of epidermal pigmentation. Protection from UV-induced erythema by melanin has been quantified for both constitutive and UV-induced pigmentation. When erythemogenicity of broadband UV was tested in different skin phototypes, darkly pigmented African-American skin (skin phototype VI) had a protection factor of about 10–15 times that of individuals with skin phototype I.[51,52] In general, average minimum erythemal doses (MEDs) are, over this tenfold range, directly correlated with skin phototype. However, there are large variations between individuals that make MED values reasonable measures of sun sensitivity, but poor predictors of skin type.[52,53] While there are large differences in UV sensitivity between individuals of different constitutive pigmentation, induction of melanization by UVR provides a relatively small protection factor. In addition, different portions of the UV spectrum have different efficacies in inducing protection from erythema. Broadband UVB induces a tan that provides a protection factor of about 2–3,[54,55] while a UVA-induced tan that is visually identical provides a protection factor of only 1.3.[54] When pigmentation was enhanced by pharmacological stimulation of the MC1R rather than by UV exposure, the protective effect of melanin was shown by reduced epidermal keratinocyte apoptosis (sunburn cell formation) after UV exposure.[56] In a similar investigation in mice, pigmentation was induced using forskolin.[57] Protection was assessed by reduced epidermal DNA damage and sunburn cell formation in forskolin-treated, hyperpigmented skin. A different study comparing white and dark human skin after UV exposure demonstrated protection from DNA damage by high constitutive melanin content of basal keratinocytes and melanocytes.[58] However, in dark skin, higher numbers of sunburn cells were registered, suggesting that melanin may be a photosensitizing agent under specific conditions.[59]

The protection factors discussed above refer of course to erythemogenicity of UV exposure only. It appears that the relative protection by dark pigmentation from the effects of chronic UV exposure, such as skin cancer, is much better than these values would indicate.[60,61] Epidemiological data support the protection by constitutive pigmentation from UV-induced carcinogenicity. For example, there is a high incidence of sun-induced skin cancers in black Africans with oculocutaneous albinism,[62] while in their normally pigmented relatives, skin cancer is an extreme rarity.[60] Similar evidence comes from the immigration of fair skinned individuals from the British Islands to Australia with its high environmental UVR levels. This skin phototype/solar UV exposure mismatch has resulted in extremely high rates of skin cancer in the Australian population of Celtic origin.[63] In contrast, the prevalence of skin cancer in the indigenous population of darkly pigmented aborigines is low.[64,65] In addition to protection from photocarcinogenesis, constitutive pigmentation appears to protect from UV-induced skin aging.[66]

This section cannot be concluded without mentioning one unwanted protective effect of melanin, namely from UV-mediated ViD conversion in the skin.[67] The importance of ViD for calcium homeostasis and bone health is well-known. The concept of ViD-mediated protection from malignancies has been put forward many years ago, and epidemiological studies have demonstrated good supportive evidence. A protective effect of higher ViD levels from internal cancers and even myocardial infarction in prospective studies has been reported more recently.[68,69]

3.2.1 Optical Properties

Two functions can be attributed to melanin – coloration and photoprotection. Despite positive evidence of melanin protection, the mechanisms are not completely understood. In contrast to most organic chromophores, which show distinctive peaks (e.g. the absorption spectra of DNA, amino acids, flavins, and carotenes), eumelanin in solution has a broadband monotonic absorption spectrum with a simple exponential decrease from the UV to the visible range.[70] This has resulted in the concept that scattering is the dominant function of melanin.[71] However, even in highly dilute, nonturbid solutions of eumelanin, the monotonous absorption curve dominates, which indicates an electronic effect at the molecular level.[72] Over 99% of the radiative energy absorbed by melanin is dissipated nonradiatively, creating heat. This is important as melanin would otherwise cause potentially damaging photochemical reactions.[72] These data have been also shown for pheomelanin.[73]

Even in solution under highly dilute conditions, scattering contributes to the overall optical properties of melanin.[71] Melanin aggregates in the native intracellular form and distribution scatter and thus attenuate incident radiation even more efficiently. This can be visualized using confocal laser scanning microscopy. In reflectance mode, this modality is based on single backscattering, and the optical properties of large melanin complexes support scattering as an important function of melanosomes in human epidermis.[74] In this setting, a focused laser beam scans a horizontal plane in the skin and the backscattered light is collected confocally, thus creating an optical section. Webb's group demonstrated that melanosomes are an excellent contrast agent for confocal microscopy.[75] Figure 3.9 illustrates this fact by comparing horizontal sections through the suprapapillary epidermis and at the midpapillary level in the skin of a phototype I and a phototype V person.[76,77] The volunteer with dark Asian skin showed an intense signal from the suprapapillary epidermis (Fig. 3.9b) and the basal layer surrounding the dermal papillae (Fig. 3.9d), while light European skin showed, at best, very weak contrast at either imaging level (Fig. 3.9a, c). The strong signal from the pigment-rich epidermal keratinocytes in Fig. 3.9b and d proves the high optical activity of melanosomes in the far-red spectrum, where melanin absorption is relatively low compared to the UV and short-wave visible range.[72] These images and data support a model where both absorption and scattering contribute *in vivo* to the attenuation of incident UVR, which results in the protection provided by melanin. Absorption still plays a dominant role, allowing for melanin-targeted laser therapies such as hair removal. In addition to its optical properties, melanin confers protection by other mechanisms.

3.2.2 Redox Properties

Eumelanin has the ability to reduce and oxidize other molecules due to the redox properties of its monomeric building blocks, namely DHI and DHICA, as well as their semiquinone and fully oxidized quinone forms.[72] Pheomelanin has analogous components that undergo stepwise oxidation. These individual components, such as

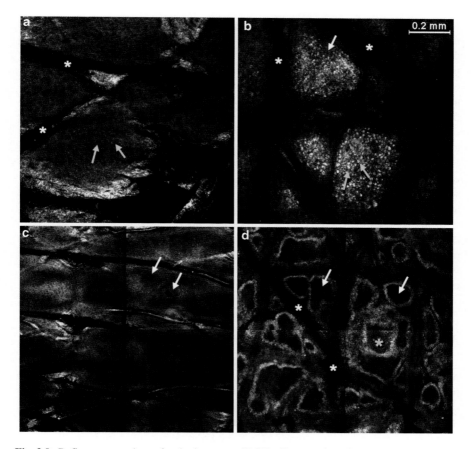

Fig. 3.9 Reflectance-mode confocal microscopy (*RCM*) allows noninvasive optical sectioning of the skin with melanin as the dominant endogenous contrast. (**a**, **c**) RCM horizontal sections of normal skin on the inner forearm of an individual with skin phototype I. Note the overall lack of contrast. (**a**) Polygonal keratinocytes (arrows) at the level of the basal layer. Keratinocytes are seen arranged in a honeycomb pattern interrupted by skin folds (asterisks). (**c**) Dermal papillary rings (arrows) at the level of the superficial dermoepidermal junction. (**b**, **d**) RCM images of normal skin on the inner forearm of an individual with skin phototype V. Note the heightened contrast due to constitutive melanin pigmentation; (**b**) pigmented keratinocytes (yellow arrows) located above dermal papillae (white arrow) at the level of the basal layer; (**d**) dermal papillae (yellow arrows) brightly refractile at the level of dermoepidermal junction. Hair follicle (yellow asterisk) and skin folds (white asterisks) can be seen. (Images courtesy of Dr. Salvador Gonzalez, Memorial Sloan Kettering Cancer Center, New York)[76]

free semiquinones, are unstable and react readily with other molecules, but within the melanin oligomers and complexes, this reactivity is reduced, likely through intramolecular interactions and steric hindrance.[78] Synthetic polymers of eumelanin and pheomelanin can act as scavengers for oxidizing as well as reducing radicals with high efficiency.[79] The significance of this ability of melanin to protect from free radical damage is unknown. It is conceivable that some cells for example postmitotic retinal pigment epithelium cells, need this property as a defense mechanism, because they perform their function under the constant threat of oxidative stress. It has been demonstrated that melanin in retinal pigment epithelium cells is able to quench reactive oxygen species. Although cutaneous melanocytes have a nearby follicular reservoir of stem cell reserves, they are also continuously exposed to oxidative stress and likely remain active in a postmitotic state for a long time. It has been shown that through radical scavenging by pheomelanin, reactive oxygen species, such as superoxide anion and hydrogen peroxide, may be formed within the cell and may become cytotoxic.[80] However, it is not clear that these findings are relevant *in vivo*.

It appears that melanin protects the function and genetic integrity of cells by a synergism of two mechanisms, namely scattering and absorption of photons and by scavenging toxic radicals, including those created by UVR exposure. Melanosomes are recognized as highly absorbing targets for a broad spectrum of radiant energy, with almost complete conversion of the light energy to heat. This creates both opportunities and obstacles for light-based therapeutic interventions. For example, eumelanin in the hair follicle makes black hair the best target for laser hair removal, while dark skin is most susceptible to the associated unwanted laser effects on the epidermis.

3.3   Regulation of Melanocyte Function

Melanocyte activity affects the pigmentary skin phenotype by contributions from total melanin, its components (eumelanin/pheomelanin), and its distribution in the skin. The stimulatory effect of pituitary hormones on amphibian melanophores has been known for about a century, when pituitary extracts darkened tadpoles. Later on, adrenocorticotropic hormone (ACTH) and α-melanocyte-stimulating hormone (α-MSH) were identified as the responsible agents in the pituitary extracts. ACTH and α-MSH were shown to increase pigmentation in human skin as well.[81] These hormones act through a specific receptor molecule, the melanocortin 1 receptor (MC1R) that is mainly expressed on melanocytes.[82] There are a total of five MCRs, but only MC1R plays a role in the regulation of pigmentation. MC1R is a member of the G–protein-coupled receptor family and has seven transmembrane domains.[83] The physiological ligands of the MC1R, α-MSH and ACTH are both derived from proopiomelanocortin (POMC) by proteolysis.[84] MC1R activation causes increased cAMP levels and signaling that results in increased melanosome formation and a shift to eumelanin synthesis.[85] The transcription factor MITF plays a central role not only during development (see above) but also in mediating melanogenic signals.[86] MITF provides positive transcriptional regulation of tyrosinase, TRP-1 and TRP-2, as well as of MC1R.[87,88] Agents that increase cAMP, such as forskolin, have shown strong melanogenic potential in vitro and *in vivo*, which supports the critical role of cAMP in melanogenesis. It was even shown that forskolin could stimulate melanogenesis in mice that were deficient in α-MSH signaling, while UV exposures failed to induce pigmentation.[57] Increased cAMP levels also lead to an increase in MC1R expression, thus likely increasing the responsiveness of the cell to external stimuli. Additional signals have been shown to modulate MC1R expression in cultured melanocytes, with upregulation by α-MSH, ET-1, basic fibroblast growth factor (bFGF), and β-estradiol.[89] MC1R exhibits considerable constitutive activity that can be downregulated by its antagonistic ligand, the agouti signaling protein (ASIP). The exact role of ASIP in humans, however, has not been clarified. It has been shown though that ASIP binding by MC1R blocks the stimulatory effect of α-MSH and even forskolin,[90] and leads to preferential pheomelanin synthesis over eumelanin production.[91]

Although the pituitary gland is the primary source of α-MSH and ACTH, localized release of mediators is likely to be more important for the regulation of melanin synthesis. Epidermal keratinocytes have been shown to have a high secretory capacity and are the source of multiple mediators that regulate melanocyte biology (Fig. 3.10). The MC1R-mediated pathway has been discussed above. The importance of this interaction between keratinocytes and melanocytes was illustrated in a study that showed that cocultures had much higher α-MSH levels than cultures of keratinocytes or melanocytes alone.[45] Additional signaling pathways include the steel factor binding to KIT, and ligand receptor interaction for bFGF, ET-1, GM-CSF, and prostaglandins.[92] Using their respective downstream pathways, these exogenous signals modulate melanocyte proliferation, differentiation, and survival, as well as dendrite formation and melanogenesis (Fig. 3.10). The effects are partially regulated through induction of MC1R expression by some of these signals, as discussed above. Most of the pathways are modulated by exposure to UVR.[93]

The MC1R gene is unusually polymorphic, and many functionally relevant natural variants have been described. In mice, specific genetic variants have been linked to altered coat color.[94] In humans, certain genetic variants were found to confer a

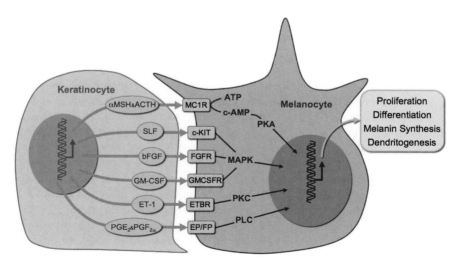

Fig. 3.10 Stimulation of a melanocyte by a keratinocyte through multiple mediators. Figure modified from Hirobe[92]

phenotype consisting of sun sensitivity, red hair color, freckling, and increased skin cancer risk.[95] Such mutations may be associated with reduced MC1R affinity for melanocortins or with diminished downstream coupling to adenylate cyclase.[96] Interestingly, MC1R gene variations may also confer melanoma risk independently of the red hair phenotype.[97] A novel aspect of MC1R polymorphism is its apparent effect on cutaneous sensitivity to psoralen phototoxicity.[98] These findings emphasize the central role of the interaction between α-MSH and MC1R, the downstream signal, c-AMP, and MITF for the maintenance of proper melanocyte function and epidermal protection.

3.3.1   UVR Effects on Pigmentation

With or without preceding sunburn, the UV portion of the solar spectrum can cause an increase in melanin formation, resulting in the delayed tanning response. Both erythemal and melanogenic responses depend on constitutive pigmentation, with baseline darker skin tanning more easily and at nonerythemogenic exposure levels.[99,100] However, there is evidence that melanogenesis does not correlate in the same way with constitutive pigmentation in East Asians.[101,102] At the clinical level, in response to UVR exposure in the range of one MED, pigmentation appears after 3–5 days and is often evaluated at 7 days. Although a tan may be visible in many subjects, the absolute increase of epidermal melanin is not dramatic. Even repeated exposures over a 3 week period do not lead to a large increase in cutaneous melanin content. As mentioned above, UV-induced melanogensis does not provide a high protection factor. That UV-induced tanning still confers significant protection is based on the redistribution of melanosomes within the epidermis and the epidermal keratinocytes.[103]

Investigative reports over the last few years have helped to elucidate the mechanisms that are involved in UV-dependent enhancement of epidermal pigmentation. Most UV-induced skin responses are tightly associated with UV-induced DNA lesions. The dominant UV photoproduct, the cyclobutane pyrimidine dimer, has been studied most extensively and has been linked to short-term UV effects, such as erythema,[104] as well as to long-term consequences of UV exposure, such as carcinogenesis.[105] Tanning is no exception and has been first tightly associated with DNA damage by work from Gilchrest's group.[106,107] They demonstrated that a variety of treatments that produce small DNA fragments cause increased melanogenesis. These include UV exposure, exogenous restriction enzyme treatment, and chemotherapy with alkylating agents that result in enzymatic DNA repair. The investigators concluded that thymidine dimers that are released by excision repair after UV exposure are likely the molecular mediators of the UV-dependent tanning response. Interestingly, upregulation of tyrosinase mRNA was observed after UV exposure.[106] Additional support for the connection between UV-induced DNA damage and tanning came from a report by Nylander et al who showed transactivation of tyrosinase and TRP-1 promoters by p53, thus identifying TRP-1 and tyrosinase as potentially p53-responsive genes.[108] Other evidence from Gilchrest's group also supported involvement of p53 in tyrosinase regulation and showed that the melanogenic response to thymidine dimers and dinucleotides depended on p53 activation.[109] Most recently, a connection was made between DNA damage-induced p53 activation and melanogenesis by showing potent stimulation of the POMC promoter by p53.[110] As described above, POMC is the source of α-MSH, ACTH, and β-endorphin, and the melanogenic response depends strongly on MC1R activation by α-MSH. The synopsis of these reports creates a scenario where DNA damage and its repair are tightly linked to the induction of melanogenesis through p53 induction. As α-MSH has been shown to protect melanocytes and keratinocytes from UVR-induced apoptosis at least in part by enhancing DNA repair,[111,112] the increased repair activity may contribute to enhanced melanogenesis through the p53-linked pathway. Also, treatment of keratinocytes with forskolin, an inducer of cAMP, increases DNA repair and protects cells from apoptosis independently of melanization.[113] These data also emphasize the central role of α-MSH in enhancement of eumelanogenesis and DNA repair while reducing apoptosis. Thus, α-MSH critically supports the survival and genetic stability of the epidermal melanocyte[93] and basal keratinocytes.[58,111] The current data also allow for the possibility that the increased melanoma risk associated with a phenotype of sun sensitivity, red hair, and freckling, and a variant of MC1R, leads to increased melanoma risk not only because of lack of eumelanin formation but also because of a deficiency in DNA repair mechanisms.

Although α-MSH and its effects on MC1R signaling play a central role in the melanogenic response after UVR exposure, other signals have been demonstrated to stimulate epidermal pigmentation. UV exposure can reduce GSH levels, which results in reduced pheomelanin synthesis favoring eumelanin production. Also, Par-2 expression is upregulated after UV exposure and has been already described in association with melanosome transfer.[114] Keratinocyte phagocytosis of latex beads and melanosomes is increased by UV exposure and by exposure to α-MSH.[45] KGF promotes the transfer of melanosomes to keratinocytes, and UV exposure has been shown to activate the KGF receptor on keratinocytes.[115]

Because of chronic stimulation of UV-inducible mechanisms, chronically sun-exposed epidermis contains higher numbers of melanocytes and greater melanin levels than unexposed skin independent of ethnic variations in skin color.[36] However, there is a continuous loss of epidermal melanocytes with increasing age at a rate of about 10% per decade.[116,117]

3.4 Racial Differences in Pigmentation

The density of melanocytes differs from one anatomic region to another. It is also affected by age, resulting in a steady decline. Chronic solar UV exposure lead to a doubling of melanocyte numbers in sun-exposed areas.[116,118] Compared to these differences, there is much less variation between light and dark skinned individuals when quantifying melanocytes in the same location.[36] A recent report even suggests that light European skin has relatively higher numbers of melanocytes than that of more darkly pigmented ethnic groups[119]; however, this is not a consistent finding.[120] This emphasizes that the density of melanocytes is not a major determinant of the degree of different pigmentation between ethnicities.

The overall melanin content is clearly an important factor in epidermal pigmentation. Chemical quantification of melanin showed about twice the amount of pigment in dark African compared to European skin.[36] In tissue culture, up to fourfold differences between light and dark skin-derived melanocytes have been reported.[93] Consistently, the amounts of the melanogenic proteins tyrosinase, TRP-1 and TRP-2, are low in light skin-derived melanocytes and high in cells from skin with dark constitutive pigmentation.[121] In addition to the total epidermal melanin content, the relative contributions from eumelanin and pheomelanin were found to impact skin color. While in black African skin, less than 15% of the pigment was alkali-soluble pheomelanin, European skin contained an average of 40%.[36] Chinese, Mexican, and Indian individuals had graded values of alkali-soluble pheomelanin between 15% and 40%.[36] Objective optical measurements of skin color may be applied to distinguish constitutive ethnic skin differences, and have been shown to correlate with skin phototyping and MED.[52,122,123]

When keratinocytes from European and Asian individuals were analyzed ultrastructurally, they were found to contain membrane-bound aggregates of multiple smaller melanosomes.[124,125] In contrast, melanosomes in dark African skin were larger and individually dispersed in the keratinocytes.[125] Keratinocytes of dark skin contain almost exclusively stage IV melanosomes, while lightly pigmented skin may have a mixture of different melanosomes with earlier stages.[126] Therefore, it appears that the size of the organelles, their maturation, and spatial arrangement are more important determinants of ethnic skin color differences than melanocyte density. Keratinocytes themselves play an important role in the transfer of melanosomes from the melanocytes, their distribution, and packaging.[127] Par-2, which has been described above for its role in melanosome transfer, is expressed on keratinocytes but not in melanocytes.[128] Par-2 is activated by trypsin, and higher levels of both trypsin and Par-2 are found in keratinocytes of dark skinned individuals.[129] To analyze which cell type contributes the ethnic component of epidermal pigment distribution, Yoshida et al grafted mixtures of keratinocytes and melanocytes from ethnically different donor skin types in chambers on the backs of immunodeficient mice.[130] In this experimental setting, the epidermal melanin content and maturation of melanosomes were significantly higher in combinations of dark skin-derived keratinocytes independently of the source of melanocytes. Emphasizing the role of keratinocytes in melanosome distribution, the ratio of individual to clustered melanosomes was also increased in recipient keratinocytes derived from dark skin.[130] This report supports the concept that keratinocytes make a significant contribution to the "ethnicity" of epidermal pigmentation.

When analyzing proteins involved in melanogenesis, no variation of tyrosinase levels but significantly higher expression of TRP-1 was seen in darkly pigmented African and Asian skin.[119] Although the function of TRP-1 is not completely understood, it is involved in regulation of melanogenesis and appears to modulate melanosome maturation. It may also determine ethnical differences in melanosome size.[119,131]

As mentioned initially, the central African origin of our common ancestry was associated with dark constitutive pigmentation. Mutations of critical steps in melanization result mostly in loss or profound dilution of pigmentation but not in natural variations of skin color. MC1R and its antagonistic ligand ASIP are important in regulating pheomelanin production, an important component of skin tone. A number of recent population-based studies tried to pinpoint additional genes that are involved in creating physiological shades of skin pigmentation.[2,132,133] They all came to similar conclusions and found polymorphisms in ASIP and OCA2 (a protein likely regulating melanosomal pH) that are involved in determining light and dark pigmentation in all populations. SLC24A5, a melanosomal calcium transporter, tyrosinase, and MATP, which is critical in tyrosinase trafficking and processing, likely played a role in the evolution of light European but not light Asian skin.[2,132,133] These data support a role for these genes in modulation of skin color, but also support evolutionary concepts of the development of lighter, less sun-protective skin pigmentation. In addition to these melanogenesis-related genes, other genetic traits that determine hair and skin color have been described.[132] Besides melanin, other chromophores, such as hemoglobin and carotenes, may contribute to skin color. These, however, have little if any influence on ethnic skin color differences and are not included in this analysis.

Several microscopic images were included to illustrate racial differences in epidermal melanin pigmentation. Figure 3.11a–c shows vertical sections of skin of

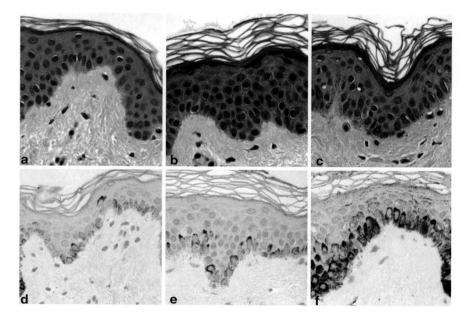

Fig. 3.11 Photomicrographs of age-matched human skin from three different skin phototypes. (**a**, **d**) European skin, (**b**, **e**) Chinese skin, and (**c**, **f**) African-American skin. The top row displays vertical sections stained with H&E, the bottom row has corresponding sections stained with the Fontana-Masson stain that highlights melanin pigment. Note the concentration of melanin granules in a cap-like distribution above the cell nuclei

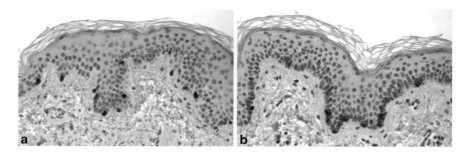

Fig. 3.12 These sections of (**a**) light European and (**b**) dark African-American skin highlight melanocytes in the basal layer of the epidermis using immunohistochemistry. An antibody against MART-1 is visualized with a red chromogen. The melanocyte density is slightly higher in (**a**). The dendrites of the melanocytes are stained and can be seen branching between the keratinocytes

racially different young adults stained by hematoxylin and eosin (H&E). All sections show brown pigment in the basal layers and variable amounts in the spinous layer. Visualization of melanin can be enhanced with the Fontana-Masson stain (Fig. 3.11d–f). Using this method, each melanin granule becomes a nidus for the reduction of a silver salt solution forming microscopic black granules. It is clearly evident that dark African-American skin contains more melanin than Chinese or European skin. In all sections, a supranuclear cap of melanosomes can be seen in several keratinocytes (Fig. 3.11). This distribution provides a protective screen to the UV-sensitive genetic material in the cell nucleus.[134] Despite the much higher epidermal melanin content in African-American skin, a very similar density of melanocytes is seen, which has been reported repeatedly. This can be readily illustrated by immunohistochemical staining for MART-1 (melanocyte antigen recognized by T cells-1), a small transmembrane protein that highlights melanocytes and their dendrites (Fig. 12). Images taken by *in vivo* confocal laser scanning microscopy demonstrate strong melanin-dependent contrast in darkly pigmented skin. Light skin is difficult to analyze by this method as it relies primarily on melanin as the endogenous contrast agent (Fig. 3.9).

3.5   Summary

Melanins determine the skin colors and protective properties of the epidermis against solar UV exposure and its hazards. The structure of melanin is not completely clarified and it functions through multiple mechanisms, including scattering and absorption of incident radiation. The complex interaction of epidermal melanocytes and keratinocytes determines constitutive skin color and adaptive responses that maintain survival and genetic integrity of the melanocytes and basal keratinocytes using cell–cell signaling and complex intracellular machinery that regulates epidermal melanization. Much of our understanding of these processes stems from genetic disorders with compromised pigmentation. An additional understanding of ethnic differences in constitutive pigmentation comes from recent population-based studies. Finally, because of chemical inertia and unique optical properties, melanin often poses a potential challenge to dermatological treatments and light-based procedures.

Acknowledgment Financial support was provided by a grant from the Dermatology Foundation (PI: Christopher R. Shea, MD). We thank Diana Bolotin, MD, PhD for critical review of the manuscript.

References

1. Harris EE, Meyer D. The molecular signature of selection underlying human adaptations. *Am J Phys Anthropol.* 2006;Suppl 43:89–130.
2. Lao O, de Gruijwwter JM, van Duijn K, Navarro A, Kayser M. Signatures of positive selection in genes associated with human skin pigmentation as revealed from analyses of single nucleotide polymorphisms. *Ann Hum Genet.* 2007;71:354–369.
3. Briollais L, Chompret A, Guilloud-Bataille M, Bressac-de Paillerets B, Avril MF, Demenais F. Patterns of familial aggregation of three melanoma risk factors: great number of naevi, light phototype and high degree of sun exposure. *Int J Epidemiol.* 2000;29:408–415.
4. Westerhof W. The discovery of the human melanocyte. *Pigment Cell Res.* 2006;19:183–193.
5. Passeron T, Mantoux F, Ortonne JP. Genetic disorders of pigmentation. *Clin Dermatol.* 2005;23:56–67.
6. Raposo G, Marks MS. Melanosomes–dark organelles enlighten endosomal membrane transport. *Nat Rev Mol Cell Biol.* 2007;8:786–797.
7. Bennett DC, Lamoreux ML. The color loci of mice–a genetic century. *Pigment Cell Res.* 2003;16:333–344.
8. Steingrimsson E, Copeland NG, Jenkins NA. Mouse coat color mutations: from fancy mice to functional genomics. *Dev Dyn.* 2006;235:2401–2411.
9. Holbrook KA, Underwood RA, Vogel AM, Gown AM, Kimball H. The appearance, density and distribution of melanocytes in human embryonic and fetal skin revealed by the anti-melanoma monoclonal antibody, HMB-45. *Anat Embryol (Berl).* 1989;180:443–455.
10. Lang D, Brown CB, Epstein JA. Neural crest formation and craniofacial development. In: Epstein C, Erickson R, Wynshaw-Boris A, eds. *Molecular Basis of Inborn Errors of Development.* San Francisco, CA: Oxford University Press; 2004:67–74.
11. Bondurand N, Pingault V, Goerich DE, et al. Interaction among SOX10, PAX3 and MITF, three genes altered in Waardenburg syndrome. *Hum Mol Genet.* 2000;9:1907–1917.
12. Hornyak TJ, Hayes DJ, Chiu LY, Ziff EB. Transcription factors in melanocyte development: distinct roles for Pax-3 and Mitf. *Mech Dev.* 2001;101:47–59.
13. Potterf SB, Furumura M, Dunn KJ, Arnheiter H, Pavan WJ. Transcription factor hierarchy in Waardenburg syndrome: regulation of MITF expression by SOX10 and PAX3. *Hum Genet.* 2000;107:1–6.
14. Widlund HR, Fisher DE. Microphthalmia-associated transcription factor: a critical regulator of pigment cell development and survival. *Oncogene.* 2003;22:3035–3041.
15. Tassabehji M, Newton VE, Read AP. Waardenburg syndrome type 2 caused by mutations in the human microphthalmia (MITF) gene. *Nat Genet.* 1994;8:251–255.
16. Wehrle-Haller B. The role of Kit-ligand in melanocyte development and epidermal homeostasis. *Pigment Cell Res.* 2003;16:287–296.
17. Toki F, Suzuki N, Inoue K, et al. Intestinal aganglionosis associated with the Waardenburg syndrome: report of two cases and review of the literature. *Pediatr Surg Int.* 2003;19:725–728.

18. Tomita Y, Suzuki T. Genetics of pigmentary disorders. *Am J Med Genet C Semin Med Genet.* 2004;131C:75–81.
19. Nordlund JJ. The melanocyte and the epidermal melanin unit: an expanded concept. *Dermatol Clin.* 2007;25:271–281,vii.
20. Marks MS, Seabra MC. The melanosome: membrane dynamics in black and white. *Nat Rev Mol Cell Biol.* 2001;2:738–748.
21. Slominski A, Tobin DJ, Shibahara S, Wortsman J. Melanin pigmentation in mammalian skin and its hormonal regulation. *Physiol Rev.* 2004;84:1155–1228.
22. Kushimoto T, Basrur V, Valencia J, et al. A model for melanosome biogenesis based on the purification and analysis of early melanosomes. *Proc Natl Acad Sci U S A.* 2001;98:10698–10703.
23. Alaluf S, Heath A, Carter N, et al. Variation in melanin content and composition in type V and VI photoexposed and photoprotected human skin: the dominant role of DHI. *Pigment Cell Res.* 2001;14:337–347.
24. Theos AC, Truschel ST, Raposo G, Marks MS. The Silver locus product Pmel17/gp100/Silv/ME20: controversial in name and in function. *Pigment Cell Res.* 2005;18:322–336.
25. Wei ML. Hermansky-Pudlak syndrome: a disease of protein trafficking and organelle function. *Pigment Cell Res.* 2006;19:19–42.
26. Kaplan J, De Domenico I, Ward DM. Chediak-Higashi syndrome. *Curr Opin Hematol.* 2008;15:22–29.
27. Ito S. The IFPCS presidential lecture: a chemist's view of melanogenesis. *Pigment Cell Res.* 2003;16:230–236.
28. del Marmol V, Beermann F. Tyrosinase and related proteins in mammalian pigmentation. *FEBS Lett.* 1996;381:165–168.
29. Smit N, Tilgmann C, Karhunen T, et al. O-methylation of L-DOPA in melanin metabolism and the presence of catechol-O-methyltransferase in melanocytes. *Pigment Cell Res.* 1994;7:403–408.
30. Lee ZH, Hou L, Moellmann G, et al. Characterization and subcellular localization of human Pmel 17/silver, a 110-kDa (pre)melanosomal membrane protein associated with 5,6,-dihydro xyindole-2-carboxylic acid (DHICA) converting activity. *J Invest Dermatol.* 1996; 106:605–610.
31. Schallreuter KU, Kothari S, Chavan B, Spencer JD. Regulation of melanogenesis–controversies and new concepts. *Exp Dermatol.* 2008;17:395–404.
32. Ito S. Reexamination of the structure of eumelanin. *Biochim Biophys Acta.* 1986;883:155–161.
33. Zajac GW, Gallas JM, Cheng J, Eisner M, Moss SC, Alvarado-Swaisgood AE. The fundamental unit of synthetic melanin: a verification by tunneling microscopy of X-ray scattering results. *Biochim Biophys Acta.* 1994;1199:271–278.
34. Clancy CM, Simon JD. Ultrastructural organization of eumelanin from Sepia officinalis measured by atomic force microscopy. *Biochemistry.* 2001;40:13353–13360.
35. Meng S, Kaxiras E. Theoretical models of eumelanin protomolecules and their optical properties. *Biophys J.* 2008;94:2095–2105.
36. Alaluf S, Atkins D, Barrett K, Blount M, Carter N, Heath A. Ethnic variation in melanin content and composition in photoexposed and photoprotected human skin. *Pigment Cell Res.* 2002;15:112–118.
37. del Marmol V, Ito S, Bouchard B, et al. Cysteine deprivation promotes eumelanogenesis in human melanoma cells. *J Invest Dermatol.* 1996;107:698–702.
38. Okulicz JF, Shah RS, Schwartz RA, Janniger CK. Oculocutaneous albinism. *J Eur Acad Dermatol Venereol.* 2003;17:251–256.
39. Menasche G, Ho CH, Sanal O, et al. Griscelli syndrome restricted to hypopigmentation results from a melanophilin defect (GS3) or a MYO5A F-exon deletion (GS1). *J Clin Invest.* 2003;112:450–456.
40. Corbeel L, Freson K. Rab proteins and Rab-associated proteins: major actors in the mechanism of protein-trafficking disorders. *Eur J Pediatr.* 2008;167:723–729.

41. Wolff K, Konrad K. Phagocytosis of latex beads by epidermal keratinocytes *in vivo*. *J Ultrastruct Res*. 1972;39:262–280.
42. Cardinali G, Ceccarelli S, Kovacs D, et al. Keratinocyte growth factor promotes melanosome transfer to keratinocytes. *J Invest Dermatol*. 2005;125:1190–1199.
43. Boissy RE. Melanosome transfer to and translocation in the keratinocyte. *Exp Dermatol*. 2003;12(Suppl 2):5–12.
44. Sharlow ER, Paine CS, Babiarz L, Eisinger M, Shapiro S, Seiberg M. The protease-2 upregulates keratinocyte phagocytosis. *J Cell Sci*. 2000;113(Pt 17):3093–3101.
45. Virador VM, Muller J, Wu X, et al. Influence of alpha-melanocyte-stimulating hormone and ultraviolet radiation on the transfer of melanosomes to keratinocytes. *Faseb J*. 2002;16:105–107.
46. Wolff K. Melanocyte-keratinocyte interactions *in vivo*: the fate of melanosomes. *Yale J Biol Med*. 1973;46:384–396.
47. Otaki N, Seiji M. Degradation of melanosomes by lysosomes. *J Invest Dermatol*. 1971;57:1–5.
48. Hori Y, Toda K, Pathak MA, Clark WHJr., Fitzpatrick TB. A fine-structure study of the human epidermal melanosome complex and its acid phosphatase activity. *J Ultrastruct Res*. 1968;25:109–120.
49. Borovansky J, Elleder M. Melanosome degradation: fact or fiction. *Pigment Cell Res*. 2003;16:280–286.
50. Honigsmann H. Erythema and pigmentation. *Photodermatol Photoimmunol Photomed*. 2002;18:75–81.
51. Cripps DJ. Natural and artificial photoprotection. *J Invest Dermatol*. 1981;77:154–157.
52. Westerhof W, Estevez-Uscanga O, Meens J, Kammeyer A, Durocq M, Cario I. The relation between constitutional skin color and photosensitivity estimated from UV-induced erythema and pigmentation dose-response curves. *J Invest Dermatol*. 1990;94:812–816.
53. Andreassi L, Simoni S, Fiorini P, Fimiani M. Phenotypic characters related to skin type and minimal erythemal dose. *Photodermatol*. 1987;4:43–46.
54. Gange RW, Blackett AD, Matzinger EA, Sutherland BM, Kochevar IE. Comparative protection efficiency of UVA- and UVB-induced tans against erythema and formation of endonuclease-sensitive sites in DNA by UVB in human skin. *J Invest Dermatol*. 1985;85:362–364.
55. Sheehan JM, Potten CS, Young AR. Tanning in human skin types II and III offers modest photoprotection against erythema. *Photochem Photobiol*. 1998;68:588–592.
56. Barnetson RS, Ooi TK, Zhuang L, et al. [Nle4-D-Phe7]-alpha-melanocyte-stimulating hormone significantly increased pigmentation and decreased UV damage in fair-skinned Caucasian volunteers. *J Invest Dermatol*. 2006;126:1869–1878.
57. D'Orazio JA, Nobuhisa T, Cui R, et al. Topical drug rescue strategy and skin protection based on the role of Mc1r in UV-induced tanning. *Nature*. 2006;443:340–344.
58. Yamaguchi Y, Takahashi K, Zmudzka BZ, et al. Human skin responses to UV radiation: pigment in the upper epidermis protects against DNA damage in the lower epidermis and facilitates apoptosis. *Faseb J*. 2006;20:1486–1488.
59. Takeuchi S, Zhang W, Wakamatsu K, et al. Melanin acts as a potent UVB photosensitizer to cause an atypical mode of cell death in murine skin. *Proc Natl Acad Sci U S A*. 2004;101:15076–15081.
60. Munyao TM, Othieno-Abinya NA. Cutaneous basal cell carcinoma in Kenya. *East Afr Med J*. 1999;76:97–100.
61. Kollias N, Sayre RM, Zeise L, Chedekel MR. Photoprotection by melanin. *J Photochem Photobiol B*. 1991;9:135–160.
62. Kromberg JG, Castle D, Zwane EM, Jenkins T. Albinism and skin cancer in Southern Africa. *Clin Genet*. 1989;36:43–52.
63. Staples MP, Elwood M, Burton RC, Williams JL, Marks R, Giles GG. Non-melanoma skin cancer in Australia: the 2002 national survey and trends since 1985. *Med J Aust*. 2006;184:6–10.
64. Cunningham J, Rumbold AR, Zhang X, Condon JR. Incidence, aetiology, and outcomes of cancer in Indigenous peoples in Australia. *Lancet Oncol*. 2008;9:585–595.

65. Condon JR, Armstrong BK, Barnes T, Zhao Y. Cancer incidence and survival for indigenous Australians in the Northern Territory. *Aust N Z J Public Health*. 2005;29:123–128.
66. Wlaschek M, Tantcheva-Poor I, Naderi L, et al. Solar UV irradiation and dermal photoaging. *J Photochem Photobiol B*. 2001;63:41–51.
67. Holick MF. The cutaneous photosynthesis of previtamin D3: a unique photoendocrine system. *J Invest Dermatol*. 1981;77:51–58.
68. Giovannucci E, Liu Y, Hollis BW, Rimm EB. 25-Hydroxyvitamin D and risk of myocardial infarction in men: a prospective study. *Arch Intern Med*. 2008;168:1174–1180.
69. Giovannucci E, Liu Y, Rimm EB, et al. Prospective study of predictors of vitamin D status and cancer incidence and mortality in men. *J Natl Cancer Inst*. 2006;98:451–459.
70. Young AR. Chromophores in human skin. *Phys Med Biol*. 1997;42:789–802.
71. Riesz J, Gilmore J, Meredith P. Quantitative scattering of melanin solutions. *Biophys J*. 2006;90:4137–4144.
72. Meredith P, Sarna T. The physical and chemical properties of eumelanin. *Pigment Cell Res*. 2006;19:572–594.
73. Riesz J, Sarna T, Meredith P. Radiative relaxation in synthetic pheomelanin. *J Phys Chem B*. 2006;110:13985–13990.
74. Rajadhyaksha M, Grossman M, Esterowitz D, Webb RH, Anderson RR. *In vivo* confocal scanning laser microscopy of human skin: melanin provides strong contrast. *J Invest Dermatol*. 1995;104:946–952.
75. Rajadhyaksha M, Anderson RR, Webb RH. Video-rate confocal scanning laser microscope for imaging human tissues *in vivo*. *Appl Opt*. 1999;38:2105–2115.
76. Rajadhyaksha M, Gonzalez S, Zavislan JM, Anderson RR, Webb RH. *In vivo* confocal scanning laser microscopy of human skin II: advances in instrumentation and comparison with histology. *J Invest Dermatol*. 1999;113:293–303.
77. Yamashita T, Akita H, Astner S, Miyakawa M, Lerner EA, Gonzalez S. *In vivo* assessment of pigmentary and vascular compartments changes in UVA exposed skin by reflectance-mode confocal microscopy. *Exp Dermatol*. 2007;16:905–911.
78. Riley PA. Radicals in melanin biochemistry. *Ann N Y Acad Sci*. 1988;551:111–119; discussion 119-120.
79. Rozanowska M, Sarna T, Land EJ, Truscott TG. Free radical scavenging properties of melanin interaction of eu- and pheo-melanin models with reducing and oxidising radicals. *Free Radic Biol Med*. 1999;26:518–525.
80. Poh Agin P, Sayre RM, Chedekel MR. Photodegradation of phaeomelanin: an in vitro model. *Photochem Photobiol*. 1980;31:359–362.
81. Lerner AB, McGuire JS. Melanocyte-stimulating hormone and adrenocorticotrophic hormone. their relation to pigmentation. *N Engl J Med*. 1964;270:539–546.
82. Abdel-Malek Z, Swope VB, Suzuki I, et al. Mitogenic and melanogenic stimulation of normal human melanocytes by melanotropic peptides. *Proc Natl Acad Sci U S A*. 1995;92:1789–1793.
83. Garcia-Borron JC, Sanchez-Laorden BL, Jimenez-Cervantes, C. Melanocortin-1 receptor structure and functional regulation. *Pigment Cell Res*. 2005;18:393–410.
84. Konig S, Luger TA, Scholzen TE. Monitoring neuropeptide-specific proteases: processing of the proopiomelanocortin peptides adrenocorticotropin and alpha-melanocyte-stimulating hormone in the skin. *Exp Dermatol*. 2006;15:751–761.
85. Hunt G, Kyne S, Wakamatsu K, Ito S, Thody AJ. Nle4DPhe7 alpha-melanocyte-stimulating hormone increases the eumelanin:phaeomelanin ratio in cultured human melanocytes. *J Invest Dermatol*. 1995;104:83–85.
86. Gaggioli C, Busca R, Abbe P, Ortonne JP, Ballotti R. Microphthalmia-associated transcription factor (MITF) is required but is not sufficient to induce the expression of melanogenic genes. *Pigment Cell Res*. 2003;16:374–382.
87. Yasumoto K, Yokoyama K, Takahashi K, Tomita Y, Shibahara S. Functional analysis of microphthalmia-associated transcription factor in pigment cell-specific transcription of the human tyrosinase family genes. *J Biol Chem*. 1997;272:503–509.

88. Aoki H, Moro O. Involvement of microphthalmia-associated transcription factor (MITF) in expression of human melanocortin-1 receptor (MC1R). *Life Sci.* 2002;71:2171–2179.
89. Scott MC, Suzuki I, Abdel-Malek ZA. Regulation of the human melanocortin 1 receptor expression in epidermal melanocytes by paracrine and endocrine factors and by ultraviolet radiation. *Pigment Cell Res.* 2002;15:433–439.
90. Suzuki I, Tada A, Ollmann MM, et al. Agouti signaling protein inhibits melanogenesis and the response of human melanocytes to alpha-melanotropin. *J Invest Dermatol.* 1997;108:838–842.
91. Abdel-Malek Z, Suzuki I, Tada A, Im S, Akcali C. The melanocortin-1 receptor and human pigmentation. *Ann N Y Acad Sci.* 1999;885:117–133.
92. Hirobe T. Role of keratinocyte-derived factors involved in regulating the proliferation and differentiation of mammalian epidermal melanocytes. *Pigment Cell Res.* 2005;18:2–12.
93. Kadekaro AL, Kavanagh RJ, Wakamatsu K, Ito S, Pipitone MA, Abdel-Malek ZA. Cutaneous photobiology. The melanocyte vs. the sun: who will win the final round? *Pigment Cell Res.* 2003;16:434–447.
94. Robbins LS, Nadeau JH, Johnson KR, et al. Pigmentation phenotypes of variant extension locus alleles result from point mutations that alter MSH receptor function. *Cell.* 1993;72:827–834.
95. Bastiaens M, ter Huurne J, Gruis N, et al. The melanocortin-1-receptor gene is the major freckle gene. *Hum Mol Genet.* 2001;10:1701–1708.
96. Ringholm A, Klovins J, Rudzish R, Phillips S, Rees JL, Schioth HB. Pharmacological characterization of loss of function mutations of the human melanocortin 1 receptor that are associated with red hair. *J Invest Dermatol.* 2004;123:917–923.
97. Kennedy C, ter Huurne J, Berkhout M, et al. Melanocortin 1 receptor (MC1R) gene variants are associated with an increased risk for cutaneous melanoma which is largely independent of skin type and hair color. *J Invest Dermatol.* 2001;117:294–300.
98. Smith G, Wilkie MJ, Deeni YY, et al. Melanocortin 1 receptor (MC1R) genotype influences erythemal sensitivity to psoralen-ultraviolet A photochemotherapy. *Br J Dermatol.* 2007;157:1230–1234.
99. Parrish JA, Jaenicke KF, Anderson RR. Erythema and melanogenesis action spectra of normal human skin. *Photochem Photobiol.* 1982;36:187–191.
100. Wagner JK, Parra EJ, L Norton H, Jovel C, Shriver MD. Skin responses to ultraviolet radiation: effects of constitutive pigmentation, sex, and ancestry. *Pigment Cell Res.* 2002;15:385–390.
101. Chung JH, Koh WS, Youn JI. Relevance of skin phototyping to a Korean population. *Clin Exp Dermatol.* 1994;19:476–478.
102. Stanford DG, Georgouras KE, Sullivan EA, Greenoak GE. Skin phototyping in Asian Australians. *Australas J Dermatol.* 1996;37(Suppl 1):S36–S38.
103. Zmudzka BZ, Hearing VJ, Beer JZ. Photobiologic role of melanin distribution in the epidermis. *J Photochem Photobiol B.* 2006;84:231.
104. Hacham H, Freeman SE, Gange RW, Maytum DJ, Sutherland JC, Sutherland BM. Do pyrimidine dimer yields correlate with erythema induction in human skin irradiated in situ with ultraviolet light (275-365 nm)? *Photochem Photobiol.* 1991;53:559–563.
105. de Gruijl FR, Rebel H. Early events in UV carcinogenesis–DNA damage, target cells and mutant p53 foci. *Photochem Photobiol.* 2008;84:382–387.
106. Eller MS, Ostrom K, Gilchrest BA. DNA damage enhances melanogenesis. *Proc Natl Acad Sci U S A.* 1996;93:1087–1092.
107. Gilchrest BA, Zhai S, Eller MS, Yarosh DB, Yaar M. Treatment of human melanocytes and S91 melanoma cells with the DNA repair enzyme T4 endonuclease V enhances melanogenesis after ultraviolet irradiation. *J Invest Dermatol.* 1993;101:666–672.
108. Nylander K, Bourdon JC, Bray SE, et al. Transcriptional activation of tyrosinase and TRP-1 by p53 links UV irradiation to the protective tanning response. *J Pathol.* 2000;190:39–46.

109. Khlgatian MK, Hadshiew IM, Asawanonda P, et al. Tyrosinase gene expression is regulated by p53. *J Invest Dermatol.* 2002;118:126–132.
110. Cui R, Widlund HR, Feige E, et al. Central role of p53 in the suntan response and pathologic hyperpigmentation. *Cell.* 2007;128:853–864.
111. Bohm M, Wolff I, Scholzen TE, et al. alpha-Melanocyte-stimulating hormone protects from ultraviolet radiation-induced apoptosis and DNA damage. *J Biol Chem.* 2005;280:5795–5802.
112. Kadekaro AL, Kavanagh R, Kanto H, et al. alpha-Melanocortin and endothelin-1 activate antiapoptotic pathways and reduce DNA damage in human melanocytes. *Cancer Res.* 2005;65:4292–4299.
113. Passeron T, Namiki T, Passeron HJ, Le Pape E, Hearing VJ. Forskolin protects keratinocytes from UVB-induced apoptosis and increases DNA repair independent of its effects on melanogenesis. *J Invest Dermatol.* 2009;129:162–166.
114. Scott G, Deng A, Rodriguez-Burford C, et al. Protease-activated receptor 2, a receptor involved in melanosome transfer, is upregulated in human skin by ultraviolet irradiation. *J Invest Dermatol.* 2001;117:1412–1420.
115. Marchese C, Maresca V, Cardinali G, et al. UVB-induced activation and internalization of keratinocyte growth factor receptor. *Oncogene.* 2003;22:2422–2431.
116. Gilchrest BA, Blog FB, Szabo G. Effects of aging and chronic sun exposure on melanocytes in human skin. *J Invest Dermatol.* 1979;73:141–143.
117. Herzberg AJ, Dinehart SM. Chronologic aging in black skin. *Am J Dermatopathol.* 1989;11:319–328.
118. Staricco RJ, Pinkus H. Quantitative and qualitative data on the pigment cells of adult human epidermis. *J Invest Dermatol.* 1957;28:33–45.
119. Alaluf S, Barrett K, Blount M, Carter N. Ethnic variation in tyrosinase and TYRP1 expression in photoexposed and photoprotected human skin. *Pigment Cell Res.* 2003;16:35–42.
120. Tadokoro T, Yamaguchi Y, Batzer J, et al. Mechanisms of skin tanning in different racial/ethnic groups in response to ultraviolet radiation. *J Invest Dermatol.* 2005;124:1326–1332.
121. Abdel-Malek Z, Swope V, Collins C, Boissy R, Zhao H, Nordlund J. Contribution of melanogenic proteins to the heterogeneous pigmentation of human melanocytes. *J Cell Sci.* 1993;106 (Pt 4):1323–1331.
122. Andreassi L, Casini L, Simoni S, Bartalini P, Fimiani M. Measurement of cutaneous colour and assessment of skin type. *Photodermatol Photoimmunol Photomed.* 1990;7:20–24.
123. Pershing LK, Tirumala VP, Nelson JL, et al. Reflectance spectrophotometer: the dermatologists' sphygmomanometer for skin phototyping? *J Invest Dermatol.* 2008;128:1633–1640.
124. Konrad K, Wolff K. Hyperpigmentation, melanosome size, and distribution patterns of melanosomes. *Arch Dermatol.* 1973;107:853–860.
125. Szabo G, Gerald AB, Pathak MA, Fitzpatrick TB. Racial differences in the fate of melanosomes in human epidermis. *Nature.* 1969;222:1081–1082.
126. Limat A, Salomon D, Carraux P, Saurat JH, Hunziker T. Human melanocytes grown in epidermal equivalents transfer their melanin to follicular outer root sheath keratinocytes. *Arch Dermatol Res.* 1999;291:325–332.
127. Cardinali G, Bolasco G, Aspite N, et al. Melanosome transfer promoted by keratinocyte growth factor in light and dark skin-derived keratinocytes. *J Invest Dermatol.* 2008;128:558–567.
128. Seiberg M, Paine C, Sharlow E, et al. The protease-activated receptor 2 regulates pigmentation via keratinocyte-melanocyte interactions. *Exp Cell Res.* 2000;254:25–32.
129. Babiarz-Magee L, Chen N, Seiberg M, Lin CB. The expression and activation of protease-activated receptor-2 correlate with skin color. *Pigment Cell Res.* 2004;17:241–251.
130. Yoshida Y, Hachiya A, Sriwiriyanont P, et al. Functional analysis of keratinocytes in skin color using a human skin substitute model composed of cells derived from different skin pigmentation types. *Faseb J.* 2007;21:2829–2839.
131. Sarangarajan R, Zhao Y, Babcock G, Cornelius J, Lamoreux ML, Boissy RE. Mutant alleles at the brown locus encoding tyrosinase-related protein-1 (TRP-1) affect proliferation of mouse melanocytes in culture. *Pigment Cell Res.* 2000;13:337–344.

132. Han J, Kraft P, Nan H, et al. A genome-wide association study identifies novel alleles associated with hair color and skin pigmentation. *PLoS Genet.* 2008;4, e1000074.
133. Norton HL, Kittles RA, Parra E, et al. Genetic evidence for the convergent evolution of light skin in Europeans and East Asians. *Mol Biol Evol.* 2007;24:710–722.
134. Kobayashi N, Nakagawa A, Muramatsu T, et al. Supranuclear melanin caps reduce ultraviolet induced DNA photoproducts in human epidermis. *J Invest Dermatol.* 1998;110:806–810.

Chapter 4
Photoprotection in Non-Caucasian Skin

Diana Santo Domingo and Mary S. Matsui

To speak about "skin of color" or "non-Caucasian skin" is to address a broadly and inexactly defined group with multiple layers of political and social implications as well as more physiological and biological parameters. For the purposes of this chapter, "skin of color" will refer to those individuals who self-identify as non-Caucasian and whose skin is characterized by a higher melanin content than "white" skin, and whose minimal erythema dose (MED) is, in general, higher than lightly pigmented individuals. Even within the narrow range of "photoprotection in skin of color," there are a number of considerations in terms of the impact of radiation in the ultraviolet radiation (UVR), visible, and infrared spectra. This chapter will survey several issues relevant to photoprotection for pigmented skin or non-Caucasian populations. In reviewing the development of sunscreens, for example, it becomes clear that these products were developed with Caucasian skin in mind. Sunscreen efficacy is still determined almost exclusively on Caucasian subjects despite growing evidence that subjects of color may differ in complicated ways related to ethnic or racial heritage rather than a simple attenuation of UVR due to melanin. Some of these differences discussed below include rates of DNA repair, the possible contribution of melanin to photodamage, variation in UVR-induced immunosuppression, the risk of postinflammatory hyperpigmentation (PIH) exacerbated by sun exposure, and the potential for vitamin D deficiency in skin of color.

The purpose of sun protection is to prevent damage to the skin that leads to melanoma and nonmelanoma cancers, photoaging, and PIH. The last is of particular concern in populations of color. It has also been suggested, with some evidence, that lentigos or "age spots" characterize photoaged skin of color rather than wrinkles, which tend to be more characteristic of Caucasian skin.

D.S. Domingo and M.S. Matsui (✉)
Department of Dermatology, University Hospitals Case Medical Center, Cleveland, OH, USA
e-mail: mmatsui@estee.com

E.D. Baron (ed.), *Light-Based Therapies for Skin of Color*,
DOI: 10.1007/ 978-1-84882-328-0_4, © Springer-Verlag London Limited 2009

4.1 Background: Cutaneous Effects of Sunlight and a Brief History of Photoprotection

The damaging effects of solar radiation on human skin have been well documented and include photoaging, DNA damage, cutaneous immunosuppression, and carcinogenesis. The UVR portion of the solar spectrum is divided into three wavelength ranges: UVC, UVB, and UVA. UVC wavelengths (200–290 nm) are absorbed by the earth's stratosphere and therefore under typical conditions have minimal relevancy for human skin. UVB wavelengths (290–320 nm) are most associated with inflammatory effects on skin such as erythemal response and direct DNA damage. Energy in the UVA region (320–400 nm) makes up 90–99% of the total reaching the earth's surface and is further divided into UVA-1 (340–400 nm) and UVA-2 (320–340 nm) based on pathologies and therapeutic modalities linked to those wavelengths. UVA is associated with the production of immediate pigment darkening (IPD), reactive oxygen species, and immunosuppression.

Since the late nineteenth century, nonthermal energy from the sun was understood to be the causative factor for tanning and sunburn and in the first decade of the twentieth century, the first publications linking malignant photodamage appeared.[1] It was not until the 1950s that there was serious interest in the development of topical agents to prevent UV-induced skin damage or sunburn. Various substances including tannins, benzyl salicylate, and red ceterinary petrolatum were tested and used as early sunscreens. Over the last several decades, public and medical community awareness of the need for photoprotection in order to prevent sunburn, skin cancer, and photoaging has led to significant advances in filtering agents and formulations of the sunscreens used today.

The development of novel photoprotective agents required reliable methods to test their efficacy. The concept of sun-protective factor or SPF was introduced by Franz Greiter in 1974. This method of classifying sunscreens was based on calculating the exposure required for induction of erythema. SPF testing is currently used by the FDA to regulate commercially available sunscreens, and it is an internationally accepted standard. One problem with this method is that although it provides good information about UVB protection, it offers minimal information about UVA protection. This is of concern because there is increasing evidence for the damaging effects of UVA wavelengths on several skin functions including the immune response. Thus, there is a need for more comprehensive safety labeling and standardization in this field and in fact, the 2007 FDA-proposed sunscreen monograph[2] requested a change in the term "sun protection factor" for SPF to "sunburn protection factor" to reflect the limits of this measurement. In particular, additional UVA in vivo and in vitro evaluation measures were proposed.

Virtually all of the photoprotection studies of the past were performed using Caucasian skin (skin types I–II). However, it has become apparent that individuals vary widely in their biological response to UVR and this suggests that non-Caucasian skin may respond differently from Caucasian skin when exposed to

UV irradiation.[3-5] Photoprotection in pigmented skin is a field with many unanswered questions. Issues of interest in non-Caucasian skin include the nature and effects of pigment, the molecular effects of UV irradiation on this type skin, and sun protection practices of non-Caucasians. This chapter will discuss the role of melanin and tanning in ethnic skin, review photoprotection studies performed on non-Caucasian skin, and discuss the importance and consequences of photoprotection in this population.

4.2   Pigmentation Differences Between Caucasian and Non-Caucasian Skin

The term non-Caucasian skin, also referred to as pigmented skin or skin of color, can be used to define the skin of many different ethnic groups including but not limited to African-American, Hispanic, Asian, Native American, and Middle Eastern.[6] It has been shown that pigmented skin differs on a biological and molecular level from white skin.[6,7] One obvious (visible) distinction between Caucasian and non-Caucasian skin is a difference in skin tone or constitutive pigmentation (the level of pigmentation that occurs in the absence of exogenous modifiers such as UVR).

Visible skin tone and color results from the interaction of epidermal thickness, blood flow (hemoglobin), and pigment found in the epidermis and dermis. Skin pigment is produced by dendritic cells called melanocytes, located in the basal layer of the epidermis. Melanocytes contain specialized organelles, melanosomes that are responsible for the synthesis and storage of melanin. Melanosomes produce two types of melanin. one type, eumelanin, is brown-black in color. It is formed when the tyrosine metabolite dopaquinone takes on a cyclic form and becomes oxidized.[6] The other type of melanin is pheomelanin. This pigment has a yellow-red color and results when dopaquinone combines with the amino acid cysteine or the tripeptide glutathione. After melanin is synthesized, the melanosomes are distributed to the neighboring keratinocytes via melanocyte dendrites.

There is not a significant difference between the number of melanocytes found in Caucasian and non-Caucasian skin.[8-10] The variation in skin color comes from a difference in the number, size, and density of melanosomes. Therefore, melanosome transfer is an important determinant affecting an individual's skin color.[11] Light skin has fewer and smaller melanosomes which are bundled together within membrane-bound complexes, whereas the melanosomes of dark skin are distributed as larger, single granules, resulting in a darker skin color.

Since the mid- to late-1970s, dermatologists have used the Fitzpatrick skin type (FST), also known as the skin phototype (SPT) system, to classify people with all skin colors into six different levels based on their erythema response to UV light. (See Table 4.1.) This is a functional classification based on an individual's constitutive skin color, and on his or her ability to tan or burn.

Table 4.1 Modified Fitzpatrick skin phototypes

Skin type	Skin color	Response to UV exposure
I	Light	Always burns
II	Light	Burns and sometimes tans
III	Light	Usually burns then tans
IV	"Olive"	Rarely burns, usually tans
V	Brown	Very rarely burns, tans darkly
VI	Dark brown	Never burns, tans black

The Fitzpatrick skin type, also known as the skin phototype system, is used to classify people into six different levels based on their response to UV light. This is a functional classification based on constitutive skin color, and on the ability to tan or burn. Types I–IV are based primarily on a physiological response, whereas classification into types V and VI is based mainly on constitutive skin pigmentation

One limitation of this system is that visualizing erythema in darker skin can be more challenging than visualizing erythema in light skin.[12] Thus, although classification into types I–IV is based on a biological response, classification into types V and VI is based mainly on constitutive skin pigmentation.

Another aspect of this skin typing method that frequently leads to confusion is that visually, many non-Caucasian individuals are automatically assumed to be in the SPT IV–VI category.[5,6] This is sometimes not the case, since the FST is a measure of sun responsiveness, not constitutive color (discussed in more detail later). This type of classification also does not address the fact that individuals with ethnic skin may be fair skinned, such as those from Arab or Asian descent, and does not acknowledge that certain ethnicities such as Hispanics may have a skin color that ranges from light to dark brown.

SPT is used as a predictor of the MED, the lowest dose of UV needed to generate visible erythema. The MED is considered to be a "biological dose" because an individual's MED is determined by their personal biological reactivity to the effects of UVR. Note that SPT does not necessarily reflect the MED of an individual with ethnic skin.[6,13,14] Studies of Asian skin[3,15] found that there is a substantial variation in the MED values within this large and diverse group. This prompted the development of a skin typing system especially designed for Asian skin types called the Japanese skin type.[16] Another study using Arab subjects,[5] all of whom were classified as having type V skin, found that there was a substantial variation between MED values despite all subjects having the same constitutive skin type.

At least two important messages arise from these studies. First, neither constitutive color nor self-identified ethnic identity is adequate predictor of an individual's response to UVR. In addition, this suggests that there are other genetically based factors, such as DNA repair rates, that contribute to an individual's tolerance for UVR exposure. Therefore, although FST is helpful in determining the appropriate dose for phototherapy, and is currently the most widely used skin typing method, it should be used with some caution, especially when considering skin of color.

4.3 Role of Melanin

Agar et al describe melanin as "a complex of insoluble eumelanin and pheomelanin monomers, the ratio of which determines final skin and hair color."[12] Melanin contributes to the color of skin and acts as a chromophore, or light-absorbing element, in the skin. Despite extensive animal and human studies, the critical function of melanin in human skin is unclear. However, it is believed that the higher melanin content in skin of color is one reason why non-Caucasian skin is resistant to some signs of photoaging and to nonmelanoma skin cancer (NMSC).

During the mid-1980s, the "sun protection" role of melanin was brought into question by Warwick Morison.[17] He theorized that the pigment from melanin provided evolutionary benefits to humans not as a photoprotector, but provided camouflage and heat conservation. Since that time, many studies have been attempted to characterize the role of melanin in skin in terms of photoprotection. Taken together, these studies seem to provide conflicting evidence – some for and some against a photoprotective benefit.

In vitro studies suggested that pheomelanin was not only not protective, but in fact detrimental. Schmitz et al demonstrated that when pheomelanin was combined with UV exposure, it had a damaging effect on the skin. This was based on the finding that UV irradiation caused pheomelanin to produce phototoxic by-products in vitro.[18] Interestingly, pheomelanin is more abundant in red haired individuals who tend to be more sensitive to UV exposure and at increased risk for skin cancer.[19] Subsequent studies done in human skin showed that the phototoxic metabolites caused by the combination of UV and pheomelanin may not be as harmful in vivo as suggested by the previous studies cited above.[11,20] The verdict on melanin given by Hill et al[21] was that of a two-edged sword. They propose that when melanin is combined with UV exposure, melanin may have both beneficial and damaging results depending on the endpoint examined.

It should be noted that melanin as photoprotection against skin cancer is unlikely to be a selection mechanism for evolutionary pressure, as UV-induced cutaneous malignancy does not often prevent reproduction. However, it has been suggested that melanin may protect folic acid, which is necessary for reproductive success, against photodegradation. Sunlight also has been shown to induce defensins and cathelicidins, cutaneous antimicrobial peptides. Therefore, melanin levels may be delicately balanced between allowing induction of antimicrobial peptides, protecting against folic acid degradation, and allowing vitamin D synthesis.

More recent studies have shown that melanin in darker skin does provide some protection from UV-induced DNA damage.[22-24] When human skin is exposed to UVR, the energy is absorbed by various chromophores in the skin. DNA in keratinocytes and other epidermal cells is the major chromophore for UVB wavelengths. When UVB energy is absorbed by DNA, the damage creates a characteristic lesion between DNA base pairs, known as cyclobutane pyrimidine dimers (CPDs).[25,26] CPDs are therefore considered a marker for UVB-induced DNA damage.

4.4   Tanning in Caucasian and Ethnic Skin

Tanning, or UVR-induced melanogenesis, is a result of UVR's environmental stress on melanocytes, and will temporarily change the color of an individual's skin. Skin darkening in response to UV exposure occurs by two distinct mechanisms, IPD and delayed tanning (DT). When fair or dark skin is exposed to UVR, there is an IPD that occurs within hours after exposure. This response is followed in all skin types by delayed melanogenesis, which takes place 48–72 h after exposure.

4.4.1   IPD and DT

IPD is primarily caused by UVA wavelengths. It is the result of oxidation of the melanin already present in the skin. IPD is also the result of a redistribution of melanosomes from a perinuclear to a peripheral dendritic location. Interestingly, IPD, which is typically grayish in color, is observed more easily in darker skin types (IV–VI).[12] IPD is believed not to offer any protection against UV damage.

DT is the result of increased melanin production. It is primarily triggered by UVB-mediated DNA damage – DNA fragments resulting from excision repair[32] – but can also result from UVA exposure. The DT caused by UVA exposure occurs through an oxygen-dependent mechanism, and it has an earlier onset than the tanning caused by DNA damage.

4.4.2   Tanning in Ethnic Skin

Increases in skin pigmentation from chronic UV exposure are caused by numerous UV-regulated physiological factors. These factors affect melanocyte growth and/or differentiation. Typically, these factors are produced by cells in the skin, including keratinocytes, fibroblasts, and even melanocytes themselves. Products of photodamaged DNA have also been implicated in stimulating pigmentation,[32-34] as discussed in more detail below. Tadokoro et al observed the effects of UVR on melanocye density and melanin content in human skin in three ethnic groups, Asian, Black, and White. Photoprotected Asian and Caucasian skin had essentially the same melanin content, while the melanin content in black skin was approximately four times higher.[10] The melanin content in skin one day after exposure to UVR was virtually unchanged from baseline. Using diffuse reflectance directly on human skin, this group noticed that 7 days after UVR exposure, the melanin content in Asian and Black skin was significantly increased when compared to White skin. They concluded that increases in pigmentation from a given dose of UV were more rapid and more intense in dark skin than in light skin.[10]

Tadokoro et al also examined the distribution of melanin in White, Asian, and Black skin using a pseudostaining technique to determine the amount of melanin within various layers of skin. They observed that 1-week post-UVR exposure, the total amount of melanin in human skin layers of all ethnicities increased by 5–10%. They also observed that there was a redistribution of melanin between the lower, middle, and upper layers of the epidermis with a decrease in the amount of melanin present in the basal layer. This effect was observed in all three races after 1 MED exposure. The most significant change was in the distribution of melanin from the lower layer upward to the middle layer of the skin, which was more dramatic in the darker skin.

Microphthalmia transcription factor (MITF) is a melanogenic protein. It regulates the expression of genes needed to transcribe several melanosome proteins and is considered a master regulator of melanocyte function. Tadokoro et al. measured the amounts of MITF in unirradiated areas of Black, White, and Asian skin and found that the highest amounts of this protein were present in Black skin. When they looked at skin that had been irradiated, they found that one day after 1 MED exposure, there was a universal increase in this regulatory protein that persisted even 7 days after exposure. Similar results were found for other melanosomal proteins including TYR, TYRP, DCT, gp100, and MART1.[10]

Agar et al suggest that because the action spectrum for erythema and melanogenesis in human skin are similar, these two phenomena share a common photochemical catalyst.[12] They further speculate that the link between erythema and CPD formation points to UVR-induced DNA photoproducts as inducers of melanogenisis.[12] Agar et al suggest that tanning (rather than burning) may be a sign of effective DNA repair. A link between tanning as an SOS response to DNA damage has been shown in several studies.[32-34] Arad et al studied the effects of T-oligos (DNA oligonucleotides substantially homologous to the telomere 3′-overhang) on DNA repair capacity after UV exposure. T-oligos can mimic the physiological signal created during DNA damage and stimulate the cellular response to telomere loop overhang fragments. In this way, T-oligos induce protective responses to DNA damage. Eller et al found that T-oligos could upregulate tyrosinase, the rate-limiting enzyme required for melanogenesis in human melanocytes in vitro.[33] In another study, ex vivo human skin was pretreated for 24 h with either T-oligos or dilutant and irradiated with UVB. Histological analysis done after irradiation at various time points showed that skin pretreated with T-oligos exhibited reduced CPDs at 24, 48, and 72 h postirradiation. In the same study, total and activated p53 protein was increased in T-oligo-pretreated skin. Both tyrosinase and the tyrosinase-related protein-1 are transcriptionally regulated by p53. This data corresponded to the finding of increased amounts of melanogenic proteins in the T-oligo-treated skin. They concluded that T-oligos are recognized by epidermal melanocytes in human skin as a physiological signal to stimulate melanogenesis, and that tanning could be interpreted as a response to DNA damage.[34]

4.5 Role of Epidermal Thickening in UVR Protection

Epidermal thickening is another adaptive response to UVR which has been shown to offer additional protection against photodamage. One study used skin from vitiligo patients and healthy Caucasians to study the photoprotective effect against erythema induction (SPF) of stratum corneum thickening versus pigmentation after UVR exposure and found that when comparing the photoprotective effect of the stratum corneum with the protection provided by pigmentation, the stratum corneum provided an estimated 57% of the total protection against erythema.[35] In another study by Hennessy et al,[36] researchers looked at the response of different ex vivo skin types to repetitive UVR exposure over 3 days and found that Caucasian skin responded with epidermal hyperplasia. Spectral absorbance data measured on samples of excised epidermis indicated that this hyperproliferation could give significant protection against photodamage. They suggested that the stratum corneum accounted for a large proportion (over two-thirds) of photoprotection in lighter colored skin and proposed that in those people with a lower degree of constitutive pigment, the primary mechanism of photoadaptation is via the nonpigmentary route. They came to this conclusion because there was no change observed in the mean thickness of Asian skin postirradiation, unlike the Caucasian epidermis. However, subsequent studies[12] were not able to reproduce these results and therefore the importance and the amount of protection provided by epidermal thickening is still uncertain.

4.6   Need for Photoprotection in Non-Caucasian Skin

Despite evidence that non-Caucasian skin is less prone to damaging effects of UV irradiation, there is a strong argument for recommending the use of sunscreen to this population. Pigmented skin is prone to the darkening and discoloration caused by PIH, and can exhibit signs of photoaging, such as atrophy, dermal collagen, and elastin damage.[37] In addition, melanin may not be protective against the immunosuppressive effects of UV exposure. Finally, despite a lower incidence of skin cancers seen among individuals with skin of color, this population is not free from skin malignancies and although this population tends to present with melanomas in sun-protected areas, studies have shown that basal cell carcinomas (BCCs) and MSC in dark skin may be related to the amount of UV exposure as well as the UV index, which is a daily prediction of the strength of the sun's UVR for a specific geographical region taking into account clouds and other local conditions that affect the amount of UVR reaching the ground.

4.7   Hyperpigmentation

Hyperpigmentation is one of the most common complaints among patients with skin of color.[38,39] Increased pigment has many causes but in skin of color, it is frequently attributed to inflammation from acne, wounding, and other inflammatory events or thought to be hormonal in nature, such as melasma. PIH is frequently the primary complaint reported among patients with skin of color seeking acne treatment. These patients often complain of blemishes, which are in fact macules left over from the inflammation (PIH) which lingers even after the original blemish has resolved.[40] (See Fig. 4.2.) Melasma is a common hypermelanosis characterized by

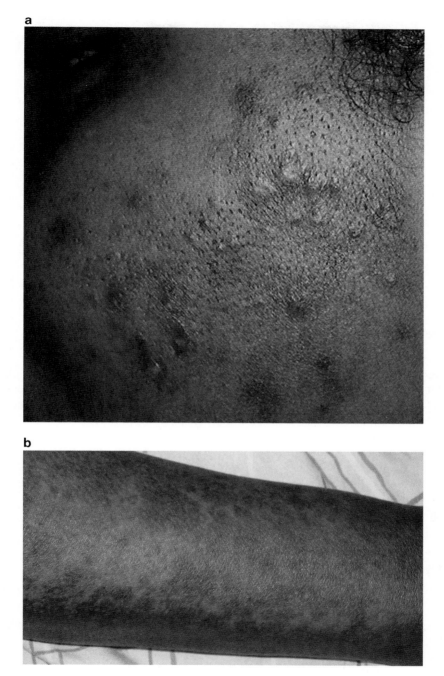

Fig. 4.2 Typical postinflammatory hyperpigmentation (*PIH*); the picture on the left shows PIH and acne. The picture on the bottom shows PIH after erythema multiforme. (Pictures courtesy of Andrew Alexis)

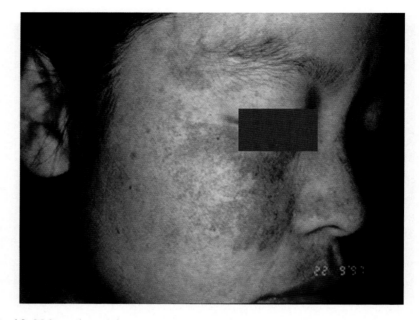

Fig. 4.3 Melasma in an Asian woman

irregular light to gray-brown macules and patches involving sun-exposed areas of skin.[41] (*See* Fig. 4.3.) This condition has a multifactorial etiology including genetic and hormonal influences, photosensitizing drugs, and exposure to UV.[41] Although melasma occurs in all skin ethnicities, it is a bigger problem for patients with skin of color and it remains a therapeutically challenging disease.[41] Because pigmentary disorders are a significant cause of distress among patients with skin of color, combined with the fact that many of the therapeutic modalities to treat hyperpigmentation are either insufficient or may subsequently cause hypo pigmented areas, broad-spectrum UV protection is recommended to this subset of patients as an adjuvant to therapy and as a way in which to prevent these problems.[38,40]

4.8 Photoaging and Other Effects of Long-Term Cumulative UV Exposure

Intrinsic or chronological aging of photoprotected skin is characterized as smooth, dry, pale, and finely wrinkled with epidermal and dermal thinning. Photoaging is distinguished from chronological aging primarily through the appearance of solar elastosis, manifested as thickening of the skin associated with a leathery texture, yellow discoloration, and deep wrinkling. In addition, photoaging is characterized by pigmentary changes that include solar keratoses and lentigos.[42,43] This general paradigm of intrinsic and photoaging holds for all pigmentary groups to a greater or lesser extent. Popular opinion supported by some published data holds that individuals with greater constitutive skin pigmentation show fewer signs of photoaging when compared to lighter skinned individuals. Studies have confirmed lower levels of several proteolytic enzymes associated with photoaging in dark skin versus light skin after UV exposure which would suggest that skin of color is at less risk of wrinkling.[24,28] Nevertheless, pigmented skin can display signs of photodamage such as epidermal atypia, atrophy, dermal collagen, and elastin damage, as well as marked hyperpigmentation.[6,37] (*See* Fig. 4.4.)

Roh et al used skin reflectance spectroscopy to compare pigmentation in Korean subjects of different ages and genders with skin types IV–V; they found that Korean skin of older individuals differed from Caucasian skin of similarly aged subjects in that facultative pigmentation and sun exposure index did not increase with aging. They concluded that although basal melanogenic regulation may be similar for Caucasians and Asians, the sun exposure index may not be representative of lifelong cumulative UV exposure in Koreans. They also speculated that genetically determined basal skin color may play an important role in predicting long-term cosmetic

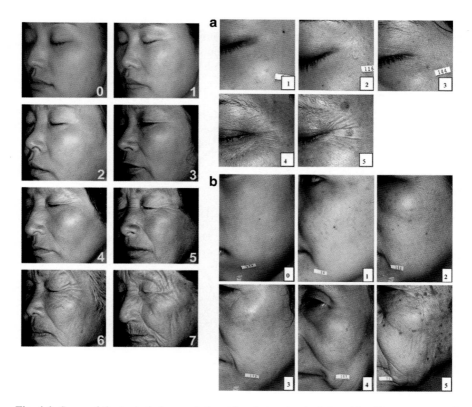

Fig. 4.4 Some of the typical changes induced by photoaging in Asian skin. (Photo courtesy of Tsukahara et al. *J Dermatol Sci.* 2007)

damage resulting from UVR. Despite a higher threshold of UV exposure needed to produce signs of photodamage, it can, however, be a consequence of UVR for people with skin of color.[44] It is also important to keep in mind that photodamage in skin of color may take on a different appearance than the deep wrinkles and furrowing which are associated with photodamaged white skin. Although a generalization, it appears that photodamaged white skin will wrinkle earlier and more severely, whereas dark ethnic skin and Asian skin tend to show pigmentary changes before serious wrinkling.[43]

4.9 Immunosuppression

UVR-induced skin cancer can be considered to develop in two stages: (1) initiated by direct DNA modification and mutagenesis and (2) subsequently promoted by suppression of the cutaneous immune system. (*See* Fig. 4.5.) In addition to DNA and structural damage, UVR has been shown to impair the cutaneous immune response.[46-48] This is best demonstrated by the increased incidence of skin cancers seen in immunosuppressed organ transplant patients.[45] Evidence for melanin's protective effect against DNA damage is strong; however, there is less of a consensus on melanin's efficacy against UV immunosuppression. There have been several studies published that explore the relationship between skin type and the ability to be immune suppressed by UVR.

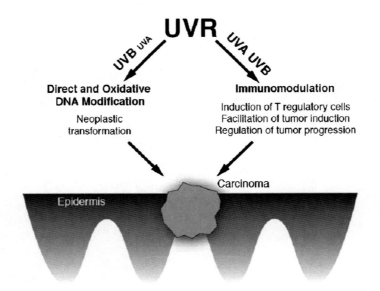

Fig. 4.5 UVR influences both the promotion and the induction of carcinogenesis. (Figure courtesy of Granstein et al. *Cutis*. 2005)

The contact hypersensitivity response (CHS) is widely used to access the integrity of cutaneous immunity. In this test, an individual is sensitized to a novel antigen not usually found in the environment such as dinitrochlorobenzene and is challenged at a later date with same antigen. The swelling of the localized reaction after challenge is used as a measure of an individual's type IV hypersensitivity response. This edematous response is usually quantified using skin calipers for measurement of skinfold thickness or the erythema is measured with a colorimeter.

Langerhans cells (LCs), known as the sentinels of the skin or the professional antigen-presenting cells, are responsible for activation of T cells by their presentation of antigen in the lymph nodes.[46,49] The morphology, function, and number of LCs are also often used as a marker of cutaneous immunity. Several studies performed in subjects with light skin have shown that UVB and UVA are able to impair cutaneous immune function and deplete LC number and function.[47,49-52]

Vermeer et al studied the effect of a low-dose UVB regimen on the CHS response to dinitrochlorobenzene of individuals with genetically melanized and heavily tanned skin.[53] Their findings showed that when subjects with dark skin (both genetically and heavily tanned) were exposed to low doses of UVB, they exhibited similar decreases in CHS and changes in LC morphology when compared to light skinned subjects. Matsuoka et al. looked at immunological responses to UVB light in dark skinned individuals. In their study, they evaluated peripheral lymphocytes of dark skinned subjects after delivering low dose of UVB irradiation and compared their observations with those found in light skinned controls. Interestingly, they observed that in light skinned subjects, the level of natural killer T cells was not affected by low-dose UVB. However, they noticed a significant increase in this cell population among dark skinned subjects after UVB exposure. The authors speculate that this increase in natural killer T cells may offer immunological protection against transformed cells and therefore help to explain the decreased incidence of skin cancer in the dark skin population.[54]

Using subjects with skin types I–VI, Selgrade et al looked at differences in the CHS response after UV irradiation. Their findings showed that neither FST nor MED was related to the degree of UV-induced CHS suppression. They observed that the slope of the erythemal dose response curve (sED) could be used to predict individuals who were susceptible to the immunosuppressive effects of UVR. Individuals with a steep curve were more likely to be suppressed, and individuals with a flat slope had such a high threshold for suppression that the UV dose needed to suppress the immune response by 50% could not be computed.[55] Interestingly, there was no correlation between FST or MED and sED slope, such that some individuals with FSTs ranging from I to V showed a steep sED, and some subjects with MEDs typically associated with FST II–III (as low as 41) as well as subjects with FST IV–VI, displayed flat dose response curves. This study confirmed the shortcomings of current skin type methods to predict certain UV responses, and confirmed that some people with darker skin types are vulnerable to UV-induced immunosuppression.

Later, studies by Kelly et al[56] demonstrated that suberythemal doses of UVR suppressed cell-mediated immunity in skin types I and II but higher erythemogenic

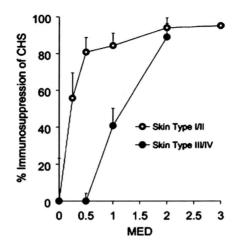

Fig. 4.6 This graph shows that skin types I–IV can be immune suppressed when given as low as a 2 MED dose of SSR. (Graph courtesy of Young et al[48])

doses were needed for suppression in skin types III and IV. Their findings suggest that darker skin types may in fact be more protected from UV-induced immunosuppression compared to lighter skin types. Similar findings were reported by Young et al.[48] (*See* Fig. 4.6.)

Rijken et al[24] examined inflammatory and immunomodulatory markers in skin of light and dark subjects after exposure to a fixed physical dose of ssUVR and assessed a range of damage markers including infiltrating neutrophils and neutrophil elastase, matrix metalloproteinases (MMP)-9 and -1, and IL-10 expression. Given equivalent physical UVR exposure, there was an absence of neutrophilic infiltrate, IL-10 positive cells, MMP-9, and MMP-1 in irradiated black skin as compared to an abundance of these cells in white skin.[24] MMP-9 and MMP-1 are part of a family proteolytic enzymes called MMPs. These endopeptidases are collectively responsible for cleavage of many of the constituents of the extracellular matrix and basement membrane. Therefore, this group of peptidases has an important role both in photoaging[57] and in the invasive growth and metastasis of primary tumors. (See review by Birkedal-Hansen et al.[58])

4.10 UVR and Skin Cancer in Ethnic Populations

Skin cancers are the most common malignancy in the USA. Skin cancers related to UV exposure in the Caucasian population are BCCs, squamous cell carcinomas (SCCs) and melanomas. BCCs and SCCs are linked to long-term chronic sun exposure, whereas melanoma is linked to intermittent intense sun exposure, especially during childhood. Skin cancers are more common among the Caucasian population with cutaneous neoplasms representing approximately 20–30% of all malignancies in whites, 2–4% of all neoplasms in Asians, and 1–2% of all malignancies in African-Americans and Asian Indians.[59]

The incidence of skin cancer (BCC, SCC, and melanoma) in the white population has been rising at a rate of approximately 5–8% per year.[59,60] Global skin cancer incidence reports show that not all ethnic groups have the same incidence for this disease as Caucasians but in addition, many of the general ethnic descriptors are too comprehensive to be meaningful.[59] For example, within a population identified as "Asian," Japanese incidence data on NMSC differ from reports from the Singapore Cancer Registry for Chinese Asians.[59] Discrepancies between the various groups might be the result of variations in cultural and social sun protection practices. However, this inexactness makes the actual incidence of NMSCs among different ethnicities difficult to estimate.[59]

Consistent diagnostic criteria of skin cancers in different racial groups can be challenging because of differences in both the clinical and the histological presentation of tumors.[59]) For example, Kikuchi et al reported that among Japanese patients, BCCs most commonly presented as pigmented lesions with a black pearly appearance.[61] This differs from the most common appearance of BCC in white skin often described as raised and pink or pearly white.

BCC is the most common skin cancer in Caucasians, Hispanics, Chinese, and Japanese Asians, while the *second* most common skin cancer in Blacks and Asian Indians. (Reviewed by Gloster and Neal)[59]. The incidence of BCC appears to be directly related to the amount of pigmentation in the skin, with fair Caucasians having the greatest incidence and African blacks having the lowest.[59] However, in all ethnicities,[59] the majority (70–90%) of BCCs are found in sun-exposed skin. This is a compelling statistic in favor of sun protection for all skin types.

While it is known that Hispanics and African-Americans have a decreased incidence of melanoma, and it is suspected that pigment plays a large role in this protection, there is also evidence that better sun-protective behavior (less high-risk behavior) may also contribute to fewer melanoma cases among these populations.[62] This is considered possible even though these populations are twice as likely to work outdoors, and therefore overall have a higher level of chronic sun exposure than Caucasians. Interestingly, it has been shown that the risk for melanoma is inversely related to chronic and occupational sun exposure.[63]

It is further difficult to compare rates of melanoma in Caucasians and Hispanics or African-Americans because it has been shown that when African-Americans and Hispanics develop cutaneous melanoma they are more likely to develop acral lengious melanoma which behaves differently from superficial spreading melanoma which is the type most commonly seen in Whites. It is also difficult to use the descriptor "Hispanic" in the debate over the protective effects of constitutive pigment because skin types in this group can vary from very fair to dark skin tones.[64]

Melanoma data from the population-based state cancer registries of states with a population of one million or more Hispanics (California, Florida, Illinois, New Jersey, New York, and Texas) allowed researchers in Miami to study a population representing 73% of the US Hispanic and 77% of the total black population in the USA. Researchers looked at the photoprotective behavior of Hispanics and African-Americans[64] and found that the rate of melanoma in both Hispanics and African-Americans increased with increasing annual UV index and/or lower latitude of residency, suggesting that darkly pigmented individuals are at a greater risk to UV carcinogenesis than previously thought.[64]

Indeed, several studies have shown that for both Hispanics and African-Americans, melanoma incidence is positively associated with the UV index.[64-66] However, in their analysis of the Surveillance Epidemiology and End Results Cancer database, Eide found that UVR does not appear to be a significant risk factor for melanoma in African-Americans and other ethnic groups who tend to develop melanoma on non-sun-exposed sites such a palmar, plantar, and mucosal surfaces.[67] There is evidence that melanin, and therefore skin with more melanin, may contribute to oxidative stress and damage by direct oxidation of melanin and the subsequent release of reactive oxygen species secondary to melanosomal damage, DNA damage, and redox metabolism.[68-70]

4.11   Habits of Non-Caucasians Versus Caucasians and Photoprotection

A study aimed at determining the sun protection practices in a wide population, including multiethnic subjects, living in Hawaii looked 932 subject surveys evaluating five photoprotective behaviors including use of sunscreen, wearing a shirt, wearing a hat, seeking shade, and wearing sunglasses. The ethnic distribution of this Hawaiian study was made up of 19.0% Caucasian, 15.4% Hawaiian or part Hawaiian, and 57.8% Asian including Japanese, Filipino, Chinese, and mixed Asian. Seven percent of the study population was classified as "other" or "mixed ethnicity."[71] This study found that the social and physical environment of an individual was more influential than specific ethic beliefs and behaviors with respect to sun protection practices.

Researchers at University of Miami speculated that differences in presentation of White Hispanics versus White non-Hispanics at the time a diagnosis of melanoma is made (White Hispanics were more likely to present with regional or distant stage disease compared to white non-Hispanics) may be a sign of differences in behavior and beliefs about sun protection between these two ethnic populations.[72] These researchers studied high school students to access differences in sun-protective behavior. They found that among high school students in Miami Dade County, white Hispanics were more than twice as likely (2.5) to use tanning beds and overall this group spent more time trying to tan than white non-Hispanics.

Both groups were similarly aware of the importance of UV exposure in skin carcinogenesis. However, White Hispanics were less aware, and therefore also less likely to perform preventative self-skin assessment examinations. White Hispanics were also less likely to report having a relative with skin cancer than White non-Hispanics. Also interesting was the finding that White Hispanics were significantly less likely to consider themselves at risk for skin cancer. This population was also significantly less likely to use sunscreen with SPF of 15 or higher, or sun-protective clothing when compared to their White non-Hispanic peers. Ma et al speculated that a lack in public education on skin cancer risk among minority populations may be responsible to these differences.[73]

4.12   Vitamin D

It is well known that vitamin D plays an important part in calcium and phosphate metabolism.[74] More recently, vitamin D and deficiency in vitamin D has been linked to several health conditions from breast and prostate cancer, cardiovascular disease, glucose intolerance, and other sequela.[75] One benefit of UVB exposure on skin is the conversion of 7-dehydrocholeserol to form vitamin D_3.[76] One evolution-based theory to explain differences in skin tone exists that is based on the hypothesis that populations originating from geographical areas with a lower UV index required lighter skin to facilitate greater vitamin D production.[77] This is due to the fact that melanin in skin prevents UVB penetration and blocks the photons from reaching the vitamin D_3 precursor.[78] There is evidence that individuals with dark skin typically have lower vitamin D levels when compared to lighter skinned people.[79,80]

In a study designed to define the relationship between UVB exposure and serum concentrations of 25-hydroxyvitamin D as a function of skin pigmentation, Armas et al[78] exposed 72 subjects with various skin tones to UVB light. In their study, skin tone was determined using a reflective meter, and subjects received doses of UVB three times a week for 4 weeks. Light skinned subjects received doses ranging from 20 to 40 mJ/cm^2, while darker skin subjects were treated with 50, 60, or 80 mJ/cm^2. Results from this study showed that therapeutically important changes in serum 25-hydroxyvitamin D were attained with minimal tanning. They also found that 80% of the variation in treatment response could be explained by UVB dose and skin tone.

Despite these findings, and others that report lower concentrations of vitamin D in dark skinned populations,[79,80] it is important to understand that skin cancer remains as an important pubic health concern for people of all skin types, and because the major cause for skin cancer is known to be excessive UVR, UV exposure should not be the preferred source for obtaining this vitamin.[81] Thus, misinterpretation of the role for UVB exposure and importance of adequate vitamin D levels have the potential to put public health in jeopardy.[81] In light of the known risks associated with UVR, alternative sources of vitamin D should be sought. These include dietary supplements and consumption of vitamin D rich foods.[78,81]

4.13   Future Studies

Despite recent studies addressing the effects of UVR on ethnic skin, many questions remain unanswered. On a clinical level, limitations in currently accepted skin typing systems warrant the development of more comprehensive and individualised skin typing guidelines and categories that include and take into consideration the various pigmentation levels of non-Caucasian individuals. On a basic science level, many of the regulatory mechanisms involved in melanin synthesis and function are yet to be explicated. Additional biological, epidemiological, and genetic studies are needed to more fully explain differences between racial groups with regards to melanoma[82] and other skin cancers and photo immunosuppression. Photoaging is popularly believed to manifest differently in skin of color when compared to white skin but there are few rigorous studies to support this. Finally, outcome studies to examine the effect of equivalent preventative education and sun protection behavior among all ethnic groups would be extremely interesting in terms of the potential to equalize relative skin cancer rates.

4.14   Conclusions

Non-Caucasian skin has distinct qualities attributed in part to its constitutive pigment. Melanin appears to protect the deeper epidermis and dermis from DNA photodamage, and induction of proteolytic enzymes such as MMPs, elastases, and collagenases. These differences explain, at least in part, why darker skin is less prone to carcinogenesis and signs of photoaging such as wrinkles and loss of elasticity. Melanin's ability to protect from UV-induced immunosuppression is less clear, and the susceptibility of dark skin to immunosuppression is a compelling indication for this population to protect themselves from UVR. Despite a need for people with skin of color to protect themselves from UVR, studies of sun-protective behaviors among ethnic groups show that this population may be not adequately protected. At this time, photoprotection through sun avoidance, protective clothing, and broad-spectrum sunscreens should be recommended to people with skin of any color. In fact, an additional reason to recommend sun-protective behavior to those with more pigmented skin is the propensity of that population to experience PIH and the possibility for sun exposure to exacerbate this pigmentation disorder.

References

1. Albert MR, Ostheimer KG. The evolution of current medical and popular attitudes toward ultraviolet light exposure: part 1. *J Am Acad Dermatol*. 2003 Nov;48(6):930–937.
2. Docket No. 1978N-0038; RIN 0910-AF43 In: Re: Sunscreen Drug Products for Over the Counter Human Use; Proposed Amendment of Final Monograph; proposed Rule.
3. Leenutaphong V. Relationship between skin color and cutaneous response to ultraviolet radiation in Thai. *Photodermatol Photoimmunol Photomed*. 1996 Oct–Dec;11(5-6):198–203.
4. Choe YB, Jang SJ, Jo SJ, Ahn KJ, Youn JI. The difference between the constitutive and facultative skin color does not reflect skin phototype in Asian skin. *Skin Res Technol*. 2006 Feb;12(1):68–72.
5. Al-Ajmi HS. A comparison of minimal erythema doses for narrowband vs. broadband ultraviolet B irradiation in darkly pigmented healthy subjects and in psoriatic patients in Kuwait. *Br J Dermatol*. 2006 Apr;154(4):795–797.

6. Taylor SC. Skin of color: biology, structure, function, and implications for dermatologic disease. *J Am Acad Dermatol.* 2002 Feb;46(2 Suppl Understanding):S41–S62.

7. Montagna W, Carlisle K. The architecture of black and white facial skin. *J Am Acad Dermatol.* 1991 Jun;24(6 Pt 1):929–937.

8. Szabo G, Gerald AB, Pathak MA, Fitzpatrick TB. Racial differences in the fate of melanosomes in human epidermis. *Nature* 1969 Jun 14 222;(5198):1081–1082.

9. Alaluf S, Atkins D, Barrett K, Blount M, Carter N, Heath A. Ethnic variation in melanin content and composition in photoexposed and photoprotected human skin. *Pigment Cell Res.* 2002 Apr;15(2):112–118.

10. Tadokoro T, Yamaguchi Y, Batzer J, Coelho SG, Zmudzka BZ, Miller SA, et al. Mechanisms of skin tanning in different racial/ethnic groups in response to ultraviolet radiation. *J Invest Dermatol.* 2005 Jun;124(6):1326–1332.

11. Tadokoro T, Kobayashi N, Zmudzka BZ, Ito S, Wakamatsu K, Yamaguchi Y, et al. UV-induced DNA damage and melanin content in human skin differing in racial/ethnic origin. *FASEB J.* 2003 Jun;17(9):1177–1179.

12. Agar N, Young AR. Melanogenesis: a photoprotective response to DNA damage? *Mutat Res.* 2005 Apr 1; 571(1-2): 121–132.

13. Jansen CT. Self-reported skin type and reactivity to UVB, UVA and PUVA irradiation. *Photodermatol.* 1989 Oct;6(5):234–236.

14. Rampen FH, Fleuren BA, de Boo TM, Lemmens WA. Unreliability of self-reported burning tendency and tanning ability. *Arch Dermatol.* 1988 Jun;124(6):885–888.

15. Youn JI, Oh JK, Kim BK, Suh DH, Chung JH, Oh SJ, et al. Relationship between skin phototype and MED in Korean, brown skin. *Photodermatol Photoimmunol Photomed.* 1997 Oct-Dec;13(5-6):208–211.

16. Kawada A, Noda T, Hiruma M, Ishibashi A, Arai S. The relationship of sun protection factor to minimal erythema dose, Japanese skin type, and skin color. *J Dermatol.* 1993 Aug;20(8): 514–516.

17. Morison WL. What is the function of melanin? *Arch Dermatol.* 1985 Sep;121(9): 1160–1163.

18. Schmitz S, Thomas PD, Allen TM, Poznansky MJ, Jimbow K. Dual role of melanins and melanin precursors as photoprotective and phototoxic agents: inhibition of ultraviolet radiation-induced lipid peroxidation. *Photochem Photobiol.* 1995 Jun;61(6):650–655.

19. Cesarini JP. Photo-induced events in the human melanocytic system: photoaggression and photoprotection. *Pigment Cell Res.* 1988;1(4):223–233.

20. Hennessy A, Oh C, Diffey B, Wakamatsu K, Ito S, Rees J. Eumelanin and pheomelanin concentrations in human epidermis before and after UVB irradiation. *Pigment Cell Res.* 2005 Jun;18(3):220–223.

21. Hill HZ, Li W, Xin P, Mitchell DL. Melanin: a two edged sword? *Pigment Cell Res.* 1997 Jun;10(3):158–161.

22. Del Bino S, Sok J, Bessac E, Bernerd F. Relationship between skin response to ultraviolet exposure and skin color type. *Pigment Cell Res.* 2006 Dec;19(6):606–614.

23. Sheehan JM, Cragg N, Chadwick CA, Potten CS, Young AR. Repeated ultraviolet exposure affords the same protection against DNA photodamage and erythema in human skin types II and IV but is associated with faster DNA repair in skin type IV. *J Invest Dermatol.* 2002 May;118(5):825–829.

24. Rijken F, Bruijnzeel PL, van Weelden H, Kiekens RC. Responses of black and white skin to solar-simulating radiation: differences in DNA photodamage, infiltrating neutrophils, proteolytic enzymes induced, keratinocyte activation, and IL-10 expression. *J Invest Dermatol.* 2004 Jun;122(6):1448–1455.

25. Pfeifer GP, You YH, Besaratinia A. Mutations induced by ultraviolet light. *Mutat Res.* 2005 Apr 1;571(1-2):19–31.

26. Wondrak GT, Jacobson MK, Jacobson EL. Endogenous UVA-photosensitizers: mediators of skin photodamage and novel targets for skin photoprotection. *Photochem Photobiol Sci.* 2006 Feb;5(2):215–237.

27. Del Bino S, Sok J, Bessac E, Bernerd F. Relationship between skin response to ultraviolet exposure and skin color type. *Pigment Cell Res.* 2006 Dec;19(6):606–614.
28. Fisher GJ, Kang S, Varani J, Bata-Csorgo Z, Wan Y, Datta S, et al. Mechanisms of photoaging and chronological skin aging. *Arch Dermatol.* 2002 Nov;138(11):1462–1470.
29. Yamaguchi Y, Takahashi K, Zmudzka BZ, Kornhauser A, Miller SA, Tadokoro T, et al. Human skin responses to UV radiation: pigment in the upper epidermis protects against DNA damage in the lower epidermis and facilitates apoptosis. *FASEB J.* 2006 Jul;20(9):1486–1488.
30. Yamaguchi Y, Beer JZ, Hearing VJ. Melanin mediated apoptosis of epidermal cells damaged by ultraviolet radiation: factors influencing the incidence of skin cancer. *Arch Dermatol Res.* 2007 Nov 6.
31. Yamaguchi Y, Beer JZ, Hearing VJ. Melanin mediated apoptosis of epidermal cells damaged by ultraviolet radiation: factors influencing the incidence of skin cancer. *Arch Dermatol Res.* 2007 Nov 6.
32. Gilchrest BA, Park HY, Eller MS, Yaar M. Mechanisms of ultraviolet light-induced pigmentation. *Photochem Photobiol.* 1996 Jan;63(1):1–10.
33. Eller MS, Gilchrest BA. Tanning as part of the eukaryotic SOS response. *Pigment Cell Res.* 2000;13 Suppl 8:94–97.
34. Arad S, Konnikov N, Goukassian DA, Gilchrest BA. T-oligos augment UV-induced protective responses in human skin. *FASEB J.* 2006 Sep;20(11):1895–1897.
35. Gniadecka M, Wulf HC, Mortensen NN, Poulsen T. Photoprotection in vitiligo and normal skin. A quantitative assessment of the role of stratum corneum, viable epidermis and pigmentation. *Acta Derm Venereol.* 1996 Nov;76(6):429–432.
36. Hennessy A, Oh C, Rees J, Diffey B. The photoadaptive response to ultraviolet exposure in human skin using ultraviolet spectrophotometry. *Photodermatol Photoimmunol Photomed.* 2005 Oct;21(5):229–233.
37. Kotrajaras R, Kligman AM. The effect of topical tretinoin on photodamaged facial skin: the Thai experience. *Br J Dermatol.* 1993 Sep;129(3):302–309.
38. Downie JB. Esthetic considerations for ethnic skin. *Semin Cutan Med Surg.* 2006 Sep;25(3):158–162.
39. Badreshia-Bansal S, Draelos ZD. Insight into skin lightening cosmeceuticals for women of color. *J Drugs Dermatol.* 2007 Jan;6(1):32–39.
40. Taylor SC. Cosmetic problems in skin of color. *Skin Pharmacol Appl Skin Physiol.* 1999 May–Jun;12(3):139–143.
41. Grimes PE. Melasma. Etiologic and therapeutic considerations. *Arch Dermatol.* 1995 Dec;131(12):1453–1457.
42. Rabe JH, Mamelak AJ, McElgunn PJ, Morison WL, Sauder DN. Photoaging: mechanisms and repair. *J Am Acad Dermatol.* 2006 Jul;55(1):1–19.
43. Chung JH. Photoaging in Asians. *Photodermatol Photoimmunol Photomed.* 2003 Jun; 19(3): 109–121.
44. Roh K, Kim D, Ha S, Ro Y, Kim J, Lee H. Pigmentation in Koreans: study of the differences from Caucasians in age, gender and seasonal variations. *Br J Dermatol.* 2001 Jan;144(1):94–99.
45. Neuburg M. Transplant-associated skin cancer: role of reducing immunosuppression. *J Natl Compr Canc Netw.* 2007 May;5(5):541–549.
46. Clydesdale GJ, Dandie GW, Muller HK. Ultraviolet light induced injury: immunological and inflammatory effects. *Immunol Cell Biol.* 2001 Dec;79(6):547–568.
47. Baron ED, Fourtanier A, Compan D, Medaisko C, Cooper KD, Stevens SR. High ultraviolet A protection affords greater immune protection confirming that ultraviolet A contributes to photoimmunosuppression in humans. *J Invest Dermatol.* 2003 Oct;121(4):869–875.
48. Young AR, Walker SL. Effects of solar simulated radiation on the human immune system: influence of phototypes and wavebands. *Exp Dermatol.* 2002;11(Suppl 1):17–19.
49. Hanneman KK, Cooper KD, Baron ED. Ultraviolet immunosuppression: mechanisms and consequences. *Dermatol Clin.* 2006 Jan;24(1):19–25.

50. Byrne SN, Spinks N, Halliday GM. The induction of immunity to a protein antigen using an adjuvant is significantly compromised by ultraviolet A radiation. *J Photochem Photobiol B.* 2006 Aug 1;84(2):128–134.
51. Schwarz T. Mechanisms of UV-induced immunosuppression. *Keio J Med.* 2005 Dec;54(4):165–171.
52. Schwarz A, Maeda A, Schwarz T. Alteration of the migratory behavior of UV-induced regulatory T cells by tissue-specific dendritic cells. *J Immunol.* 2007 Jan 15;178(2):877–886.
53. Vermeer M, Schmieder GJ, Yoshikawa T, van den Berg JW, Metzman MS, Taylor JR, et al. Effects of ultraviolet B light on cutaneous immune responses of humans with deeply pigmented skin. *J Invest Dermatol.* 1991 Oct;97(4):729–734.
54. Matsuoka LY, McConnachie P, Wortsman J, Holick MF. Immunological responses to ultraviolet light B radiation in Black individuals. *Life Sci.* 1999;64(17):1563–1569.
55. Selgrade MK, Smith MV, Oberhelman-Bragg LJ, LeVee GJ, Koren HS, Cooper KD. Dose response for UV-induced immune suppression in people of color: differences based on erythemal reactivity rather than skin pigmentation. *Photochem Photobiol.* 2001 Jul;74(1):88–95.
56. Kelly DA, Young AR, McGregor JM, Seed PT, Potten CS, Walker SL. Sensitivity to sunburn is associated with susceptibility to ultraviolet radiation-induced suppression of cutaneous cell-mediated immunity. *J Exp Med.* 2000 Feb 7;191(3):561–566.
57. Fisher GJ, Wang ZQ, Datta SC, Varani J, Kang S, Voorhees JJ. Pathophysiology of premature skin aging induced by ultraviolet light. *N Engl J Med.* 1997 Nov 13;337(20):1419–1428.
58. Birkedal-Hansen H, Moore WG, Bodden MK, Windsor LJ, Birkedal-Hansen B, DeCarlo A, et al. Matrix metalloproteinases: a review. *Crit Rev Oral Biol Med.* 1993;4(2):197–250.
59. GlosterJr. HM, NealK. Skin cancer in skin of color. *J Am Acad Dermatol.* 2006 Nov;55(5): 741–760; quiz 761-764.
60. Coups EJ, Manne SL, Heckman CJ. Multiple skin cancer risk behaviors in the U.S. population. *Am J Prev Med.* 2008 Feb;34(2):87–93.
61. Kikuchi A, Shimizu H, Nishikawa T. Clinical histopathological characteristics of basal cell carcinoma in Japanese patients. *Arch Dermatol.* 1996 Mar;132(3):320–324.
62. Saraiya M, Hall HI, Uhler RJ. Sunburn prevalence among adults in the United States, 1999. *Am J Prev Med.* 2002 Aug;23(2):91–97.
63. MacKie RM, Aitchison T. Severe sunburn and subsequent risk of primary cutaneous malignant melanoma in Scotland. *Br J Cancer* 1982 Dec;46(6):955–960.
64. Hu S, Ma F, Collado-Mesa F, Kirsner RS. UV radiation, latitude, and melanoma in US Hispanics and blacks. *Arch Dermatol.* 2004 Jul;140(7):819–824.
65. Hu S, Soza-Vento RM, Parker DF, Kirsner RS. Comparison of stage at diagnosis of melanoma among Hispanic, black, and white patients in Miami-Dade County, Florida. *Arch Dermatol.* 2006 Jun;142(6):704–708.
66. Tsai T, Vu C, Henson DE. Cutaneous, ocular and visceral melanoma in African Americans and Caucasians. *Melanoma Res.* 2005 Jun;15(3):213–217.
67. Eide MJ, Weinstock MA. Association of UV index, latitude, and melanoma incidence in nonwhite populations – US Surveillance, Epidemiology, and End Results (SEER) Program, 1992 to 2001. *Arch Dermatol.* 2005 Apr;141(4):477–481.
68. Meyskens Jr. FL, McNulty SE, BuckmeierJA, TohidianNB, SpillaneTJ, KahlonRS, et al. Aberrant redox regulation in human metastatic melanoma cells compared to normal melanocytes. *Free Radic Biol Med.* 2001 Sep 15;31(6):799–808.
69. MeyskensJr. FL, FarmerPJ, Anton-CulverH. Etiologic pathogenesis of melanoma: a unifying hypothesis for the missing attributable risk. *Clin Cancer Res.* 2004 Apr 15;10(8):2581–2583.
70. Meyskens, Jr. FL, FarmerPJ, Anton-CulverH. Diet and melanoma in a case-control study. *Cancer Epidemiol Biomarkers Prev.* 2005 Jan;14(1):293.
71. Glanz K, Lew RA, Song V, Cook VA. Factors associated with skin cancer prevention practices in a multiethnic population. *Health Educ Behav.* 1999 Jun;26(3):344–359.
72. Ma F, Collado-Mesa F, Hu S, Kirsner RS. Skin cancer awareness and sun protection behaviors in white Hispanic and white non-Hispanic high school students in Miami, Florida. *Arch Dermatol.* 2007 Aug;143(8):983–988.

73. Ma F, Collado-Mesa F, Hu S, Kirsner RS. Skin cancer awareness and sun protection behaviors in white Hispanic and white non-Hispanic high school students in Miami, Florida. *Arch Dermatol.* 2007 Aug;143(8):983–988.

74. Heaney RP. Functional indices of vitamin D status and ramifications of vitamin D deficiency. *Am J Clin Nutr.* 2004 Dec;80(6 Suppl):1706S–1709S.

75. Holick MF. Sunlight and vitamin D for bone health and prevention of autoimmune diseases, cancers, and cardiovascular disease. *Am J Clin Nutr.* 2004 Dec;80(6 Suppl):1678S–1688S.

76. Glerup H, Mikkelsen K, Poulsen L, Hass E, Overbeck S, Thomsen J, et al. Commonly recommended daily intake of vitamin D is not sufficient if sunlight exposure is limited. *J Intern Med.* 2000 Feb;247(2):260–268.

77. Jablonski NG, Chaplin G. The evolution of human skin coloration. *J Hum Evol.* 2000 Jul;39(1):57–106.

78. Armas LA, Dowell S, Akhter M, Duthuluru S, Huerter C, Hollis BW, et al. Ultraviolet-B radiation increases serum 25-hydroxyvitamin D levels: the effect of UVB dose and skin color. *J Am Acad Dermatol.* 2007 Oct;57(4):588–593.

79. Harris SS, Dawson-Hughes B. Seasonal changes in plasma 25-hydroxyvitamin D concentrations of young American black and white women. *Am J Clin Nutr.* 1998 Jun;67(6):1232–1236.

80. Nesby-O'Dell S, Scanlon KS, Cogswell ME, Gillespie C, Hollis BW, Looker AC, et al. Hypovitaminosis D prevalence and determinants among African American and white women of reproductive age: third National Health and Nutrition Examination Survey, 1988-1994. *Am J Clin Nutr.* 2002 Jul;76(1):187–192.

81. Lim HW, Carucci JA, Spencer JM, Rigel DS. Commentary: A responsible approach to maintaining adequate serum vitamin D levels. *J Am Acad Dermatol.* 2007 Oct;57(4):594–595.

82. Zell JA, CinarP, MobasherM, ZiogasA, MeyskensJr. FL, Anton-CulverH. Survival for patients with invasive cutaneous melanoma among ethnic groups: the effects of socioeconomic status and treatment. *J Clin Oncol.* 2008 Jan 1;26(1):66–75.

Chapter 5
Light Treatment of Follicular Disorders in Dark Skin

Bassel H. Mahmoud and Iltefat H. Hamzavi

5.1 Introduction

On the one hand, the majority of the published data on the topic of cosmetic dermatology and laser surgery have been focused on the Caucasian population; on the other hand, statistics in the United States showed significantly shifting demographics in the past decade. Hispanics and Asians accounted for 40% of the total growth of the US population, African Americans for 12%, and non-Hispanic Caucasians for somewhat over 2%. According to the 2000 census, 29% of the United States population, representing approximately 85 millions, is not Caucasian but are individuals of color.[1] By the year 2056 it is expected that more than 50% of the US population will be of non-European descent and will likely include a large number of ethnic patients with cosmetic needs.[2] Most of the current literature remains devoted to examining laser procedures performed on individuals with fair skin tones (Fitzpatrick skin phototypes I–II) and protocols have largely been defined on the basis of the more extensive clinical experience that has accumulated surrounding these patients, even though Asians, Hispanics, and African Americans are showing increased demand for dermatologic laser surgery.[3]

> Statistics in United States showed significant shifting demograph
>
> By the year 2056, more than 50% of the US population will be of non-European descent

To select an appropriate modality, it is imperative that the dermatologists not only be aware of the unique needs of those with darker skin but also be knowledgeable of the latest laser technology, including the risks and benefits of cutaneous laser procedures as they relate to the specific needs of the ethnic patient.[4]

B.H. Mahmoud (✉) and I.H. Hamzavi
Multicultural Dermatology Center, Department of Dermatology,
Henry Ford Hospital, Detroit, MI, USA
e-mail: bmahmou1@hfhs.org

E.D. Baron (ed.), *Light-Based Therapies for Skin of Color,*
DOI: 10.1007/ 978-1-84882-328-0_5, © Springer-Verlag London Limited 2009

5.2 Follicular Disorders in Dark Skin Treated with Light Therapy

Table 5.1 shows the variety of follicular disorders that can be treated with the different types of light therapy.

5.2.1 Hirsutism and Hypertrichosis

5.2.1.1 Does the theory of selective photothermolysis need to be modified?

One of the greatest advancements in laser technology has been in the area of laser-assisted hair removal. To achieve effective results with laser-assisted hair removal, modification of the theory of selective photothermolysis may be needed.[5] This theory states that by using the appropriate wavelength, pulse duration, and fluence, thermal injury can be confined to the chromophore, protecting the surrounding tissue.[6] The target chromophore in laser-assisted hair removal is the melanin rich hair shaft and bulb. Due to the fact that melanin pigments have a wide absorption spectrum ranging from 250 to 1,200 nm, melanin can be specifically targeted by all visible-light and near-infrared dermatologic lasers currently in use.[7]

> To achieve effective results with laser hair removal, the theory of selective photothermolysis needs to be modified.

> Melanin pigments have a wide absorption spectrum ranging from 250 to 1,200 nm

Different sites of the hair follicles are targeted by light therapy, which represents a challenge for realization of the theory of selective photothermolysis, which is largely based on the fact that it remains vague as to which portion of the follicle is the preferred target to effect hair destruction.[8] On the basis of the original theory of selective photothermolysis, the pulse duration should be shorter than or equal to the thermal relaxation time of the hair shaft to ensure that the thermal damage is

Table 5.1 Follicular disorders amenable for light treatment and types of light sources

Follicular disorders	Light sources
1-Hirsutism and Hypertrichosis	1-Laser
2-Pseudofolliculitis Barbae	a-red-light (694-nm ruby)
3-Acne Keloidalis Nuchae	b-infrared-light (755-nm alexandrite, 800-nm diode, and
4-Dissecting cellulitis	1,064-nm Nd:YAG)
5-Hidradenitis Suppurativa	2-Intense pulsed light (590- to 1,200-nm)

localized to the selective target, which in the case of hair removal, is the hair follicle. To achieve the selective destruction of target chromophores, appropriate pulse duration must be determined for laser or intense pulsed light-assisted photoepilation.[9] The thermal relaxation time (TRT) is defined as the time taken for an increase in temperature to reduce by 1/2 of its peak value. A pulse time substantially longer than the TRT reduces heat conduction from the target to adjacent tissue, whereas too short a pulse time is likely to develop an epidermal burn. The TRT of epidermal melanosomes is 1–2 ms, and that of the hair shaft is estimated to be in the range of 10–100 ms[10]; therefore, a pulse time between that of epidermal melanin and hair follicles is probably most effective for selectively destroying hair follicles without damaging surrounding tissues. The ability of the laser to selectively destroy melanin within the hair follicle while protecting that within the epidermis is possible through thermokinetic selectivity, based on the theory of selective photothermolysis.[5] Smaller structures (epidermal melanocytes) will dissipate their heat more quickly than larger structures of the same chromophore with greater surface-to-volume ratio (hair follicle) when both are heated with laser energy. The ability of these smaller structures to dissipate heat more quickly acts as a protective mechanism. However, the concept of an appropriate pulse time for hair removal is still a controversy. To achieve permanent hair reduction, the heat must diffuse through the bulb, hair shaft, and also the entire surrounding tissue of the hair follicle. For heat to diffuse from the hair shaft through the entire hair follicle, longer pulse durations in the milliseconds are necessary to achieve the targeted thermal destruction of the entire hair follicle.[5] Within the follicular unit, the laser targets are the melanocytic outer root sheath, shaft, and the matrix. In addition, stem cells are crucial for hair development and growth. To permanently inhibit hair growth, lasers must thermally destroy not only the entire hair follicle, but also these progenitor cells.[11] Dierickx disputed that the actual target during hair removal is not the pigmented structure, but rather the components removed from a pigmented structure, like the follicular stem cells that lie in the hair follicle outer root sheath. Pulses longer than the TRT of hair shafts allow the propagation of thermal damage through the entire volume of hair, as well as damage to follicular stem cells. The study also shows that the longer pulse width applications produced better permanent hair removal results for the same number of treatments.[12]

TRT of epidermal melanosomes is 1–2 ms, and that of the hair shaft is estimated to be in the range of 10–100 ms

TRT is defined as the time taken for an increase in temperature to reduce by 1/2 of its peak value.

Longer pulse durations in the ms are necessary to achieve the targeted thermal destruction of the entire hair follicle

---

There are two stem cells reservoirs in the human anagen hair follicle. The first is located in the proximal outer root sheath. These stem cells are amelanotic

epidermis and is converted to heat, which can lead to epidermal blistering, dyspigmentation, and scarring. Epidermal melanin absorption of laser light, especially in dark–skinned individuals, causes less light to reach its intended chromophores and consequently less tissue effects. However, darker skin types can be treated with minimal side effects using longer wavelengths, longer pulse durations, and more efficient cooling devices. By manipulating laser parameters, new generation laser hair removal devices can provide the safety necessary to effectively treat darker ethnic skin.[5] Figure 5.1 shows the chin area of an African American female patient before (a) and after treatment (b) with long pulsed NdYAG laser.

> Light absorbed within the pigmented epidermis is converted to heat, which leads to epidermal blistering dyspigmentation, and scarring

Several pigment–specific laser systems with relatively long (millisecond) pulse durations have demonstrated safety and efficacy in darker skin phototypes, including the 755–nm alexandrite, 810–nm diode, and 1,064–nm NdYAG.[3] Studies looking at IPL treatment of hirsutism in patients with darker skin phototypes have been limited.[17] Alster and colleagues[8] demonstrated significant long–term hair reduction after a series of three monthly long–pulsed 1,064–nm NdYAG laser treatments in 20 women with skin phototypes IV–VI. Adverse effects were limited to transient pigmentary alteration without fibrosis or scarring. NdYAG laser irradiation has demonstrated the lowest incidence of side effects caused by nonspecific epidermal melanin absorption since its wavelength is relatively less absorbed by melanin than any other laser–assisted hair–removal modality currently available.[18]

> Nd: YAG laser has demonstrated the lowest incidence of side effects

Although difficult, effective laser therapy in patients with darker skin phototypes can be achieved, since the absorption coefficient of melanin decreases exponentially as wavelengths increase[19] (Fig. 5.2). Epidermal melanin absorbs about four times as much energy when irradiated by a 694–nm ruby laser as when exposed to the 1,064–nm beam generated by the NdYAG laser, leading to greater penetration of the longer wavelength into the dermis. Consequently, laser systems generating wavelengths that are less efficiently absorbed by endogenous melanin can often provide a greater margin of safety while still achieving satisfactory results.[20] Following wavelength, the second important parameter is the pulse duration. As the main cause for laser–induced side–effects is epidermal thermal damage, longer pulse durations allow for more efficient cooling of the epidermis. The more slowly light energy is deposited into the skin, the slower the epidermis heats, making cooling of the skin more efficient. The risk for thermal–damage–induced epidermal side–effects is minimized by removing the heat from the epidermis. Longer pulse durations are also safer for darker skin types based on the theory of thermokinetic selectivity. The theory states that smaller structures (e.g., epidermal melanin) will lose heat faster than larger structures (dermal hair follicles). The quicker dissipation of heat of the epidermal melanocytes in comparison to the larger hair follicle serves as a

a

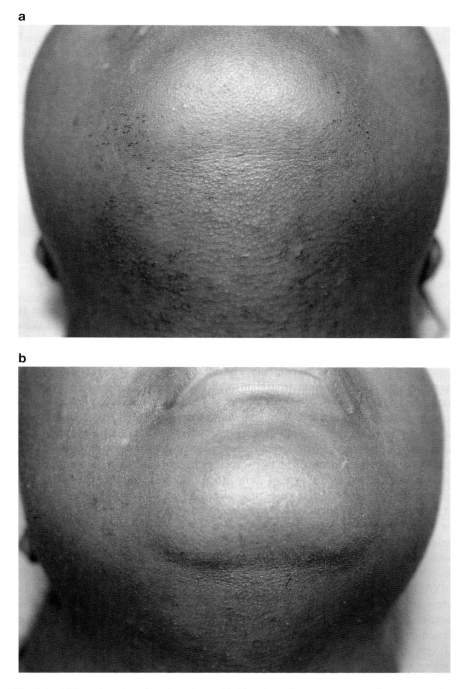

b

Fig. 5.1 African-American female patient with hirsutism of the beard area before (**a**) and after treatment (**b**) with long pulsed Nd/YAG laser

when fluence levels and exposure duration remain constant.[25] Conservative power settings (the minimal threshold fluences necessary to produce the desired tissue effect in a given individual as determined through irradiation test spots) should be employed initially to minimize the extent of collateral tissue damage. Moderate to severe pain is another indicator that the fluence may be too high. This is particularly helpful for patients who state that pain is worse than what had been experienced in prior treatments. The discomfort patients feel from laser hair removal is very subjective, but in general, should be tolerable for most patients. A topical anesthesia is often used when discomfort is not acceptable, but most patients can be treated without any topical anesthesia.[5]

Test spots are the best way to determine the appropriate fluence and right pulse duration

Evaluation of epidermal tissue response, through performing test spots, is the best way to determine the appropriate fluence and right pulse duration for a particular candidate. Test spots should be performed in a similar area that is to be treated, in order to closely match the skin color, sun exposure, and hair density level. The choice of where to perform test spots is crucial not only to closely simulate the area to be treated, but also to minimize the patients dissatisfaction if a side–effect occurs.[5]

Test spots should start with the safest parameters (lower fluences and longer pulse durations), and slowly progress to higher fluences and shorter pulse durations. Classically, two to four fluences are tested, followed by a waiting time of at least 48 h (optimally 3 weeks) after performing the test spots before safe treatment fluence can be determined. This time frame is ideal because patients with darker skin types can have a one– to two–day delay in demonstrating cutaneous side effects. Test spots should be conducted with the intent to simulate actual treatment, with a minimal of four overlapping test spots for every fluence/pulse duration parameter tested. On the basis of the results from the test spots, the safest fluence parameter can be determined to use for initiating treatment.[5] Figure 5.3 shows a posttest spots laser treatment on the right cheek and mandibular area of a dark skinned patient.

A waiting time of least 48 hours, optimally 3 weeks, after performing the test spots before determining the safe treatment fluence

In high hair density areas, such as the beard and upper back, lower fluences should be initially used to decrease the risk of thermal damage caused by the pooling of heat from the heat diffusion from close adjacent hairs. Similar to treating lighter skin types, perifollicular edema and mild erythema are immediate clinical outcome, which can be hoped for. However, this epidermal response is not always observed, because of the lower fluence often used for darker skin. Permanent hair reduction can still be achieved even if this response is not visible. Laser–induced perifollicular erythema and edema generally last from few minutes to few hours. If these reactions last longer, this should serve as a warning of being close to the epidermal thermal damage threshold and the fluence may need to be adjusted downward.

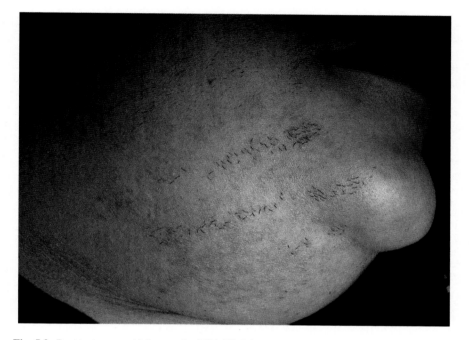

Fig. 5.3 Post test spots with long pulsed Nd: YAG laser

In high hair density areas lower fluences should be used to decrease the risk of thermal damage.

5.2.1.5 Patient selection

Ideal candidates for laser–assisted hair removal have conventionally included individuals with pale skin tones and dark terminal hair. The safest hair removal laser systems to treat phototypes IV–VI are the long pulsed NdYAG (1,064 nm). Long pulse (≥100 ms) diode (810 nm) lasers can also be used to safely treat darker skin types, but adjunct aggressive cooling is essential to safely treat skin type VI. There are very few contraindications for laser–assisted hair removal. Photosensitizing drugs activated by ultraviolet A wavelengths have often been considered a contraindication. However, hair removal lasers are in the visible and near–infrared wavelength spectrum, and, therefore, are generally felt to be safe to use on patients taking these medications.[5]

The safest hair removal laser to treat phototypes IV–VI are the long pulsed Nd: YAG (1,064 nm)

People with a history of keloids or hypertrophic scarring should be treated cautiously. Also, it has been long held that like other laser procedure, laser hair removal would increase the risk of delayed healing, keloid formation, and scarring in patients undergoing isotretinoin therapy and should be off the medication for at least six months prior to treatment. There have been no studies showing that there is an increased incidence of laser–assisted side effects on patients who are on or have recently been on Accutane. In theory, laser hair removal should not affect collagen in the dermis and healing process as it works based on the principle of the theory of selective photothermolysis, targeting melanin in the hair follicle. Khatri[26] showed in a study to evaluate the side effects of Diode laser hair removal in patients undergoing isotretinoin treatment that there was no erythema, pigmentary change, swelling, or scarring at any follow–up visits after these 36 treatments. However, patients should still wait three to six months, to be on the safe side, after stopping Accutane prior to initiating laser hair removal.[5]

Prophylaxis antivirals are necessary for people with chronic or active herpetic infections

Prophylaxis antiviral medications are necessary for people with chronic or active herpetic infections, especially if they occur in the desired treatment area. Prophylaxis is typically started one day before continuing for a total of five to seven days.[5]

5.2.1.6 Preoperative discussion of patients with darker skin types

Patient's expectations are important prior to laser–assisted hair removal. Patients should understand that multiple treatment sessions are necessary to achieve permanent hair reduction. It usually takes a minimum of five laser treatments, and often more, to reach the patient's desired hair reduction expectation. With each treatment, there is a decrease of between 10% and 20% in the hair count, color, and diameter of the hair. Because patients with darker skin types need lower fluences and longer pulse durations, more treatments maybe required compared with those with lighter skin type lighter skin types. The frequency of treatment is still controversial, and is based on many factors, particularly the growth rate and body region of the hair to be treated. Patients with facial hair should be treated approximately every four weeks. Facial hair is usually finer and lighter than hair on the rest of the body making it one of the most recalcitrant areas to treat. Therefore, more than the usual number of treatments may be necessary. It is generally agreed upon that more–frequent treatments are better than less–frequent ones to treat again before the damaged hair has had a chance to fully revitalize and strengthen. The treatments should usually be performed for four to eight weeks, depending upon the site to be treated.[5]

> With each treatment there is a decrease of between 10 and 20% in the hair count

To maximize the amount of pigmented hair chromophore in the skin, the patient should not wax or pluck hairs prior to or in between treatments. Shaving, bleaching, or utilizing depilatory creams are preferable methods for hair removal between treatment sessions. Some level of discomfort during the procedure maybe felt, often times described as a small rubber band snapping against the skin.

A topical anesthetic preparation (e.g., 4–5% lidocaine) and cooling (e.g., air cooling) helps to decrease the pain during the procedure. After the treatment, there may be immediate perifollicular edema and mild erythema lasting from minutes to hours. Regardless of the ethnicity or skin color of the patient, there should be no crusting, blistering, or scabbing posttreatment. In the event of any thermal damage-related cutaneous side-effects, a topical antibiotic or corticosteroids may be required.[5]

5.2.1.7   Treatment Protocol

Before the treatment session, the area treated must be wiped clean, and the hairs must be closely shaven. The topical anesthetic must be removed prior to treatment. A gentle alcohol cleanse should be performed to make sure that no residual makeup or anesthetic remains on the skin, followed by a final wipe with water to the area to make sure that no residual alcohol is left on the skin. Appropriate protective goggles, based on the wavelength of the laser, must be worn by everyone in the room. The patient should be wearing occlusive goggles for added protection. Individual pulses should overlap by 10–30%, depending on the type of system used.[5]

> When treating high-density, a relatively lower fluence should be used until the hair density has thinned

When treating high-density areas (e.g., the beard or upper back), a relatively lower fluence should be used until the hair density has thinned. If higher fluences are used, thermal damage could ensue due of the pooling and accumulation of heat from the diffusion of heat of the closely situated adjacent hairs. Similarly, more conservative fluences should be used on the neck in females as there is a higher incidence of scarring. When treating the face, it is better to be very conservative, utilizing lower fluences, to fully minimize any risk of epidermal injury. In treating the upper lip and chin, the enamel of the teeth should be protected using gauze overlaying the teeth or having the patient place their tongue over the teeth during treatment. It is important to closely shave the hair prior to treatments, especially for the upper lip (Fig. 5.4) and sideburns areas since they can heat up and cause superficial side effects (e.g., blistering and discoloration).[5]

Immediate icing of the treated area after treatment reduces discomfort, erythema, edema, and epidermal side effects. A topical corticosteroid can be used twice a day

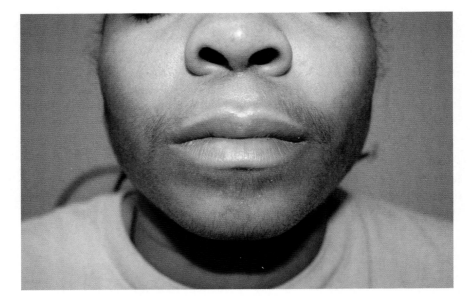

Fig. 5.4 Female patient with increased hair density of the upper lip

for 48 h if prolonged erythema, edema, or irritation occurs. Additional treatments are performed four to eight weeks apart, depending on the area treated. If there were no epidermal side effects from the previous treatment, the same parameters can be used, or one can moderately increase the fluence. Caution should be applied when increasing the fluence since small increases can tip the scale beyond the patient's epidermal thermal damage threshold, creating side effects. If the previous treatment has produced any unfortunate epidermal side-effects, the fluence should be adjusted downward and longer pulse durations should be used. If there were no adverse effects, but perifollicular edema and erythema lasted more than a few hours, the fluence should be slightly decreased.[5]

5.2.1.8 Laser-induced side effects

With the long pulse diode and NdYAG laser system, the risk of any adverse events is extremely rare.[27] Epidermal thermal damage can cause crusting, scabbing, blistering, pigmentary alterations, and scarring. The risk of infection is remote with laser-assisted hair removal, but a "folliculitis" type reaction can take place, and should be treated with antibiotics and/or corticosteroids. Herpetic infections occur in individuals with a history of chronic infections.[5]

Excessive hair growth, whether from hirsutism or hypertrichosis, in women or men can create a major medical and cosmetic problem. Conventional treatments, such as waxing, plucking, electrolysis, or shaving, have high incidence of epidermal side effects in patients with darker skin types. Laser hair removal treatments provide patients who have darker skin types with a safe and successful therapeutic option.

Pigmentary alterations and epidermal side effects affiliated with conventional methods of hair removal dramatically improve with each consecutive laser treatment. Patients satisfaction does not depend only on permanent hair reduction, but also the improvement of skin texture and pigmentary disorders.[5]

Postinflammatory hyperpigmentation is attributable to the labile response of melanocytes to irritation or inflammation.[28] Fortunately, this hyperpigmentation is transient and usually amenable to treatment with a bleaching agent and sun protection.[29] In a study done by Aldraibi et al.,[30] they found that the effect of betamethasone dipropionate cream in minimizing the incidence of hyperpigmentation was more notable in skin types IV and V. They applied the cream 10 min prior to laser application to begin its antiinflammatory effect to decrease the incidence of potential side effects.

Topical steroids minimize the incidence of hyperpigmentation in dark skin

Transient hypopigmentation is believed to be related to the reversible suppression of melanogenesis in the epidermis rather than destruction of melanocytes.[31] Aldraibi et al.[30] observed that hypopigmentation occurred mainly in areas where crusts formed indicating that the loss of melanin-rich keratinocytes in the epidermis plays a role in pathogenesis. At one month, three of their patients with skin types V and VI had hypopigmentation in the laser only areas. At 6 months, all areas were completely repigmented.

Laser hair removal can lead to an increase in hair in some patients as a paradoxical effect. Postlaser hypertrichosis is defined as occurring if patients developed a definite increase in hair density, color, coarseness, or a combination of these at treated sites when compared with baseline clinical photographs in the absence of any other known cause of hypertrichosis. Small proportion of patients have reported an increased hair growth at sites of previous laser epilation, and patients with darker skin (types III–V) may be at more increased risk for developing paradoxical hypertrichosis. One possible explanation may relate to the concept that the process of laser epilation may serve to synchronize the cycling of those hairs growing within the laser treatment sites.[32] In addition the heat from laser ablation may convert vellus hairs into terminal hairs.

5.2.2   Pseudofolliculitis Barbae

Pseudofolliculitis barbae (PFB) (razor bumps) is a foreign body inflammatory reaction surrounding in-grown facial hair that results from shaving, waxing, or plucking. It is a condition with a high incidence in the African-American population. Many black patients face a difficult challenge of the removal of unwanted hair and many are diagnosed with PFB. It is a common dermatological condition that occurs in persons with curly hair, with over 50% incidence in black men. Figure 5.5 shows a severe case of PFB of the beard of a middle age African-American male. This condition can also affect black women with a history of hirsutism.[33]

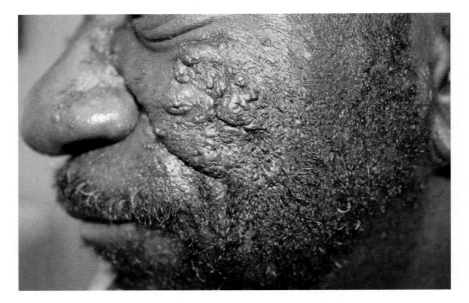

Fig. 5.5 Pseudofolliculitis barbae in an African-American male

Hair removal is the precipitating factor of PFB, especially close shaving in individuals with tightly curled coarse hair. The condition occurs when strongly curved hairs emerging parallel with the skin surface are cut obliquely in the process of shaving, giving them sharp points. These sharp, knife-like points then begin to curve in a 180° arc toward the epidermis and penetrate the skin within a short distance of the follicle. The hair shaft becomes ensheathed with epithelial cells, forming a pseudofollicule. As a result, a foreign body reaction provoked by the ingrown hair develops and is manifested by inflammatory papules and pustules. The chronic presentation of papules and pustules is often accompanied by fibrotic scarring and hyperpigmentation.[33] This is particularly seen in areas such as the beard, neck, and face of men, or in the underarms or bikini area of women who shave. Like hirsutism, conventional methods of treatment are not effective, leading to a high incidence of side effects.[34]

Management for controlling PFB includes topical steroids, antibiotics, and exfoliating agents. Although these agents are sometimes helpful in the treatment and management of PFB, the positive effects are often short-lived. Present therapies include chemical depilatories, retinoids, topical corticosteroids, topical antibiotics, eflornithine hydrochloride cream, and laser. Clipping the hair above the skin surface often results in improvement. Other physical modalities such as shaving with conventional razors or electric razors, depilatory creams, electrolysis, and plucking are ineffective in the treatment of PFB and may cause further problems for the patient such as scarring and hyperpigmentation. Electrolysis has also been used in treatment, but this technique, in addition to being tedious, can cause pigmentation abnormalities, scarring, and residual keratin abscesses from fragmentary destruction of the hair follicle.[35] For some patients with PFB, the best treatment is maintaining a neatly trimmed "beard" with an average "above the surface" hair length of about 1/8 in.[34] The most effective treatment in the past was to allow the beard to grow. Many occupations, however, prohibit beards, and this certainly would not be the best treatment for the female patient. The military, for example, has protocols specifically addressing this condition due to their grooming standards: the presence of refractory PFB can lead to discharge from the service.[36]

> Best treatment maintaining neatly trimmed "beard" with an average "above the surface" hair length of about 1/8 inch

More recently, laser treatment has been shown to reduce hair density and decrease the severity of PFB. Laser-assisted hair removal is a successful treatment for PFB. Temporarily or permanently removing the hair from the PFB lesion dramatically improves the condition, leading to resolution of the papular and pustular condition, and improvement of the skin's texture and associated postinflammatory hyperpigmentation.[34] Figure 5.6 shows an African-American male patient with PFB of the beard before (a) and after treatment (b) with long pulsed NdYAG laser. In treating the beard area of men, the goal should be both to improve the papular and pigmentary disorder conditions to provide the patient with a cosmetic pleasing appearance. Lower fluences and longer pulse durations can be used to provide a hair delay management approach. Most male patients who have beard PFB are most affected in the lower neck area.[5]

Nanni, Brancaccio, and Cooperman[37] reported the use of a long-pulsed alexandrite laser, but noted that hair reduction was temporary. They also suggested that part of the decrease in papules and pustules might be due to a gentle exfoliative effect often observed after treatment. The 810-nm wavelength diode laser proved to be an effective method of hair removal for patients with dark pigmented skin, and also an excellent treatment for patients diagnosed with PFB.[27] Rogers and Glaser[38] reported the effective use of a Q-switched NdYAG laser and topical carbon suspension in the reduction of inflammatory papules and pustules. Chui et al.[39] used a normal mode ruby laser in a white patient with PFB and observed improvement even 10 months after the last of three treatments. Battle et al. have reported the use of a novel long-pulsed 800-nm laser (20–200 ms) in darker skin types (up to type VI). They achieved safe and effective hair reduction by combining lower fluences with longer pulses.[40] Most recently, Kauvar[41] has showed reduction in the severity and number of shaving bumps with a more traditional 800-nm diode laser using pulse durations ranging from 20 to 30 ms.

Jacques and McAuliffe[42] showed that the relative absorption for 1,064-nm radiation for black coarse hair is about 1.5 times that of a very dark epidermis. For black thick hair and brown skin (typical patient with PFB), there is a ratio of relative light absorption that allows for sufficient hair heating without epidermal damage, particularly if epidermal cooling is applied. The ratio of melanin absorption for 800 and 1,064 nm is about 3:1. This does not mean that the same hair reduction could be achieved without epidermal damage in darker skin by simply reducing the incident fluences for 800 nm or other even shorter wavelengths, due to the scattering properties of the turbid dermis. Scattering losses as a function of depth are decreased for longer wavelengths, so that there is greater penetration into the dermis as shown by

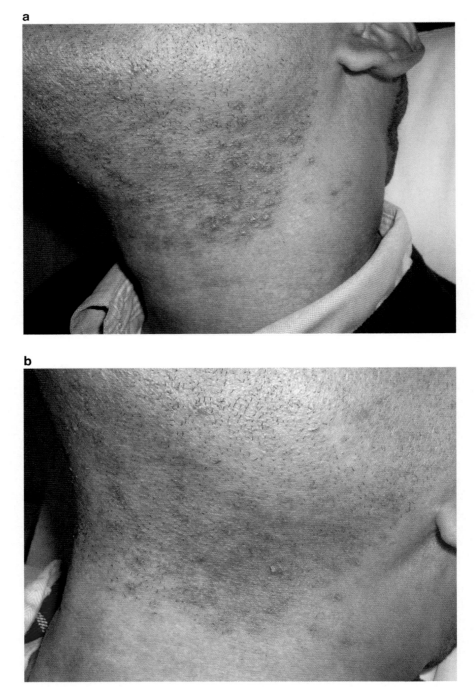

Fig. 5.6 African-American male with Pseudofolliculitis barbae before (**a**) and after treatment (**b**) with long pulsed NdYAG laser, showing the improvement of the inflammatory papules

Zhao and Fairchild,[43] who found that in black skin, the penetration of 1,064 nm light was three times higher than 700-nm light at 3.3 mm deep in the dermis, which represent the typical depth of a hair bulb.

> Ratio of melanin absorption for 800 and 1,064 nm is about 3:1
>
> Penetration of 1,064 nm light was 3 times higher than 700-nm light at 3.3 mm deep in the dermis

On the one hand, in individuals with Fitzpatrick type VI skin, NdYAG laser has been demonstrated to be safe and effective.[8] This wavelength theoretically allows for the greatest ratio of hair bulb to epidermal heating.[44] On the other hand, when there is thick black hair with high density (normal male beard), the 1,064 nm laser tends to produce significant discomfort that requires topical anesthesia.[45] The 810 nm diode laser has been applied in a few PFB studies.[27] With the longer-pulse modes (30–500 ms), an acceptable degree of efficacy and safety has been shown in some darker skin types (V and lighter type VI), but blistering and subsequent pigmentation changes have been reported in patients with very dark type VI skin. Of the wavelengths available for laser hair reduction, 1,064 nm offers the greatest ratio of threshold fluences for efficacy to epidermal damage.[44] However, by combining extended pulse widths and optimized surface cooling, we can minimize side effects induced by 810 nm in very dark skin.[46]

> 1,064 nm offers the greatest ratio of threshold fluences for efficacy to epidermal damage

Using this very long pulse strategy for PFB, delayed hair growth is the goal, especially in very dark skin. Permanent hair reduction might not be achieved in very dark skin because maximum tolerated fluence appears to be insufficient to predictably cause long-term reduction. In PFB, however, simply delaying hair growth reduces the frequency and vigor of shaving and therefore can reduce the severity of the disease.[45] In reviewing side effects and efficacy in this study, lighter-skinned patients corresponding clinically to roughly type V and lighter type VI skin responded more favorably. With increased pigmentation in the darkest-skinned blacks, the power and fluence restrictions lessened the response to treatment. In reviewing the responses, the fluence thresholds for efficacy and epidermal damage were very similar for dark skin. For lighter black skin or darker Hispanic skin, the fluence threshold for crusting exceeded that for efficacy. Because hair color in the patients was similar regardless of skin type, the thresholds for efficacy would be predicted to be similar. In short, even when the 810 nm device was optimized for treating dark skin, the ratio of minimum damaging fluences to minimum effective fluences was only about 1.2:1 (for very dark skin). In contrast, for very dark skin, the NdYAG laser offers a greater window of safety, where the fluence ratio of safety to efficacy is about 1.5–2:1.[34] This study demonstrates that a super long-pulse diode laser can improve PFB, particularly in individuals with type V skin treated at higher fluences. The benefit to safety ratio was less well defined in very dark type VI patients, and the device, although capable of reducing shaving bumps, must be used with more caution in these patients and with the expectation of less improvement and/or more treatment sessions.[45] NdYAG laser, although less absorbed by melanin, offers better laser penetration affecting all portions of the hair follicles and more safety profile.

Nd:YAG laser offers greater window of safety, where the fluence ratio of safety to efficacy is about 1.5 to 2:1

Nanni et al.[37] reported the use of a 755-nm laser for the treatment of pseudofolliculitis but noted that the hair and papule/pustule reduction was temporary. More recently, Ross et al.[34] reported the use of a 1,064-nm long-pulse NdYAG laser for the treatment of PFB in dark skin types. The results showed safe and efficacious PFB and hair reduction. Similar to the study device used by Ross, the laser system used in this study, the 1,064-nm long-pulse NdYAG laser, provides a unique long wavelength that penetrates to the depth of the hair bulb while sparing the epidermis.

The long-pulse 1,064-nm NdYAG laser appears to have a distinct advantage over other shorter wavelengths for the treatment of PFB; 1,064-nm light is able to exploit the differences in melanin concentration between the hair bulb and epidermis in patients with skin types V and VI. The absorption coefficient for 1,064-nm light and black hair is roughly $27 \, cm^{-1}$ while for a very dark epidermis is estimated to be $18 \, cm^{-1}$. There exists a ratio of absorption for thick black hair and brown skin that allows for the 1,064-nm light to heat sufficiently the hair bulb and bulge without damage to the epidermis, especially if (MS PAGE NO 25) contact cooling is applied.[44] The ratio of melanin (major chromophores for hair removal) absorption for 800-nm and 1,064-nm light is roughly 3:1. Zhing-Quan and Fairchild[47] showed that in black skin the penetration of 1,064-nm light was three times higher than of 700-nm light at 3.3-mm depth in the dermis (typical depth of hair bulb). The 1,064-nm wavelength penetrates far enough into the dermis to disrupt the follicular mechanism of hair growth while sparing the epidermis from heat absorption. As the wavelength is shortened, melanin absorption is increased, leading to increased heat absorption on the surface of the skin. Dark skin treated with the long-pulse alexandrite laser (755 nm) using relatively large fluences has been known to produce severe epidermal damage such as blistering and dyspigmentation.[48] This confirms that the ratio of dermal (hair bulb) to epidermal temperature (and subsequent thermal damage) increases with increasing wavelength.[44] In other words, as the wavelength gets longer, there exists a greater percentage change in temperature between the hair bulb and the surface of the skin. This can be greatly enhanced with the use of external cooling to the epidermis. This emphasizes the value of the NdYAG laser for the treatment of PFB in dark-skinned patients. This study has demonstrated the use of the long pulse 1,064-nm NdYAG laser with continuous contact cooling for the treatment of PFB to be both a safe and effective means of treatment. The treatment has provided an observable objective positive result and has been met with encouraging investigator and patient satisfaction.[33]

Absorption coefficient for 1,064-nm black hair is roughtly $27 \, cm^{-1}$ while for a very dark epidermis is estimated to be $18 \, cm^{-1}$

5.2.3 Acne Keloidalis Nuchae

Acne keloidalis nuchae is most frequently seen in African-Americans and rarely occurs in women; in either case, its occurrence has a significant impact on the patient's quality of life.[49] It is characterized by persistent follicular and perifollicular papules and plaques, which often lead to scarring and keloidal thickening located on the occipital area of the scalp.[5] Figure 5.7 shows acne keloidalis nuchae in an African-American male patient. Treatment with conventional methods is difficult with marginal results. In early lesions, there is usually evidence of an entrapped hair, and laser-assisted hair removal is a somewhat helpful adjunctive therapy. Lower fluences and longer pulse durations should be initially used to minimize permanency and provide more of a hair delay approach. However, for more chronic changes associated with long-standing acne keloidalis nuchae, such as scarring, foreign body reaction, and decreased hairs, modest fluences with longer pulse durations are necessary. The goal is to destroy the tufted like hair that acts as a foreign body in hopes of decreasing further scarring. The clinical outcome in chronic cases is not as satisfactory.[5] If there is keloid formation or hypertrophic scars, debulkment with a CO_2 laser followed by triamcinolone injections are beneficial.[49] Our multicultural dermatology center, at Henry Ford Hospital, has significant experience treating this condition with the long pulsed NdYAG laser. Figures 5.8 shows the result of one of our patients before (a) during the course of laser (b) and after treatment (c) with long pulsed NdYAG laser.

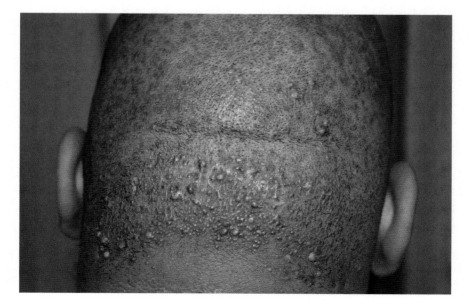

Fig. 5.7 Acne keloidalis nuchae in an African-American male

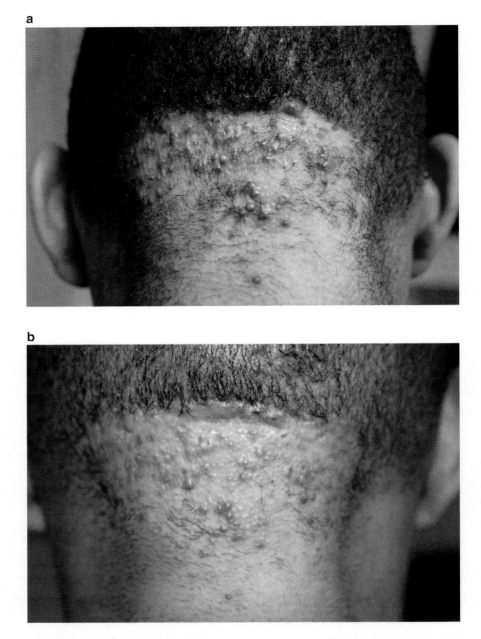

Fig. 5.8 African-American male with acne keloidalis nuchae before (**a**), during (**b**) and after treatment (**c**) with long pulsed NdYAG laser, showing the resolution of the inflammation following laser

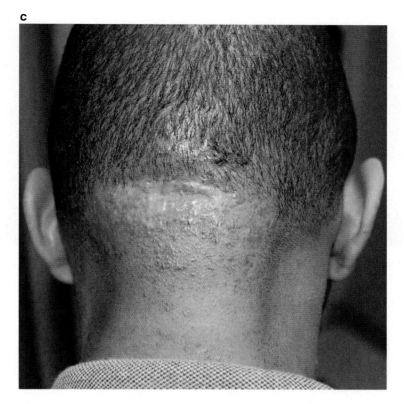

Fig. 5.8   (continued)

5.2.4   Dissecting Cellulitis

Dissecting cellulitis is a chronic progressive inflammatory condition of the scalp characterized by recurrent eruptions of pustular nodules, sinus tract formation, and a resultant cicatricial alopecia (Fig. 5.9). This condition is most common in black men 20–40 years of age, with an onset typically in the second to fourth decades of life.[50] It can rarely occur in males of other races and in women or girls. Familial cases have been reported. Dissecting cellulitis usually starts on the scalp vertex or occiput (Fig. 5.10) as a folliculitis. It expands into patches of perifollicular pustules, nodules, abscesses, and sinuses. Nodules may be firm or fluctuant and pus and serous fluid can be expressed. The course is typically chronic and relapsing.[51] Different lesions can be present simultaneously and healing occurs with scarring alopecia, which may be patchy or confluent. Often, keloidal scars form in areas of inflammation. Dissecting cellulitis can occur with acne conglobata, hidradenitis suppurativa, and pilonidal cysts, a syndrome referred to as the follicular occlusion triad or tetrad. Each of these conditions includes an occlusion of the follicular orifice with secondary inflammation

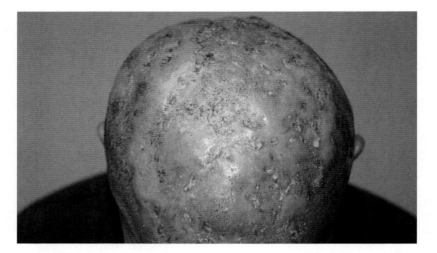

Fig. 5.9 Dissecting cellulitis in an African-American male patient showing pustules, nodules, crustations, discharging sinus tracts and scarring

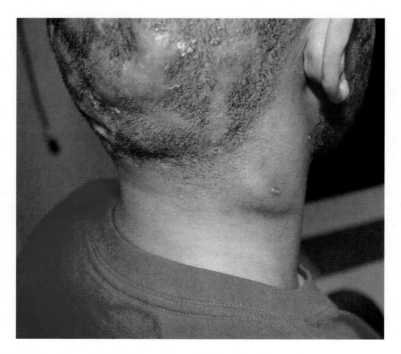

Fig. 5.10 Dissecting cellulitis of the occiput and right side of the neck

and pus formation, development of sinus tracts, and scarring.[51] The pathophysiology involves follicular blockage in all these conditions. As material accumulates in the follicle, the follicle dilates and then ruptures. Keratin and bacteria from the ruptured follicles can initiate a neutrophilic and granulomatous response. It likely represents a primary inflammatory process with secondary bacterial infection (usually with *Staphylococcus aureus* or *Staphylococcus epidermidis*).[50]

> Dissecting cellulitis can occur with acne conglobata, hidradenitis suppurativa and pilonida cysts (follicular occlusior triad or tetrad)

Multiple therapeutic modalities include antibiotics, isotretinoin, incision and drainage, intralesional steroids, X-ray epilation.[52] Surgery is also a possible therapy, where incision and drainage of lesions is a common first step in treating these lesions. Surgical excision of lesions should be considered in severe or recalcitrant cases. Wide excision of the affected areas and split thickness skin grafting has advocates. Combined treatment using tissue expansion, radical excision, and isotretinoin has been used successfully.

Medical therapies include antibiotics, antibiotic soaps (chlorohexidine, benzoyl peroxide), dapsone, intralesional kenalog 10–40 mg/cc, zinc supplements, tetracycline-type antibiotics and prednisone 40–60 mg/day. The follicular occlusion triad in a young woman has been successfully treated with high dose oral antiandrogens and minocycline. Various combination therapies have been used. Isotretinoin 1 mg/kg/day is reported as an effective treatment for this condition.[51] Dissecting cellulitis remains a difficult condition to treat. Recognition of this condition allows for the early institution of therapy, which is the best chance for effective intervention. New laser therapies seem particularly promising for this recalcitrant condition.[51]

Because the pathophysiology of cellulitis centers around the dysfunction of the pilosebaceous unit, hair follicle destruction via laser hair removal devices, either by diode laser (800 nm)[51] or by long-pulsed ruby laser (694 nm)[39], is used as a treatment option with some efficacy. Side effects including dyspigmentation and permanent alopecia from laser treatments, however, have been noted.[53] The long-pulsed NdYAG (1,064-nm) laser has been effectively employed in hair removal for darkly pigmented skin due to the laser–tissue interactions offering both an increased depth of penetration and a decreased melanin chromophore specificity.[8] Krasner et al.[52] treated patients with dissecting cellulitis with the long pulsed NdYAG laser to determine the capabilities and limitations of this treatment modality with respect to reduce pus formation, enable the termination of systemic treatments, investigate the side-effect profile including dyspigmentation and scarring alopecia, and terminate the disease process. Figure 5.11 shows a patient with dissecting cellulitis before treatment (a) and after 6 sessions of long pulsed NdYAG laser (b).

In dark-skinned patients with dissecting cellulitis, however, hair melanin must be destroyed while sparing epidermal melanin to avoid transient or permanent dyspigmentation.[52] In laser therapy, matching pulse duration to the appropriate cutaneous target is important. A pulse duration of 40–70 ms was chosen based on

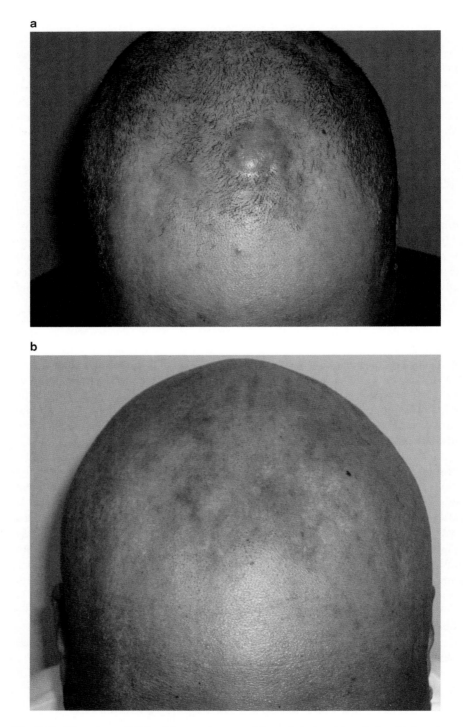

Fig. 5.11 Dissecting cellulitis of the anterior part of the scalp before (**a**) and after (**b**) 6 sessions of long pulsed NdYAG laser

the observation that longer pulse durations tend to target larger structures and thus, to a degree, spare epidermal damage from thermal injury.[34] Krasner et al.[52] performed initial test spots using longer pulse durations and only proceeded with treatment when it was clear that these were found to be safe. The 1,064-nm-wavelength laser has the weakest absorption by melanin of all hair removal systems. Because of this weak absorption, the NdYAG is one of the safer hair removal lasers for all skin types with respect to number and duration of side effects.[54] Ross and colleagues[34] noted that increased cooling time reduced the risk of hypopigmentation and scarring. The need for cooling, however, must be balanced against the hygiene of exposing the cooling tip to lesional contents upon irradiating the skin with laser energy. Laser therapy also has less morbidity than surgical excision and grafting (along with incision and drainage) of the scalp because surgery has the certain risk of infection and the assured result of permanent scarring. The monthly NdYAG laser therapy may reduce pain and pus formation, allows patients to discontinue or maintain lower doses of systemic medications, and thus may slow disease progression by obliterating diseased follicles. As stated earlier, however, the use of the NdYAG is still not without risk of irreversible dyspigmentation and scarring.[52]

> 1,064-nm wavelength laser has the weakest absorption by melanin of all hair removal systems
>
> Laser therapy has less morbidity than surgical excision and grafting

5.2.5   Hidradenitis Suppurativa

Hidradenitis suppurativa (HS) is a complex skin condition characterized by recurring inflammation and suppuration of the "inverse areas of the skin." The disease is initiated by inflammation surrounding the hair follicles, followed by acne-like comedone formation leading to a cascade of destructive events including rupture of the follicular infundibulum, abscess formation, and ultimately sinus tract formation and scarring affecting mainly the axilla, inframammary, and groin areas (Figs. 5.12–5.14).[55] Although originally proposed to be a disorder of the apocrine glands, recent histological studies by Sellheyer and Krahl[56] have suggested that the primary event in HS is follicular hyperkeratosis and obstruction. HS is included in the follicular occlusion tetrad, in conjunction with acne conglobata, dissecting cellulitis, and pilonadal sinuses.[55]

> Primary event in HS is follicular hyperkeratosis and obstruction

Light-based modalities have been used with varying success rates in the treatment of HS. Recently, Iwasaki et al.[57] have published a recent report regarding the utilization of a nonablative radiofrequency device in the treatment of HS, highlighting the importance of deep dermal/subcutaneous heating in the treatment of the

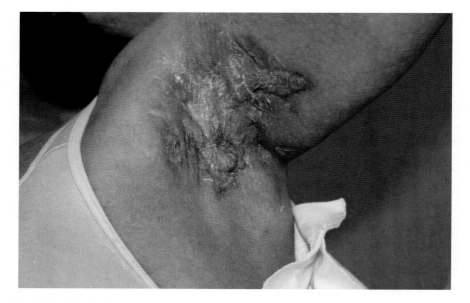

Fig. 5.12 Hidradenitis suppurativa of the left axilla in an African-American female showing nodules, fistulae, and severe scarring

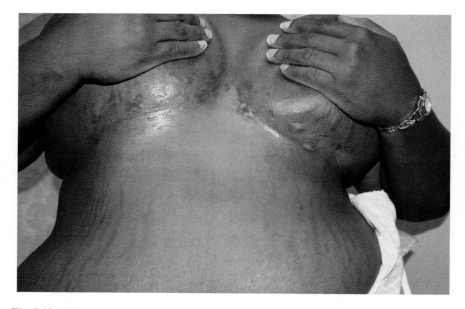

Fig. 5.13 Hidradenitis suppurativa affecting the inframammary areas

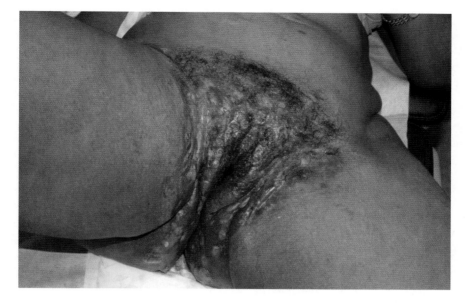

Fig. 5.14 Hidradenitis suppurativa of the groin, buttocks, and pubic areas showing discharging pustules and nodules

condition. Downs et al.[58] reported the use of the 1,450 nm diode laser for HS, where partial improvement was noted after four laser treatments; however, longstanding HS cases with established sinuses and thick scar tissue were not improved. Gold et al.[59] in 2004 published a case series of ALA-PDT utilized to treat four patients with recalcitrant HS. After three or four treatments at 1- to 2-week intervals, clearance was noted in 75–100% of the patients at the 3-month follow-up period; however, no quantitative scale of lesion counts was utilized to evaluate improvement. In 2005, Strauss et al.[60] reported a study of 4 patients with recalcitrant HS treated with MAL-PDT (utilizing broadband light (570–640 nm) and a diode laser (633 nm), where no improvement and worsening of the disease process after treatment was noted. In a study by Lapins et al.,[61] patients with Hurley stage II HS with chronic fistulating lesions were treated with CO_2 laser stripping secondary intention healing, where at 4 weeks posttreatment, 22 out of 24 patients (91.7%) had no recurrences in the site of surgery.

A new exciting study is soon to be published by the authors addressing the safety and efficacy of NdYAG laser for the treatment of HS. Treatment response was measured using the Hidradenitis Suppurativa Lesion, Area and Severity Index (HS-LASI) for HS originally described by Sartorius et al.[62] on the basis of the recommendation of the HS European Research Group (HS-LASI). In addition, a modification to the HS-LASI scoring system (modified HS-LASI) was calculated whereby scores were added at each session for the extent of erythema, edema, pain, and purulent discharge of each anatomic site (scale: 0–3, for each clinical indicator).

Our results showed that the percent change in HS severity after 3 months of treatment was: −65.3% over all anatomic sites: −73.4% inguinal, −62.0% axillary, and −53.1% inframammary. Furthermore, the change in HS severity from baseline to month 3 was statistically significant at the treated sites ($p < 0.02$) but not at the control sites ($p > 0.05$). Our study demonstrated the efficacy of the long-pulsed 1,064 nm NdYAG laser, a device utilized primarily for laser hair epilation.[63] Figure 5.15 shows female patient with affection of the left axilla before (a) and after (b) NdYAG laser treatment. The efficacy of a laser hair removal device in HS further emphasizes the theory that HS is a primary follicular disease.

Efficacy of Nd: YAG laser hair removal in HS emphasizes the theory that HS is a primary follicular disease

5.2.6 Intense pulsed light

The currently used photoepilation devices include ruby, alexandrite, longpulsed NdYAG, diode lasers, and intense pulsed light (IPL).[5] IPL is a high-intensity polychromatic light. Unlike laser systems, these flashlamps work by using incoherent light in the wavelength range 515–1,200 nm[12], and by using different filters, a wide range of wavelengths are possible for IPL systems. The latter can be a good alternative to laser systems in treating different types of skin problems with only one machine. However, because of the lack of monochromaticity, the spectrum may not be consistent from pulse to pulse. Various studies have reported that 33–80% hair reduction is achieved over follow-up periods ranging from 12 weeks to 21.1 months.[12] However, direct comparison among studies is not possible, because of differences in treatment device, wavelength application, and treatment conditions.

The management of dark skin phenotypes remains problematic for laser and IPL-assisted treatments.[8] An increasing number of studies have confirmed the long-term hair removal efficacies of IPL systems that emit a broad spectrum of longer wavelengths.[64,65] Flashlamp-assisted hair removal enables a wide choice of emitting wavelengths to be chosen simply by choosing different cut-off filters, and thus this modality may be effective in a wide range of skin types, especially in darker skins.[5]

IPL may be effective in a wide range of skin types, especially in darker skins

Lee et al.[66] used two devices in their study, one that emits a wavelength in the range of 600–950 nm (average wavelength 800 nm), and the other one emits a wavelength in the range of 645–950 nm (average wavelength 830 nm). The 830 nm device applicator was fitted with a lower cut-off filter (at 645 nm), and thus eliminated shorter wavelengths (600–645 nm) absorbed by epidermal melanin pigment. This probably reduced epidermal absorption and caused the treatment to be less

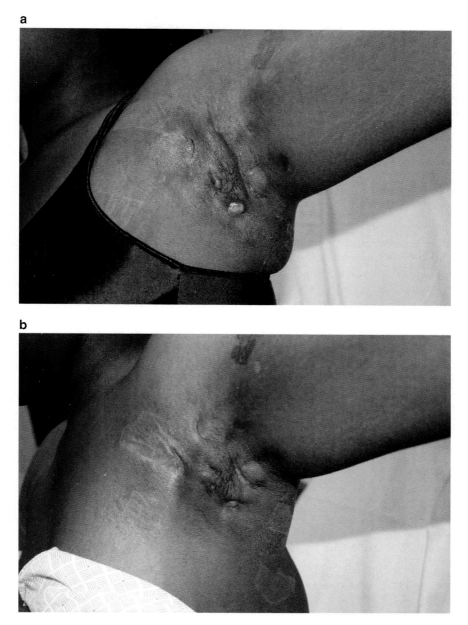

Fig. 5.15 Hidradenitis suppurativa of the left axilla before (**a**) and after (**b**) treatment with long pulsed NdYAG laser, showing regression of the inflammatory nodules

painful. They showed that with the same wavelengths and pulse width applications, applied fluence may be the most important factor of hair removal efficiency, which concurs with the report by Liew and colleagues.[67] The main limitation that prevents clinicians from applying higher fluences is pain occurring during the procedure, because as applied fluence is increased, treatment pain also increases. Pain levels documented by volunteers were significantly higher during the 800 nm than 830 nm treatment, which implies that wavelengths shorter than 600–645 nm are better absorbed by epidermal melanin and may produce more pain to patients.[66]

5.3   Conclusions

Until recently, most published studies in laser surgery have excluded those with darker skin, therefore, additional research is needed to better elucidate the efficacy, and safety in ethnic skin. Appropriate patient selection and thorough physician training lead to a safer treatment for patients of color. The balance between efficacy and side effects is critical when performing laser treatment in patients with darker skin. Conservative laser parameters such as lower energy settings and longer pulse duration minimize the occurrence of side effects in dark skin. The ongoing development of laser technologies to protect epidermal surface from thermal damage will lead to improved outcomes.

The safest and most effective lasers to treat darker skin types are either the diode or NdYAG-based laser systems. Because of the longer wavelength, the NdYAG system is the safest, while the diode wavelength is more effective as it is absorbed more by the follicular pigments.

References

1. Taylor SC, Cook-Bolden F. Defining skin of color. *Cutis.* 2002;69:435–437.
2. Projections of the resident population by race, Hispanic origin, and nativity: middle series, 2006 to 2010. Washington, DC: US Census Bureau; 2000.
3. Bhatt N, Alster TS. Laser surgery in dark skin. *Dermatol Surg.* 2008;34:184–94; discussion 94–95.
4. Jackson BA. Lasers in ethnic skin: a review. *J Am Acad Dermatol.* 2003;48:S134–S138.
5. Battle EF, Jr., Hobbs LM. Laser-assisted hair removal for darker skin types. *Dermatol Ther.* 2004;17:177–183.
6. Anderson RR, Parrish JA. Selective photothermolysis: precise microsurgery by selective absorption of pulsed radiation. *Science.* 1983;220:524–527.
7. Tanzi EL, Alster TS. Cutaneous laser surgery in darker skin phototypes. *Cutis.* 2004;73:21–24, 7–30.
8. Alster TS, Bryan H, Williams CM. Long-pulsed Nd:YAG laser-assisted hair removal in pigmented skin: a clinical and histological evaluation. *Arch Dermatol.* 2001;137:885–889.
9. van Gemert MJ, Welch AJ. Time constants in thermal laser medicine. *Lasers Surg Med.* 1989;9:405–421.

10. Sadick NS, Weiss RA, Shea CR, Nagel H, Nicholson J, Prieto VG. Long-term photoepilation using a broad-spectrum intense pulsed light source. *Arch Dermatol.* 2000;136:1336–1340.
11. Commo S, Gaillard O, Bernard BA. The human hair follicle contains two distinct K19 positive compartments in the outer root sheath: a unifying hypothesis for stem cell reservoir? *Differentiation.* 2000;66:157–164.
12. Dierickx CC. Hair removal by lasers and intense pulsed light sources. *Semin Cutan Med Surg.* 2000;19:267–275.
13. Cotsarelis G, Sun TT, Lavker RM. Label-retaining cells reside in the bulge area of pilosebaceous unit: implications for follicular stem cells, hair cycle, and skin carcinogenesis. *Cell.* 1990;61:1329–1337.
14. Nanni CA, Alster TS. A practical review of laser-assisted hair removal using the Q-switched Nd:YAG, long-pulsed ruby, and long-pulsed alexandrite lasers. *Dermatol Surg.* 1998;24:1399–1405; discussion 405.
15. Olsen EA. Methods of hair removal. *J Am Acad Dermatol.* 1999;40:143–55; quiz 56–57.
16. Jackson BA. Laser resurfacing in ethnic skin. *Facial Plast Surg Clin North Am.* 2002;10:397–404.
17. Johnson F, Dovale M. Intense pulsed light treatment of hirsutism: case reports of skin phototypes V and VI. *J Cutan Laser Ther.* 1999;1:233–237.
18. Lanigan SW. Incidence of side effects after laser hair removal. *J Am Acad Dermatol.* 2003;49:882–886.
19. Ho C, Nguyen Q, Lowe NJ, Griffin ME, Lask G. Laser resurfacing in pigmented skin. *Dermatol Surg.* 1995;21:1035–1037.
20. Tanzi EL, Lupton JR, Alster TS. Lasers in dermatology: four decades of progress. *J Am Acad Dermatol.* 2003;49:1–31; quiz-4.
21. Fuchs M. Thermokinetic selectivity—a new highly effective method for permanent hair removal: experience with the LPIR Alexandrite laser. *Derm Prakt Dermatologie.* 1997;5.
22. Nanni CA, Alster TS. Laser-assisted hair removal: side effects of Q-switched Nd:YAG, long-pulsed ruby, and alexandrite lasers. *J Am Acad Dermatol.* 1999;41:165–171.
23. Goldberg DJ, Samady JA. Evaluation of a long-pulse Q-switched Nd:YAG laser for hair removal. *Dermatol Surg.* 2000;26:109–113.
24. Parrish JA. New concepts in therapeutic photomedicine: photochemistry, optical targeting and the therapeutic window. *J Invest Dermatol.* 1981;77:45–50.
25. Anderson RR. Laser-tissue interactions in dermatology. In: Arndt K Dover J, Olbricht S, eds. *Lasers in Cutaneous and Aesthetic Surgery.* Philadelphia: Lippincott-Raven; 1997: 28.
26. Khatri KA. Diode laser hair removal in patients undergoing isotretinoin therapy. *Dermatol Surg.* 2004;30:1205–1207; discussion 7.
27. Greppi I. Diode laser hair removal of the black patient. *Lasers Surg Med.* 2001;28:150–155.
28. Grimes PE, Stockton T. Pigmentary disorders in blacks. *Dermatol Clin.* 1988;6:271–281.
29. McBurney EI. Side effects and complications of laser therapy. *Dermatol Clin.* 2002;20:165–176.
30. Aldraibi MS, Touma DJ, Khachemoune A. Hair removal with the 3-msec alexandrite laser in patients with skin types IV–VI: efficacy, safety, and the role of topical corticosteroids in preventing side effects. *J Drugs Dermatol.* 2007;6:60–66.
31. Liew SH. Laser hair removal: guidelines for management. *Am J Clin Dermatol.* 2002;3:107–115.
32. Alajlan A, Shapiro J, Rivers JK, MacDonald N, Wiggin J, Lui H. Paradoxical hypertrichosis after laser epilation. *J Am Acad Dermatol.* 2005;53:85–88.
33. Weaver SM, 3rd, Sagaral EC. Treatment of pseudofolliculitis barbae using the long-pulse Nd:YAG laser on skin types V and VI. *Dermatol Surg.* 2003;29:1187–1191.
34. Ross EV, Cooke LM, Timko AL, Overstreet KA, Graham BS, Barnette DJ. Treatment of pseudofolliculitis barbae in skin types IV, V, and VI with a long-pulsed neodymium:yttrium aluminum garnet laser. *J Am Acad Dermatol.* 2002;47:263–270.
35. Halder RM. Pseudofolliculitis barbae and related disorders. *Dermatol Clin.* 1988;6:407–412.
36. Alexander AM, Delph WI. Pseudofolliculitis barbae in the military. A medical, administrative and social problem. *J Natl Med Assoc.* 1974;66:459–464, 79.
37. Nanni C, Brancaccio R, Cooperman M. Successful treatment of pseudofolliculitis barbae with a long pulsed alexandrite laser. *Lasers Surg Med.* 1999;Suppl 11:21.

38. Rogers CJ, Glaser DA. Treatment of pseudofolliculitis barbae using the Q-switched Nd:YAG laser with topical carbon suspension. *Dermatol Surg.* 2000;26:737–742.
39. Chui CT, Berger TG, Price VH, Zachary CB. Recalcitrant scarring follicular disorders treated by laser-assisted hair removal: a preliminary report. *Dermatol Surg.* 1999;25:34–37.
40. Battle E, Suthamjariya K, Alora M, Pali K, Anderson R. Very long pulses (20–200 ms) diode laser for hair removal on all skin types. *Lasers Surg Med.* 2000;12 (suppl):21.
41. Kauvar AN. Treatment of pseudofolliculitis with a pulsed infrared laser. *Arch Dermatol.* 2000;136:1343–1346.
42. Jacques SL, McAuliffe DJ. The melanosome: threshold temperature for explosive vaporization and internal absorption coefficient during pulsed laser irradiation. *Photochem Photobiol.* 1991;53:769–775.
43. Zhao Z, Fairchild P. Dependence of light transmission through human skin on incident beam diameter at different wavelengths. *Proc Soc Photo-instrumentation Eng.* 1998;2681:468–477.
44. Ross EV, Ladin Z, Kreindel M, Dierickx C. Theoretical considerations in laser hair removal. *Dermatol Clin.* 1999;17:333–355, viii.
45. Smith EP, Winstanley D, Ross EV. Modified superlong pulse 810 nm diode laser in the treatment of pseudofolliculitis barbae in skin types V and VI. *Dermatol Surg.* 2005;31:297–301.
46. Altshuler GB, Anderson RR, Manstein D, Zenzie HH, Smirnov MZ. Extended theory of selective photothermolysis. *Lasers Surg Med.* 2001;29:416–432.
47. Zhing-Quan Z, Fairchild P. Dependence of light transmission through human skin on incident beam diameter at different wavelengths. *SPIE Proc* 1998;3254:354–360.
48. Narurkar V. The safety and efficacy of the long pulse alexandrite laser for hair removal in various skin types. *Lasers Surg Med.* 1998;10.
49. Quarles FN, Brody H, Badreshia S, Vause SE, Brauner G, Breadon JY, et al. Acne keloidalis nuchae. *Dermatol Ther.* 200 z7;20:128–132.
50. Chicarilli ZN. Follicular occlusion triad: hidradenitis suppurativa, acne conglobata, and dissecting cellulitis of the scalp. *Ann Plast Surg.* 1987;18:230–237.
51. Boyd AS, Binhlam JQ. Use of an 800-nm pulsed-diode laser in the treatment of recalcitrant dissecting cellulitis of the scalp. *Arch Dermatol.* 2002;138:1291–1293.
52. Krasner BD, Hamzavi FH, Murakawa GJ, Hamzavi IH. Dissecting cellulitis treated with the long-pulsed Nd:YAG laser. *Dermatol Surg.* 2006;32:1039–1044.
53. Campos VB, Dierickx CC, Farinelli WA, Lin TY, Manuskiatti W, Anderson RR. Hair removal with an 800-nm pulsed diode laser. *J Am Acad Dermatol.* 2000;43:442–447.
54. Littler CM. Hair removal using an Nd:YAG laser system. *Dermatol Clin.* 1999;17:401–430, x.
55. Lam J, Krakowski AC, Friedlander SF. Hidradenitis suppurativa (acne inversa): management of a recalcitrant disease. *Pediatr Dermatol.* 2007;24:465–473.
56. Sellheyer K, Krahl D. "Hidradenitis suppurativa" is acne inversa! An appeal to (finally) abandon a misnomer. *Int J Dermatol.* 2005;44:535–540.
57. Iwasaki J, Marra DE, Fincher EF, Moy RL. Treatment of hidradenitis suppurativa with a nonablative radiofrequency device. *Dermatol Surg.* 2008;34:114–117.
58. Downs A. Smoothbeam laser treatment may help improve hidradenitis suppurativa but not Hailey-Hailey disease. *J Cosmet Laser Ther.* 2004;6:163–164.
59. Gold M, Bridges TM, Bradshaw VL, Boring M. ALA-PDT and blue light therapy for hidradenitis suppurativa. *J Drugs Dermatol.* 2004;3:S32–S35.
60. Strauss RM, Pollock B, Stables GI, Goulden V, Cunliffe WJ. Photodynamic therapy using aminolaevulinic acid does not lead to clinical improvement in hidradenitis suppurativa. *Br J Dermatol.* 2005;152:803–804.
61. Lapins J, Marcusson JA, Emtestam L. Surgical treatment of chronic hidradenitis suppurativa: CO_2 laser stripping-secondary intention technique. *Br J Dermatol.* 1994;131:551–556.
62. Sartorius K, Lapins J, Emtestam L, Jemec GBE. Suggestions for uniform outcome variables when reporting treatment effects in hidradenitis suppurativa. *Br J Dermatol* 2003;149(1): 211–213.
63. Lorenz S, Brunnberg S, Landthaler M, Hohenleutner U. Hair removal with the long pulsed Nd:YAG laser: a prospective study with one year follow-up. *Lasers Surg Med.* 2002;30:127–134.

64. Weiss RA, Weiss MA, Marwaha S, Harrington AC. Hair removal with a non-coherent filtered flashlamp intense pulsed light source. *Lasers Surg Med.* 1999;24:128–132.
65. Gold MH, Bell MW, Foster TD, Street S. Long-term epilation using the EpiLight broad band, intense pulsed light hair removal system. *Dermatol Surg.* 1997;23:909–913.
66. Hee Lee J, Huh CH, Yoon HJ, Cho KH, Chung JH. Photo-epilation results of axillary hair in dark-skinned patients by intense pulsed light: comparison between different wavelengths and pulse width. *Dermatoi Surg.* 2006;32:234–240.
67. Liew SH, Grobbelaar A, Gault D, Sanders R, Green C, Linge C. Hair removal using the ruby laser: clinical efficacy in Fitzpatrick skin types I–V and histological changes in epidermal melanocytes. *Br J Dermatol.* 1999;140:1105–1109.

Chapter 6
Phototherapy for Vitiligo

Camile L. Hexsel, Richard H. Huggins, and Henry W. Lim

6.1 History

The roots of vitiligo phototherapy can be traced to before 1500 BC. Indian Hindus with depigmented patches had plant extract applied to these lesions and were subsequently exposed to sunlight. A similar form of heliotherapy (i.e. therapy using sunlight) was performed in ancient Egypt. Extracts from the plants *Ammi majus* and *Psoralen corylifolia* were used in these historical treatments.[1] In 1947, these plants were found by Fahmy et al. to contain 8-methoxypsoralen (8-MOP) and 5-MOP.[2] The use of phototherapy in combination with *A. majus* or psoralens (i.e. photochemotherapy) was introduced by El Mofty in 1948.[3]

The modern history of phototherapy began in 1801 when the German scientist JW Ritter isolated ultraviolet (UV) radiation. This knowledge was first utilized for dermatological therapeutic purposes in 1893 when Danish dermatologist Finsen used filtered sunlight to treat lupus vulgaris. The first employment of an artificial UV radiation source for the treatment of skin diseases came in 1894 when Lahman in Germany utilized the combination of a carbon arc lamp and a parabolic mirror to successfully treat lupus vulgaris. The transition from heliotherapy to phototherapy was solidified in 1901 when Finsen, who had replaced filtered sunlight with the carbon arc lamp for the treatment of lupus, published his results. Finsen won the Nobel Prize for medicine in 1903 for his work. He is recognized as the founder of modern phototherapy.[2] Montgomery was the first to treat vitiligo with phototherapy in 1904 in the form of a Finsen light.[3]Although phototherapy had been established by this time as a legitimate therapeutic modality for some disorders, the low output of carbon arc lamps limited their usefulness. The journey toward a radiation source capable of higher output began with the development of the quartz lamp by the German Küch in 1906. The concept of using the quartz lamp for therapeutic

C.L. Hexsel, R.H, Huggins, and H.W. Lim (✉)
Multicultural Dermatology Center, Department of Dermatology, Henry Ford Medical
Center – New Center One, Detroit, MI, 48202, USA
e-mail: hlim1@hfhs.org

E.D. Baron (ed.), *Light-Based Therapies for Skin of Color*,
DOI: 10.1007/ 978-1-84882-328-0_6, © Springer-Verlag London Limited 2009

purposes was spearheaded by Hagelschmidt in 1911. A quartz lamp with a high UV output was developed by Kromayer in 1912. The greatly increased UV output of this device significantly expanded the range of skin diseases that could be treated with phototherapy.

The development of UVB phototherapy began in the early 1900s with Goeckerman. The first version of Goeckerman's regimen for the treatment of psoriasis consisted of the topical application of tar, a photosensitizer, followed by exposure to a mercury quartz lamp. In 1988, Van Weelden and Green introduced narrowband UVB (NB-UVB) phototherapy as a treatment for psoriasis.

The evolution of psoralen plus UVA (PUVA) photochemotherapy began in the middle of twentieth century. In 1960, the action spectrum of 8-MOP in the UVA range was identified by Buck in the UK and by Pathak and Fellman in the USA. The first reports of combining UV radiation with 8-MOP were given by Allyn (topical 8-MOP) in 1962 and by Oddoze (oral 8-MOP) in 1967. Vitiligo was first treated with this combination in 1969 by Fulton who used "black light" UVA tubes and topical 8-MOP as a repigmentation therapy. This treatment modality combination was modified for whole body treatment in 1970 when Mortazawi and Oberste-Lehn used an array of "black light" UVA tubes in a cabin following topical 8-MOP application. However, to this point, the UVA output of the radiation sources used was sufficient for use with topical 8-MOP, but not for oral administration. This changed in 1974, when Parish utilized a then-recently developed, high-intensity UVA tube. The combination of this higher output tube and orally administered 8-MOP resulted in significantly more efficacious treatment of psoriasis. With this began modern-day PUVA therapy.[2]

6.2 Mechanism of Action and Rationale for the Treatment of Vitiligo

Vitiligo represents a complete or subtotal absence of melanocytes in affected skin. Melanocytes in the bulb and infundibulum of the hair follicle are destroyed in vitiliginous skin, although inactive cells in the middle and lower parts of the follicle and the outer root sheath are spared.[3] Considering this, as would be expected, proliferation of melanocytes is an important mechanism of vitiligo phototherapy. Although UV radiation has an overall antiproliferative effect, there is substantial evidence that it selectively induces replication of melanocytes. UVB irradiation has long been known to increase human skin pigmentation through enhancement of the number of DOPA-positive melanocytes, synthesis of melanin by melanocytes, and transfer of melanin from melanocytes to keratinocytes. More recently, an increase in human melanocyte DNA synthesis has been demonstrated following UVB radiation exposure.[4] Furthermore, UVB radiation-induced melanocyte proliferation has been demonstrated in exposed as well as shielded skin of human subjects.[5] This suggests a soluble melanocyte mitogen which has a systemic effect of pigmentation.

There is strong evidence suggesting that basic fibroblast growth factor (bFGF) is this substance. Cultured keratinocytes, proliferating following UVB exposure, have been found to produce increased amounts of bFGF. Observed increases in DNA synthesis in UVB-exposed melanocytes cultured in the absence of keratinocytes suggest that there is also another mechanism involved. Because of melanocytes' dependence on the proper medium as well as cAMP, it is thought that UVB radiation also allows for melanogenesis by directly increasing melanocyte intracellular cAMP levels.[4]

PUVA is known to inhibit DNA synthesis in keratinocytes.[6] However, sera from vitiligo patients treated with PUVA were shown to stimulate melanocyte growth in vitro.[7] The identity of the PUVA-induced factor(s) is not known at this time, though it may be the same bFGF induced by UVB exposure. Although vitiligo lesions are usually devoid of melanocytes, a reservoir of DOPA-negative melanocytes which lack all of the enzymatic proteins and many of the structural proteins necessary for melanogenesis has been demonstrated in the outer shaft of hair follicles. During repigmentation, the cells in the outer root sheath proliferate, mature, and migrate up the hair follicle into the epidermis and spread centrifugally.[3,8] Furthermore, repigmentation can occur from migration of melanocytes from perilesional skin[3] or rarely from remaining epidermal melanocytes spared from the depigmentation process.[9]

Although the etiology of vitiligo has not yet been definitively established, autoimmunity is the most favored hypothesis. UV radiation causes substantial alterations in the immune response. The UVB spectrum in particular is felt to be the most important in mediating immunosuppression. In fact, long-term low-dose UVB has been shown to result in decreased immune responsiveness.[10] Clearly, an immune-mediated disease would benefit from such an effect. Additionally, there is significant evidence supporting cell-mediated autoimmunity specifically as the major culprit. NB-UVB phototherapy results in the destruction of T-cell lymphocytes.[6] In vitro studies have shown T-cell apoptosis primarily resulting from UVB-induced T-cell DNA damage.[11] In vitro, T-cell apoptosis has also been found to occur as a result of CD95L-independent activation of the CD95 molecule following UVB exposure.[12] UVB radiation-induced alterations in the cytokine milieu result in a diversion toward the B-cell-dominated Th2 response and away from the T-cell-mediated Th1 response. NB-UVB exposure has been shown in vitro to suppress the Th1 cytokines IFN-γ and IL-12 and increase the Th2 cytokine IL-4.[13] IL-10 is a known antagonist of IFN-γ. Some studies have shown elevated IL-1 levels in suction blister fluid taken from normal skin sites following UVB irradiation, though conflicting results have been observed.[10] UVA exposure may also result in significant immunomodulation in vitiligo patients. T-cell apoptosis has also been shown to be induced by UVA irradiation in vitro. The T-cell destruction is mediated through increased CD95L expression resulting from singlet oxygen formation. This is in contrast to the CD95L-independent T-cell apoptosis induced by UVB exposure. UVA phototherapy is also known to downregulate lesional expression of IFN-γ from T-helper cells, which also decreases the Th2-type immune response.[14]

6.3   Phototherapy of Vitiligo

Whole body phototherapy is the main treatment option available for the treatment of vitiligo with over 10% body surface area involved. Phototherapy consists of exposure to UV radiation two to three times a week. With this treatment protocol, initial repigmentation, for those who respond, is expected during the first 30 treatments. After initial repigmentation is observed, the definitive number of treatments is determined on an individual basis and location of vitiliginous lesions. In general, face and neck are the most responsive locations to phototherapy, which are areas with large number of hair follicles. Acral sites, nipples, lips, and large areas of vitiligo or disease are the least responsive. Once maximal response is obtained, phototherapy is usually tapered and discontinued.

For patients with localized vitiligo with less than 10% body surface area of involvement, topical therapy with topical immunomodulators, topical corticosteroids, targeted phototherapy, and topical PUVA have all been used. For localized vitiligo, targeted phototherapy allows for selective treatment of lesional skin, thus avoiding side effects in unaffected areas, and allowing higher doses to be achieved as well as larger dose increments. Different targeted devices have been introduced and studied, including 308-nm excimer laser and several broadband UVA- and UVB-targeted light sources.[15]

6.3.1   Review of the Literature and Levels of Evidence

The evidence of the different phototherapy modalities with and without a combined topical agent, for the treatment of vitiligo, is reviewed and presented. Although a large number of reputable studies have been published, this chapter focuses on studies with the highest levels of evidence, which are summarized in Table 6.1. The level of evidence was graded on the following five-point scale[16,17]:

I– At least one properly designed randomized controlled trial.

II-1 – Well-designed controlled trial without randomization.

II-2 – Well-designed cohort or case-control analytic study, preferably from more than one center or research group.

II-3 – Multiple time series with or without intervention or dramatic results from uncontrolled studies.

III– Clinical experience, descriptive studies, or reports of experts committees.

6.3.1.1   NB-UVB Versus PUVA

NB-UVB is widely available, simpler to be administered than PUVA photochemotherapy, and has been demonstrated to be superior to PUVA in the induction of repigmentation in patients with vitiligo in several prospective clinical trials.

Table 6.1 Summary of studies on phototherapy and photochemotherapy for vitiligo

Author, year	Study design	Level of evidence	Results	Dosage protocols
NB-UVB/PUVA				
Yones et al, 2007	RCT	I	>50% improvement in body surface area affected by vitiligo at 48 treatments: 53% of patients on the NB-UVB group (n = 21), 23% on the PUVA group (n = 13)	NB-UVB: Initial dose, 100 mJ/cm²; dose increments, 20% as tolerated, max 2 J/cm²; frequency, 2×/week; median number of treatments, 97 (16–200) PUVA: Initial dose, 0.5 J/cm²; dose increments, 0.25 J/cm² as tolerated, max 5 J/cm²; frequency, 2×/week; median number of treatments, 49 (3–196)
Bathnegar et al, 2007	RCT	I	Mean degree of repigmentation: 52.2% in the NB-UVB group (n = 25), 44.7% in the PUVA group (n = 25); after excluding hands and feet, 67.57% (n = 25) in the NB-UVB group and 54.2% (n = 25) in the PUVA group	NB-UVB: Initial dose, 280 mJ/cm²; dose increments, 20% as tolerated; frequency, 3×/week tapered to 2×/week after >75% repigmentation achieved; mean duration 6.3 months PUVA: Initial dose, 2 J/cm², dose increments, 0.5 J/cm² as tolerated; frequency, 3×/week tapered to 2×/week after >75% repigmentation; mean duration 5.6 months
Westerhof and Nieuweboer-Krobotoval, 2007	Controlled clinical trial	II-1	At 4 months, 46% of the patients (n = 13) treated with topical PUVA showed repigmentation compared to 67% (n = 52) of the patients treated with NB-UVB	NB-UVB: Initial dose, 75 mJ/cm²; dose increments, 20% as tolerated; frequency, 2×/week PUVA: Initial dose, 0.5 J/cm², dose increments, 20% as tolerated; frequency, 2×/week
El Mofty et al, 2006	Controlled clinical trial	II-1	Percent of patients with 60–75% repigmentation: 57% (n = 8) in both PUVA- and NB-UVB-treated sides; 38.9% (n = 7) of the patients had 60–75% repigmentation in both NB-UVB- and NB-UVB + 8-MOP-treated sites	NB-UVB: initial dose, 740 mJ/cm²; dose increments, 15% as tolerated; frequency, 3×/week for 48 treatments PUVA: initial dose, 1 J/cm²;dose increments, 0.5 J/cm² as tolerated, frequency, 3×/week, 48 treatments

(continued)

Table 6.1 (continued)

Author, year	Study design	Level of evidence	Results	Dosage protocols
NBUVB/308 nm				
Cassaci et al, 2007	RCT	I	Mean repigmentation scores of 2.68 in the 308-nm excimer light group, 2.12 in NB-UVB group; >75% repigmentation in 37.5% ($n = 6$) of the lesions treated with 308-nm excimer light and 6% ($n = 1$) of the lesions treated with NB-UVB	Initial dose, 70% of the MED on normally pigmented skin; dose increments, 20–40% as tolerated; frequency, 2×/week for 6 months
BB-UVB				
Don et al, 2006	Prospective study	II-3	Arrest in the progression of actively spreading vitiligo in all patients ($n = 9$); repigmentation induced after 8–12 treatments, 51–100% repigmentation induced after 2–8 months of treatment in all patients ($n = 9$)	BB-UVB + vitamin C 500 mg, vitamin B_{12} 1000 μg and folic acid 5 mg twice daily. Initial dose, 20–30 mJ/cm²; dose increments, 10–20 mJ/cm² as tolerated; 2–3 times per week for 2–11 months
BB-UVA				
El Mofty et al, 2006	RCT	I	>60% repigmentation in 50% ($n = 5$) of patients treated with 15 J/cm² and 0% ($n = 1$) of patients treated with 5 J/cm² regimen	Dose, 15 J/cm² vs 5 J/cm²; frequency, 3×/week for 48 sessions
308-nm Excimer laser or monochromatic light				
Hofer et al, 2006	RCT	I	>75% repigmentation in 25% ($n = 7$) of lesions on the high-responder location group (face, trunk, arm, and/or leg) vs 2% ($n = 1$) of lesions on the low-responder location group (elbow, wrist, dorsum of the hand, knee, and/or dorsum of the foot)	Initial dose, 50 mJ/cm² less than the MED in vitiliginous skin; dose increments, 50–200 mJ/cm² as tolerated; frequency, 3×/week for 6–10 weeks
Hofer et al, 2005	RCT	I	At 12 weeks, 7 patients completed treatment, repigmentation rates were 60% (1×/week), 79% (2×/week), and 82% (3×/week) treatment frequency regimens	Initial dose, 50 mJ/cm² less than the MED in vitiliginous skin; dose increments, 50–100 mJ/cm² as tolerated; frequency, 1–3× /week groups for 6–12 weeks

Hadi et al, 2004	Retrospective chart review	II-3	>75% repigmentation: 52.8% ($n = 29$) of excimer laser-treated lesions, mean of 23 treatments	Initial dose, 1 MED (100 mJ/cm²) first and second treatment; dose increments, 0.5 MED (50 mJ/cm²) as tolerated; frequency, 2×/week; mean of 23 treatments
Tacrolimus with phototherapy				
Passeron et al, 2005	RCT	I	>75% repigmentation: 70% of 308-nm excimer laser and tacrolimus-treated lesions ($n = 16$), 20% of 308-nm excimer laser-treated lesions ($n = 4$)	Initial dose, 50 mJ/cm² less than MED in vitiliginous skin; dose increments, 12 mJ/cm² every second session; frequency, 2×/week, maximum of 24 treatments
Fai et al, 2007	Prospective trial	II-3	>50% repigmentation in 42% of lesions ($n = 168$), 73% of the face lesions ($n = 64$), 68% of the limbs lesions ($n = 57$), 53.5% of the trunk lesions ($n = 47$). Lesions of the extremities and genital areas lacked repigmentation greater than 25%	Initial dose, 400 mJ/cm²; dose increments, 100 mJ/cm²; every other week if tolerated, maximum of 910 mJ/cm²
Topical calcipotriene (calcipotriol) with phototherapy				
Goldinger et al, 2007	RCT	I	Mean overall repigmentation at 24 sessions was 22.4% ($n = 9$), no significant difference between excimer laser with and without calcipotriol	24 treatments; initial dose, 100 mJ/cm², dose increments, 50 mJ/cm² as tolerated; frequency, 3×/week for 8 weeks
Arca et al, 2006	RCT	I	Mean repigmentation percentage at 30 treatments: 45.01 ± 19.15% with NB-UVB + calcipotriol and 41.6 ± 19.4% with NB-UVB ($n = 40$)	Initial dose, 100 mJ/cm²; dose increments, 50 mJ/cm² as tolerated; frequency, 3×/week for 30 treatments
Kullavanijaya and Lim, 2004	Prospective controlled clinical trial	I-1	Appreciably better response on the NB-UVB and calcipotriol side compared to NB-UVB alone in 53% ($n = 9$) of patients by 29–114 treatments	Initial dose, 280 mJ/cm², dose increments 10–15% as tolerated; frequency, 3×/week
Gotkas et al, 2006	Prospective controlled clinical trial	I-1	Repigmentation: 51 ± 19.6% on NB-UVB with calcipotriol side, 39 ± 18.9% on NB-UVB monotherapy. 24 patients total	Initial dose, 140 mJ/cm², dose increments, 25 mJ/cm² if tolerated; maximum of 740 mJ/cm²

(continued)

Table 6.1 (continued)

Author, year	Study design	Level of evidence	Results	Dosage protocols
Ermis et al, 2001	RCT	I	>75% repigmentation: 63% ($n = 17$) of calcipotriol + PUVA-treated lesions, 15% of placebo + PUVA-treated lesions ($n = 4$)	Initial dose, based on MED of pigmented skin + dosimetry chart published; dose increments based on chart, frequency, 2×/week for 27–39 treatments
Polypodium leucotomos with phototherapy				
Middlekamp-Hup et al, 2007	RCT	I	No significant differences in body areas other than head and neck. Repigmentation of the head and neck after NB-UVB: *P. leucotomos* group 44% vs 19% placebo in patients attending more than 80% of required NB-UVB sessions	Initial dose, 210–360 mJ/cm^2, according to skin type, gradually increased, frequency, 2×/week for 25–26 weeks

NB-UVB narrowband ultraviolet B, *PUVA* psoralen + ultraviolet A, *RCT* randomized controlled trial, *mJ* millijoules, *J* Joules, *max* maximum, *8-MOP* methoxypsoralen, *MED* minimal erythemal dose, BB-UVB broadband UVB

In 1997, Westerhof and Nieuweboer-Krobotova were the first group that reported the efficacy of NB-UVB for vitiligo. They performed an observer-blinded prospective study comparing NB-UVB with topical PUVA. At 4 months, 46% ($n = 13$) of the patients treated with topical PUVA showed repigmentation compared to 67% ($n = 52$) of the patients treated with NB-UVB.[18]

Yones et al published the first double-blind, randomized clinical trial comparing NB-UVB with PUVA.[17,19] At the end of all treatments, both treatment modalities induced a reduction in percentage of body surface area affected by vitiligo with a tendency for better efficacy in the NB-UVB-treated group. Because of a larger average total number of treatments in the NB-UVB-treated compared to the PUVA-treated group (97 vs 47 treatments, respectively), a comparison was done at the end of 48 treatments; greater than 50% improvement in body surface area affected by vitiligo at 48 treatments occurred in 53% of patients on the NB-UVB group ($n = 21$), compared to 23% of patients on the PUVA group ($n = 13$). In addition, 100% of NB-UVB-treated patients ($n = 97$) had excellent color match compared to 44% ($n = 11$) of PUVA patients; NB-UVB treatment was also associated with a lower incidence of side effects.

Bathnagar et al performed a randomized clinical trial comparing NB-UVB and PUVA.[20] Mean degree of repigmentation was 52.2% in the NB-UVB group ($n = 25$) and 44.7% in the PUVA group ($n = 25$). After excluding treatment-resistant sites, such as hands and feet, the mean degree of repigmentation was 67.57% in the NB-UVB group ($n = 25$) and 54.2% in the PUVA group ($n = 25$). Thus, this trial demonstrated superiority of NB-UVB in repigmentation with the exception of treatment resistant sites.

El Mofty et al performed a left–right comparison trial in two groups: NB-UVB versus PUVA ($n = 15$) and NB-UVB versus 8-MOP NB-UVB ($n = 20$).[21] In the NB-UVB versus PUVA group, at 60 sessions, 57% ($n = 8$) of the patients had 60–75% repigmentation in both PUVA- and NB-UVB-treated sides. In the NB-UVB versus NB-UVB and 8-MOP, 38.9% ($n = 7$) of the patients had 60–75% repigmentation in both NB-UVB-treated and NB-UVB + 8-MOP-treated sites, but phototoxicity was significantly higher in the NB-UVB + 8-MOP-treated side.

6.3.1.2 Stability of Pigmentation and Predictors of Response to NB-UVB Phototherapy

Sitek et al investigated to what degree the NB-UVB treatment-induced repigmentation remains stable for up to 2 years posttreatment in an open prospective clinical trial.[22] In 31 patients with generalized vitiligo, 35% ($n = 11$) of patients developed repigmentation ≥ 75%. Two years after cessation of the treatment program of up to 1 year of NB-UVB therapy, 5 of those 11 patients (45%) retained ≥75% stable repigmentation.

Nicaloudiou et al assessed the efficacy of NB-UVB phototherapy and the predictors of response in an open clinical trial of 70 patients.[23] Over 75% repigmentation was achieved in 34.4% ($n = 21$) of patients with lesions on the face and in 7.4% ($n = 5$) of patients with lesions on the body. Repigmentation was stable in 14.3% ($n = 3$) of patients 4 years after cessation of treatment. Patients with darker Fitzpatrick skin phototypes (III to V), patients who responded in the first month of treatment, and patients with vitiligo on the face were more likely to achieve 75% or greater repigmentation.

Anbar et al performed an open clinical trial on patients with both segmental and nonsegmental vitiligo treated with NB-UVB.[24] They reported that patients with nonsegmental vitiligo and patients treated early in the disease course had better repigmentation rates. Repigmentation rates were higher on the face followed by trunk and limbs

6.3.1.3   NB-UVB Versus 308-nm Monochromatic Excimer Light

Cassaci et al compared 308-nm monochromatic excimer light to NB-UVB in randomized, investigator-blinded and half-side comparison trial; treatment was started at 70% of the minimal erythema dose (MED) of the pigmented skin, with increments ranging from 20% to 40% until erythema was observed.[25] The lesions treated with 308-nm monochromatic excimer light had significantly higher mean repigmentation scores than the symmetrical lesions treated with NB-UVB (2.68 vs 2.12, respectively); repigmentation of ≥75% was achieved in 37.5% ($n = 6$) of the lesions treated with 308-nm monochromatic excimer light and 6% ($n = 1$) of the lesions treated with NB-UVB; repigmentation of ≥50% was obtained in 25% ($n = 4$) of the lesions treated with 308-nm monochromatic excimer light and 31% ($n = 5$) treated with NB-UVB.

6.3.1.4   BB-UVB Versus NB-UVB and PUVA

Since broadband UVB has been largely replaced by NB-UVB, very limited evidence exists on the treatment of vitiligo with BB-UVB. A meta-analysis by Njoo et al[26] compared data on BB-UVB, NB-UVB, and PUVA. Treatment was considered successful when more than 75% repigmentation was achieved. The highest success rates were achieved with NB-UVB (63%, with a 95% confidence interval ranging from 50–76%), followed by BB-UVB (57%, with a confidence interval ranging from 29–82%), and PUVA (51%, with a 95% confidence interval ranging from 46–56%).

Don et al performed an open trial with nine patients with actively spreading progressive vitiligo who received BB-UVB two to three times a week in combination with vitamin C 500 mg, vitamin B$_{12}$ 1,000 µg, and folic acid 5 mg twice daily.[27] The treatment regimen arrested the progression of vitiligo in all patients, induced repigmentation after 8–12 treatments (6–8 weeks), and induced 51–100% repigmentation after 2–8 months of treatment in all patients.

6.3.1.5   Broadband UVA

El Mofty et al assessed the efficacy of broadband UVA three times a week in a randomized, double-blinded controlled study.[28] Patients with symmetrical vitiligo with ≥30% body surface area affected were randomized to two constant dosing regimens, 5 and 15 J/cm². Over 60% repigmentation occurred in 50% ($n = 5$) of patients on the 15 J/cm² regimen, and in 10% ($n = 1$) of patients on the 5 J/cm² regimen.

6.3.1.6   Targeted UVB Phototherapy

Hofer et al assessed efficacy of the 308-nm excimer laser on a controlled prospective trial.[29] After 10 weeks of treatment (30 treatments), repigmentation of more than 75% was observed in 25% ($n = 7$) of lesions of the high-responder location group (face, trunk, arm, and/or leg), and 2% ($n = 1$) of lesions of the low-responder location group (elbow, wrist, dorsum of the hand, knee, and/or dorsum of the foot). Lesion repigmentation started after a mean of 13 and 22 treatments in the high- and the low-responder location groups, respectively. In most cases, laser-induced repigmentation was persistent at 12 months after the end of treatment. Hofer et al also performed a randomized controlled trial comparing the efficacy of once a week, twice a week, and thrice a week regimens.[17,30] Repigmentation was fastest with thrice a week regimen; on the other hand, repigmentation initiation depended on the total number of treatments rather than frequency of treatment. At 12 weeks, repigmentation rates were 60% (1×/week), 79% (2×/week), and 82% (3×/week).

In a retrospective study of 32 patients with 55 vitiliginous lesions treated with 308-nm excimer laser by Hadi et al, 52.8% ($n = 29$) of the lesions showed 75% or more repigmentation with an average number of 23 treatments.[17,31] When stratified by body sites, ≥75% repigmentation was observed in 71.5% ($n = 15$) of the lesions on the face, 60% ($n = 3$) on the neck and scalp, 50% ($n = 2$) on the genitalia, 46.7% ($n = 7$) on the extremities, 40% ($n = 2$) on the trunk, and 0% on the hands and feet.

6.3.1.7   Phototherapy in Combination with Topical Tacrolimus

Calcineurin inhibitors tacrolimus and pimecrolimus inhibit the synthesis and release of proinflammatory cytokines and vasoactive mediators from basophiles and mast cells.[15] They are one of the first line treatments for vitiligo localized to up to 10% body surface area, as their efficacy is comparable to topical corticosteroids but provides a better side effects profile.[32]

A number of studies have investigated whether topical tacrolimus in combination with phototherapy is more effective than phototherapy alone.

A randomized controlled study by Passeron et al reported that repigmentation of ≥75% was observed in 70% ($n = 16$) of lesions treated with 308-nm excimer laser in combination with tacrolimus 0.1% ointment versus 20% ($n = 4$) of lesions treated with 308-nm excimer laser monotherapy.[17,33] Response was further analyzed based in UV-sensitive areas (face, neck, trunk, and limbs) and in classically UV-resistant sites (bony prominences and extremities). This greater efficacy of combination treatment was observed in both UV-sensitive areas [repigmentation of ≥75% was observed in 77% ($n = 10$) of group lesions on combination therapy and 57% ($n = 4$) of lesions on laser monotherapy] and in classically UV-resistant lesions [repigmentation of ≥75% was observed in 60% ($n = 6$) of lesions on combination therapy and none of lesions on laser monotherapy].

In an open labeled prospective study of 110 patients with chronic stable vitiligo refractory to conventional treatments, treated with NB-UVB in combination with tacrolimus ointment, 0.1% to the body and 0.03% to the face, Fai et al reported more than 50% repigmentation in 42% of lesions ($n = 168$).[34] When stratified by site, more than 50% repigmentation was observed in 73% of the lesions on the face ($n = 64$), 68% on the limbs ($n = 57$), and 53.5% on the trunk ($n = 47$). None of the lesions of the extremities and genital areas had more than 25% repigmentation.

While studies have shown the promising efficacy results of combination treatment, it should be noted that in vitro, calcineurin inhibitors have been shown to inhibit the removal of cyclobutane pyrimidine dimers following UVB radiation and to inhibit UVB-induced apoptosis.[35] Therefore, it is advisable to warn patients of the potential theoretical increased risk of skin cancer until time allows for long-term studies to determine the clinical relevance of these in vitro findings.

6.3.1.8 Phototherapy in Combination with Topical Calcipotriol/Calcipotriene

Calcipotriol is a synthetic analogue of vitamin D_3. Vitamin D_3 stimulates melanocyte and keratinocyte growth and differentiation by binding to vitamin D receptors in the skin, possibly stimulating melanogenesis via the 1-α-dihydroxyvitamin D_3 receptors present in melanocytes.[15] Calcipotriol as monotherapy for the treatment of vitiligo has limited efficacy; therefore, it has also been studied in combination with topical corticosteroids and phototherapy. It can be safely used in combination with phototherapy.

There are reports of both efficacy and lack of added efficacy when combining calcipotriol with phototherapy.

Goldinger et al performed a right/left comparative, single-blinded trial comparing 308-nm excimer laser three times a week alone or in combination with calcipotriol ointment in nine patients.[36] After 24 sessions, there was no significant difference in repigmentation between both sides; one patient did not have any repigmentation. Mean overall repigmentation at 24 weeks was 22.4%. A randomized controlled clinical trial by Arca et al showed no statistically significant difference between NB-UVB in combination with topical calcipotriol ointment (0.005%) and NB-UVB monotherapy at the end of a mean of 30 treatments.[17,37] Kullavanijaya et al reported, in a prospective controlled clinical trial, that 53% ($n = 9$) of patients had an appreciably better response on the NB-UVB and calcipotriol side compared to NB-UVB alone by 29–114 treatments.[17,38] Similarly, Goktas et al reported on a prospective controlled clinical trial with 24 patients that repigmentation was significantly higher in the NB-UVB with calcipotriol-treated side than NB-UVB alone, with mean repigmentation of $51 \pm 19.6\%$ and $39 \pm 18.9\%$ for each group, respectively.[39] The median cumulative UVB dose was higher and the number of UVB exposures for initial repigmentation was lower on the side that received combination therapy.

6.3.1.9   Phototherapy in Combination with *Polypodium leucotomos*

A randomized, double-blind clinical trial assessing the combination of NB-UVB and *Polypodium leucotomos* (250 mg twice daily) in 50 patients by Middelkamp-Hup reported higher mean repigmentation in the head and neck area in the *P. leucotomos* group than in the placebo group (50% vs 19%, $P < 0.002$) in patients attending more than 80% of required NB-UVB sessions; no significant differences were seen in the other body areas.[40]

6.4   Treatment Protocols

6.4.1   Nb-uvb

Generally, the starting dose for phototherapy for vitiligo is the dose equivalent to 50–70% of the MED to NB-UVB of Fitzpatrick skin phototype I. The MED of Fitzpatrick skin type I to NB-UVB is in the range of 400 mJ/cm^2; thus, 70% of the MED is equivalent to 280 nm and 50% of the MED is 200 mJ/cm^2.[41] Dose increments of up to 5–20% are safe. Maximum dose is dependent on individual tolerance. Dosing protocols vary by institution and clinical trials. Table 6.1 describes the dosing protocols used by the different studies cited in this chapter. A study comparing NB-UVB with monochromatic excimer light has used the MED on normally pigmented skin to guide therapy[25] as vitiliginous skin does not provide large enough surface areas for phototests.

In our center, we use a starting dose of 280 mJ/cm^2, which is equivalent to 70% of the MED for Fitzpatrick skin type I and dose increments of 10–15% as tolerated. Once symptomatic erythema develops, the dose is then decreased to the previously tolerated dose and is maintained unless the patient develops tolerance (photoadaptation) and increasing doses are tolerated. We use a maximum dose of 3 J/cm^2 for the body, 1 J/cm^2 for the face and neck in patients with Fitzpatrick skin types I and II, 1.5 J/cm^2 for patients with Fitzpatrick skin types III and IV, and 2 J/cm^2 for patients with Fitzpatrick skin types V and VI.

6.4.2   PUVA Photochemotherapy

Prior to, or within a month of the initiation of treatment, an eye examination should be obtained and repeated annually. The recommended dose of 8-MOP for photochemotherapy is 0.4–0.6 mg/kg with a maximum dose per treatment of 70 mg; the dose of

5-MOP is 1.2 mg/kg. Psoralen should be taken with a low-fat meal 1 h prior to treatment. Patients should avoid sun exposure for at least 8 h after the ingestion of psoralen, preferably 24 h, and special photoprotection measures should be undertaken, such as photoprotective clothing, hats, UV protective sunglasses, and a broad-spectrum sunscreen with both UVB and UVA coverage. In indoor setting, unless the patient is exposed to high-intensity UVA (such as sitting next to a brightly lighted window for extensive period of time), photoprotective eyewear does not have to be used.

UVA dosing protocols vary by institution and clinical trials. Table 6.1 describes the dosing protocols used by the different studies cited. We recommend an initial dose of $0.5–1$ J/cm^2, followed by dose increments of $0.25–0.5$ J/cm^2 as tolerated, that is, using a protocol that we use for Fitzpatrick skin phototype I. Once symptomatic erythema develops, the dose should be decreased to the previously tolerated dose and maintained unless the patient develops tolerance (photoadaptation) and increasing doses are tolerated. We recommend a maximum dose of 4 J/cm^2 for the face, and the following for the rest of the body, depending on the skin type: 8 J/cm^2 for skin types I and II, 12 J/cm^2 for skin types III and IV, and 20 J/cm^2 for skin types V and VI.

Topical 8-MOP can be used for localized vitiligo. 8-MOP topical lotion, 0.1% in Lubriderm™, is applied 20–30 min before irradiation and is washed off immediately after the treatment.

Other less commonly used form of photochemotherapy include oral and topical PUVAsol, which is the application of psoralens orally or topically and gradually increasing amount of sun exposure or exposure to a solar simulator. This form of therapy is being largely replaced especially by NB-UVB, PUVA, and targeted phototherapy in which the doses are delivered in a controlled and safer manner.

6.4.3 Targeted Phototherapy with 308-nm Excimer Laser

In our Center, we use a starting dose of 150 mJ/cm^2 with dose increments of 5–15% as tolerated, a maximum dose of 3 J/cm^2 for the body and 1 J/cm^2 for the face.

6.5 Side Effects of Therapy

6.5.1 Acute Effects

Acute side effects of phototherapy include sunburn-like reaction with erythema,[42] which, depending on the severity, may be accompanied by tenderness, pruritus, and less commonly peeling and blistering of the skin. Tanning, xerosis, reactivation of herpes simplex, and injury to the eyes if appropriate UV protective goggles are not worn during treatment and are also immediate side effects common to both UVB[42,43] and UVA phototherapy.[42]

PUVA has additional acute side effects which include nausea, headache, dizziness, and sunburn-like erythema reactions and acute ocular reaction secondary to additional sun exposure in the 24 h following treatment if photoprotection and UVA-protective eyewear is not worn.[42]

6.5.2   Long-Term Side Effects

Photoaging, actinic keratosis, and photocarcinogenesis are long-term side effects of phototherapy and photochemotherapy.[42,43]

In the first 10 years of follow-up of the PUVA cohort of patients treated for psoriasis indicated a 12-fold greater risk of squamous cell carcinoma in patients who received more than 259 treatments compared to patients who received less than 160 treatments. A modest increase in the incidence of basal cell carcinoma was observed compared to the normal population, in patients who received at least 200 treatments.[44] Research from such cohort has additionally demonstrated that the risk for squamous cell carcinoma persists, and the risk of basal cell carcinoma continues to increase 15 years after cessation of PUVA.[42,45]

From 1975 to 1990, the risk of melanoma in the cohort psoriasis patients treated with PUVA was nearly identical to the Caucasian general population. However, beginning 15 years after the first exposure to PUVA or after 1991, a dose-dependent increase in melanoma incidence has been observed.[46]

Strict photoprotection of the skin and eyes is recommended for 24 h after PUVA. Baseline and routine ophthalmological evaluation is recommended in patients treated with PUVA. Because of its long-term side effects, PUVA should be used with caution in individuals younger than 18 years. While psoralens are not teratogens, PUVA is contraindicated in women who are pregnant or breast-feeding.[42]

6.6   Conclusion

Phototherapy has repigmentation and immunosuppressive properties that are valuable in the treatment of vitiligo. Evidence points to NB-UVB as the treatment of choice for vitiligo affecting >10% body surface area, with PUVA as a second alternative. Overall, NB-UVB has less side effects than PUVA. Targeted phototherapy is an alternative to topical therapy and more practical than whole body phototherapy for patients with vitiligo with ≤10% body surface area affected.

References

1. Millington GW, Levell NJ. Vitiligo: the historical curse of depigmentation. *Int J Dermatol.* 2007;46:990–995.
2. Roelandts R. The history of phototherapy: something new under the sun? *J Am Acad Dermatol.* 2002;46:926–930.
3. Kovacs SO. Vitiligo. *J Am Acad Dermatol.* 1998;38:647–666; quiz 667-668.

4. Halaban R, Langdon R, Birchall N, et al. Basic fibroblast growth factor from human kerati-nocytes is a natural mitogen for melanocytes. *J Cell Biol.* 1988;107:1611–1619.

5. Stierner U, Rosdahl I, Augustsson A, Kagedal B. UVB irradiation induces melanocyte increase in both exposed and shielded human skin. *J Invest Dermatol.* 1989;92:561–564.

6. Fitzpatrick TB. Mechanisms of phototherapy of vitiligo. *Arch Dermatol.* 1997;133:1591–1592.

7. Abdel-Naser MB, Hann SK, Bystryn JC. Oral psoralen with UV-A therapy releases circulat-ing growth factor(s) that stimulates cell proliferation. *Arch Dermatol.* 1997;133:1530–1533.

8. Horikawa T, Norris DA, Johnson TW, et al. DOPA-negative melanocytes in the outer root sheath of human hair follicles express premelanosomal antigens but not a melanosomal anti-gen or the melanosome-associated glycoproteins tyrosinase, TRP-1, and TRP-2. *J Invest Dermatol.* 1996;106:28–35.

9. Falabella R. Surgical approaches for stable vitiligo. *Dermatol Surg.* 2005;31:1277–1284.

10. Duthie MS, Kimber I, Norval M. The effects of ultraviolet radiation on the human immune system. *Br J Dermatol.* 1999;140:995–1009.

11. Kulms D, Poppelmann B, Yarosh D, Luger TA, Krutmann J, Schwarz T. Nuclear and cell membrane effects contribute independently to the induction of apoptosis in human cells exposed to UVB radiation. *Proc Natl Acad Sci U S A.* 1999;96:7974–7979.

12. Aragane Y, Kulms D, Metze D, et al. Ultraviolet light induces apoptosis via direct activation of CD95 (Fas/APO-1) independently of its ligand CD95L. *J Cell Biol.* 1998;140:171–182.

13. Walters IB, Ozawa M, Cardinale I, et al. Narrowband (312-nm) UV-B suppresses interferon gamma and interleukin (IL) 12 and increases IL-4 transcripts: differential regulation of cytokines at the single-cell level. *Arch Dermatol.* 2003;139:155–161.

14. Morita A, Werfel T, Stege H, et al. Evidence that singlet oxygen-induced human T helper cell apoptosis is the basic mechanism of ultraviolet-A radiation phototherapy. *J Exp Med.* 1997;186:1763–1768.

15. Grimes PE. New insights and new therapies in vitiligo. *JAMA.* 2005;293:730–735.

16. Harris RP, Helfand M, Woolf SH, et al. Current methods of the US Preventive Services Task Force: a review of the process. *Am J Prev Med.* 2001;20:21–35.

17. Lim HW, Hexsel CL. Vitiligo: to treat or not to treat. *Arch Dermatol.* 2007;143:643–646.

18. Westerhof W, Nieuweboer-Krobotova L. Treatment of vitiligo with UV-B radiation vs topical psoralen plus UV-A. *Arch Dermatol.* 1997;133:1525–1528.

19. Yones SS, Palmer RA, Garibaldinos TM, Hawk JLM. Randomized double-blind trial of the treatment of vitiligo: efficacy of psoralen-UV-A therapy vs. narrowband UV-B therapy. Arch Dermatol. 2007.

20. Bhatnagar A, Kanwar AJ, Parsad D, De D. Comparison of systemic PUVA and NB-UVB in the treatment of vitiligo: an open prospective study. *J Eur Acad Dermatol Venereol.* 2007;21:638–642.

21. El Mofty M, Mostafa W, Esmat S, et al. Narrow band Ultraviolet B 311 nm in the treatment of vitiligo: two right-left comparison studies. *Photodermatol Photoimmunol Photomed.* 2006;22:6–11.

22. Sitek JC, Loeb M, Ronnevig JR. Narrowband UVB therapy for vitiligo: does the repigmenta-tion last. *J Eur Acad Dermatol Venereol.* 2007;21:891–896.

23. Nicolaidou E, Antoniou C, Stratigos AJ, Stefanaki C, Katsambas AD. Efficacy, predictors of response, and long-term follow-up in patients with vitiligo treated with narrowband UVB phototherapy. *J Am Acad Dermatol.* 2007;56:274–278.

24. Anbar TS, Westerhof W, Abdel-Rahman AT, El-Khayyat MA. Evaluation of the effects of NB-UVB in both segmental and non-segmental vitiligo affecting different body sites. *Photodermatol Photoimmunol Photomed.* 2006;22:157–163.

25. Casacci M, Thomas P, Pacifico A, Bonnevalle A, Paro Vidolin A, Leone G. Comparison between 308-nm monochromatic excimer light and narrowband UVB phototherapy (311–313 nm) in the treatment of vitiligo – a multicentre controlled study. *J Eur Acad Dermatol Venereol.* 2007;21:956–963.

26. Njoo MD, Westerhof W, Bos JD, Bossuyt PM. A systematic review of autologous transplantation methods in vitiligo. *Arch Dermatol.* 1998;134:1543–1549.
27. Don P, Iuga A, Dacko A, Hardick K. Treatment of vitiligo with broadband ultraviolet B and vitamins. *Int J Dermatol.* 2006;45:63–65.
28. El-Mofty M, Mostafa W, Youssef R, et al. Ultraviolet A in vitiligo. *Photodermatol Photoimmunol Photomed.* 2006;22:214–216.
29. Hofer A, Hassan AS, Legat FJ, Kerl H, Wolf P. The efficacy of excimer laser (308 nm) for vitiligo at different body sites. *J Eur Acad Dermatol Venereol.* 2006;20:558–564.
30. Hofer A, Hassan AS, Legat FJ, Kerl H, Wolf P. Optimal weekly frequency of 308-nm excimer laser treatment in vitiligo patients. *Br J Dermatol.* 2005;152:981–985.
31. Hadi SM, Spencer JM, Lebwohl M. The use of the 308-nm excimer laser for the treatment of vitiligo. *Dermatol Surg.* 2004;30:983–986.
32. Lepe V, Moncada B, Castanedo-Cazares JP, Torres-Alvarez MB, Ortiz CA, Torres-Rubalcava AB. A double-blind randomized trial of 0.1% tacrolimus vs 0.05% clobetasol for the treatment of childhood vitiligo. *Arch Dermatol.* 2003;139:581–585.
33. Passeron T, Ostovari N, Zakaria W, et al. Topical tacrolimus and the 308-nm excimer laser: a synergistic combination for the treatment of vitiligo. *Arch Dermatol.* 2004;140:1065–1069.
34. Fai D, Cassano N, Vena GA. Narrow-band UVB phototherapy combined with tacrolimus ointment in vitiligo: a review of 110 patients. *J Eur Acad Dermatol Venereol.* 2007;21:916–920.
35. Yarosh DB, Pena AV, Nay SL, Canning MT, Brown DA. Calcineurin inhibitors decrease DNA repair and apoptosis in human keratinocytes following ultraviolet B irradiation. *J Invest Dermatol.* 2005;125:1020–1025.
36. Goldinger SM, Dummer R, Schmid P, Burg G, Seifert B, Lauchli S. Combination of 308-nm xenon chloride excimer laser and topical calcipotriol in vitiligo. *J Eur Acad Dermatol Venereol.* 2007;21:504–508.
37. Arca E, Tastan HB, Erbil AH, Sezer E, Koc E, Kurumlu Z. Narrow-band ultraviolet B as monotherapy and in combination with topical calcipotriol in the treatment of vitiligo. *J Dermatol.* 2006;33:338–343.
38. Kullavanijaya P, Lim HW. Topical calcipotriene and narrowband ultraviolet B in the treatment of vitiligo. *Photodermatol Photoimmunol Photomed.* 2004;20:248–251.
39. Goktas EO, Aydin F, Senturk N, Canturk MT, Turanli AY. Combination of narrow band UVB and topical calcipotriol for the treatment of vitiligo. *J Eur Acad Dermatol Venereol.* 2006;20:553–557.
40. Middelkamp-Hup MA, Bos JD, Rius-Diaz F, Gonzalez S, Westerhof W. Treatment of vitiligo vulgaris with narrow-band UVB and oral *Polypodium leucotomos* extract: a randomized double-blind placebo-controlled study. *J Eur Acad Dermatol Venereol.* 2007;21:942–950.
41. Zanolli M, Farr P. Phototherapy with UVB: broadband and narrowband. In: LimH W, Honigsmann H, Haek JLM. Photodermatology. New York, NY: Informa Healthcare USA; 2007:319–334.
42. Naldi L, Griffiths CE. Traditional therapies in the management of moderate to severe chronic plaque psoriasis: an assessment of the benefits and risks. *Br J Dermatol.* 2005;152:597–615.
43. Ibbotson SH, Bilsland D, Cox NH, et al. An update and guidance on narrowband ultraviolet B phototherapy: a British Photodermatology Group Workshop Report. *Br J Dermatol.* 2004;151:283–297.
44. Stern RS, Lange R. Non-melanoma skin cancer occurring in patients treated with PUVA five to ten years after first treatment. *J Invest Dermatol.* 1988;91:120–124.
45. Nijsten TE, Stern RS. The increased risk of skin cancer is persistent after discontinuation of psoralen + ultraviolet A: a cohort study. *J Invest Dermatol.* 2003;121:252–258.
46. Stern RS. The risk of melanoma in association with long-term exposure to PUVA. *J Am Acad Dermatol.* 2001;44:755–761.

Chapter 7
Lasers and Light Therapies for Pigmentation

Malcolm S. Ke

With the ever-increasing interest in minimally invasive cosmetic procedures and the growing non-Caucasian population of the USA, demand for research in photorejuvenation for darker skin tones is high. Lasers, specifically, have progressed tremendously in the last 20 years, becoming more elegant, efficient, and most of all, safer for all skin tones. They are no longer reserved just for fair skin, and can safely and effectively treat the ailments of individuals with dark skin.

The use of lasers and light sources for pigmentation is generally based on wavelengths targeting melanin or pigment as the chromophore. Patients with darker skin tones present a challenge because light therapies are limited by their potential to cause postinflammatory dyspigmentation. Any therapy resulting in robust inflammation may induce this unwanted response. Although oftentimes temporary, postinflammatory hyperpigmentation may persist for many months, oftentimes becoming even more pronounced when approaches are taken to treat it. Strict perioperative use of topical bleaching agents and sun-protective measures are valuable in optimizing outcomes. Inciting factors such as sun exposure and other topicals need to be identified and discontinued to prevent further dyspigmentation during and after surgical treatment. Test spotting a representative lesion 4 weeks before treating the entire area is always recommended.

Nonablative light sources, such as the intense pulsed light (IPL) system, have been used safely and effectively to treat patients with darker skin. Various Q-switched (QS) lasers that deliver pulses in the nanosecond range are commonly used to treat pigmentary disorders. They include the 532 nm Nd:YAG, 694 nm ruby, 755 nm alexandrite, and 1,064 nm Nd:YAG. Given increased melanin absorption at shorter wavelengths, the use of longer wavelength lasers is generally preferred in treating darker skinned patients. However, ablative lasers such as the 2,940 nm Erbium:YAG and 10,600 nm CO_2 carry a significant risk of postinflammatory hyper- or hypopigmentation. They are reserved for selective resistant cases and should be used with caution. A relatively new modality called fractional photothermolysis

M.S. Ke
Division of Dermatology, University of California, Los Angeles, CA 90095, USA
e-mail: mke@mednet.ucla.edu

E.D. Baron (ed.), *Light-Based Therapies for Skin of Color*,
DOI: 10.1007/ 978-1-84882-328-0_7, © Springer-Verlag London Limited 2009

(FP) may prove to be the happy medium between ablative and nonablative techniques.

7.1   Clinical Applications

7.1.1   *Lentigines*

Often referred to as "liver spots" or "age spots," lentigines are hyperpigmented macules that manifest on sun-exposed areas. Multiple lesions are often seen and some lesions can enlarge to patches. Histologically, increased melanin is seen in the basal layer of the epidermis, while underlying solar elastosis can typically be seen in the papillary dermis. Since lentigines occur on visible parts of the body and can be viewed as a sign of photoaging, patients often seek cosmetic treatment for these lesions.

Therapy consists of topical bleaching agents and different cosmetic procedures including cryotherapy, chemical peels, lasers, and light sources. Additionally, in order to achieve and maintain resolution of lentigines, the use of broad-spectrum sunscreens and sun-protective habits are critical. Various topical therapies, such as hydroquinone, tretinoin, adapalene, and combination mequinol and tretinoin have been used successfully and safely to lighten lentigines.[1-3] However, they can take time to attain optimal results.

Advancements in laser technology targeting the broad absorption spectrum of melanin have rendered newer systems more effective and safe for the treatment lentigines. Again, pretreatment and concomitant use of a bleaching agent and sunscreens can minimize postinflammatory hyperpigmentation and optimize results.[4-6] In addition, careful clinical assessment of the nature of the pigmented lesion before treatment is paramount. Clinically atypical lesions require further evaluation to rule out possible malignancy. Treatment failure and recurrence should prompt a reexamination of the original diagnosis, as illustrated in the case of repigmentation after QS ruby laser treatment of a lentigo. This was later biopsied as lentigo maligna melanoma.[7]

Lasers used to improve lentigines include the pulsed dye (595 nm), copper vapor (511 nm), krypton (520–530 nm), frequency-doubled Nd:YAG (532 nm), diode (532–630 nm), QS ruby (684 nm), QS alexandrite (755 nm), QS Nd:YAG (1,064 and 532 nm), and CO_2 (10,600 nm) lasers. As opposed to treatment in lighter skin types, not all lasers used in darker skin types have a sufficient therapeutic window of effectiveness before side effects preclude their use. This is particularly true with continuous wave lasers. QS lasers, such as the QS Nd:YAG and ruby lasers, have been utilized to treat lentigines (Fig. 7.1a, b).[8,9] These devices emit very short pulses of energy that induce both photothermal and photomechanical reactions after preferential absorption by melanin.

Other lasers and light sources, in addition to the QS lasers, have been employed to treat lentigines in ethnic skin. Kono et al reported the 595-nm long-pulsed dye laser to improve lentigines in a study of 18 Asian patients of skin types III–IV.[10] Using glass compression and no cryogen cooling, the long-pulsed dye laser cleared

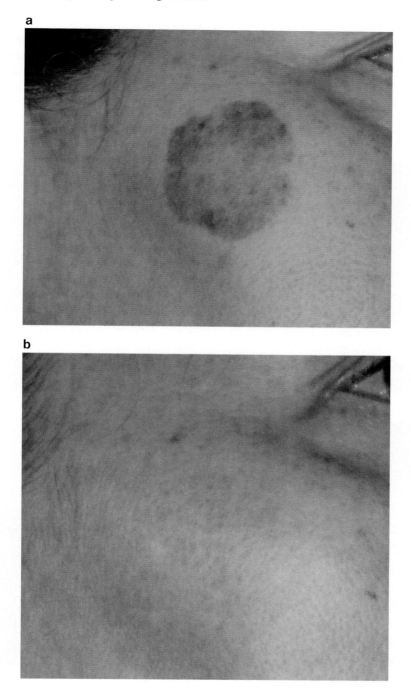

Fig. 7.1 (**a**) Baseline. (**b**) Status post Q-switched laser

83% of lesions compared with 70% with the QS ruby laser. No hyperpigmentation was noted in the areas treated with the long-pulsed dye laser as opposed to four patients with the QS ruby laser. A validation study of 54 Asian patients using similar settings (595-nm long-pulsed dye laser with 7-mm spot size, 1.5-ms pulse duration, 9–13 J/cm^2, compression) revealed a 70% excellent, 24% good, and 4% fair response.[11] Only one patient suffered hyperpigmentation. Our experience in Los Angeles is similar in the Asian population (Fig. 7.2a–d). Likewise, a long-pulsed

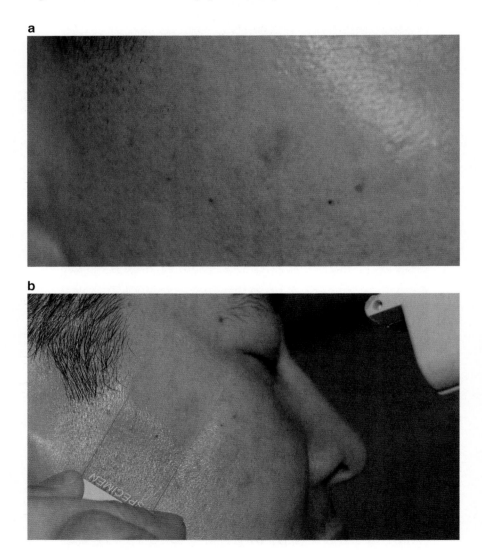

Fig. 7.2 (**a**) Baseline. (**b**) Demonstration of glass slide compression. (**c**) One day status post compression pulsed dye laser (*PDL*) treatment. (**d**) One week status post compression PDL treatment

c

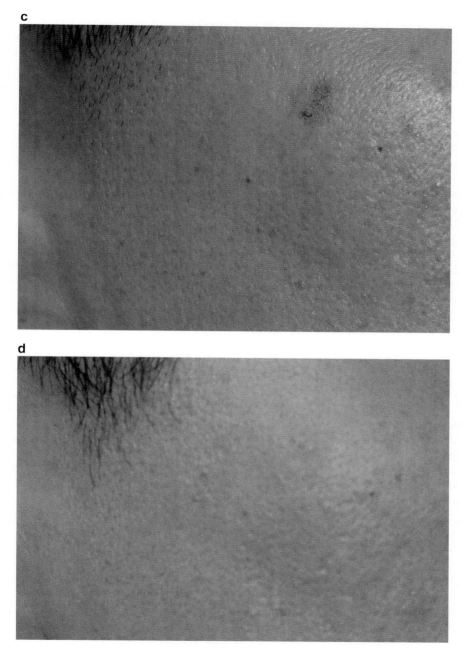

d

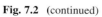

Fig. 7.2 (continued)

532-nm Nd:YAG laser has been successfully used in Asian patients with facial lentigines. Chan et al compared the long-pulsed dye laser with a conventional QS 532 nm laser showing no significant difference in degree of clearing.[12] Hyperpigmentation was the most common complication and cleared with topical bleaching agents and glycolic acid creams.

IPL, which emits broadband visible light from a noncoherent light source, has also been used. Multiple treatments at 2- to 4-week intervals are often required to achieve maximal results. This treatment modality offers the advantage of minimal to no downtime for the patient. There are several studies showing its efficacy and safety in Asian patients.[6,13] A study reported a greater than 50% improvement in 40% of patients with lentigines after an average of four IPL treatments at 2–3 weeks intervals. No hyperpigmentation or scarring occurred.[13] However, lower efficacy compared with other modalities is generally cited. A recent split-face study comparing IPL versus pulsed dye laser in ten Asian patients revealed a 62% versus 81% improvement in lentigines, respectively, and no difference in wrinkles.[14]

A study comparing TCA 35% peel and QS Nd:YAG (532 nm, 10 ns, 2 mm spot) laser therapy in 20 patients with skin types III–IV with facial lentigines demonstrated greater improvement with laser therapy. Sixty-five percent of patients showed better improvement on the laser-treated areas, 14% had superior improvement on the TCA-treated areas and 21% showed similar improvements with both treatments. No scarring or dyspigmentation was seen.[15]

7.1.2   Café au Lait Macules

Café au lait macules (CALMs) are "coffee" colored birthmarks that occur anywhere on the body and frequently darken with age. Although multiple lesions can be markers for underlying diseases such as neurofibromatosis, isolated CALMs are commonly encountered. Around 10–20% of the population has them, with an increased prevalence in darker skin types.[8] On histopathology, the melanin is found in giant melanosomes mainly within the basal layer of the epidermis.

Laser therapy is the main treatment modality. Multiple laser treatments are necessary to achieve clearance of lesions. The QS laser systems have generally been considered safe; however, the effect of treatment can be inconsistent as some CALMs may even darken after treatment. Thus, a test spot should be performed. The treatment area is reevaluated 4–8 weeks later for clinical response and adverse effects. Hyperpigmentation can occur but usually improves with topical bleaching regimens and the tincture of time. Hypopigmentation is a potential risk particularly with the shorter wavelength lasers.

The QS ruby, alexandrite, and Nd:YAG lasers have been shown to treat CALMs with varying degrees of efficacy. Grossman et al found variable response in treating CALMs with a 694 nm QS ruby laser and a 532 nm frequency-doubled QS Nd:YAG laser.[16] Nine lesions were treated; half with each laser. At 6 months, five of the lesions showed lightening and one resolved. One lesion resolved after the first month, but recurred at the 3-month follow-up, while two lesions darkened 1 month after the first treatment. Clinical experience with multiple QS laser treatments has yielded inconsistent results with 50% of the cases achieving total clearance and repigmentation occurring in the other half.[9] Other reports suggest that a single laser treatment may lighten up to 50% of café au lait spots and almost clear 20–50% of lesions. However, one-third of these showed repigmentation.[17-19]

Longer pulsed lasers have been used in treating CALMs, but have also yielded inconsistent long-term results. The 510 nm pulsed dye laser has been used to treat CALMs. A report described its use to successfully treat a facial CALM in a patient with Fitzpatrick skin type V using the following parameters: 2.5 J/cm², 300 ns, with single, nonoverlapping laser pulses every 2 months for six treatments.[20] In another study using the QS alexandrite laser to treat CALMs, nine of ten patients had 60–100% response after a mean of 6.7 treatments. Three patients had partial or complete recurrence. One patient had postinflammatory hyperpigmentation and another had hypertrophic scarring. A preliminary study described a lower risk of recurrence with the normal-mode ruby laser (42% recurrence) in 33 patients with café au lait patches compared with the QS ruby laser (82% recurrence).[5] The data was limited to a 3-month follow-up after a single treatment. The authors proposed that the longer pulse width may reduce the recurrence rate by affecting the follicular melanocytes.

7.1.3   Nevus of Ota

Nevus of Ota is a benign pigmentary disorder that usually manifests as blue-brown or gray patches over facial skin innervated by the first and second trigeminal nerve. Associated lesions include scleral melanocytosis as well as involvement of the nasopharynx, auricular mucosa, tympanic membrane, palate, and dura. It is seen most commonly in Asians and is typically congenital or acquired by adolescence. The use of the QS lasers is the current treatment of choice for the cutaneous component (Fig. 7.3a, b).

Several studies have reported successful clearing after multiple treatments using various QS laser systems. A study of 114 patients with Ota's nevi treated with the QS ruby resulted in good to excellent clearing after three or more treatment sessions.[21] Transient hyperpigmentation after the first treatment was the most common complication. A Japanese study also reported the safe and successful use of the QS ruby laser in treating nevi of Ota in 106 adults and 46 children using the following parameters: 30 ns pulse duration, 4 mm spot size, and 5–7 J/cm² fluence at 3- to 4-month intervals.[22] They found that the average number of sessions to achieve significant clearing was less in the younger age group (3.5 sessions) than the older age group (5.9 sessions).

In a study of 55 Korean patients with Ota's nevi treated with the QS alexandrite laser for three sessions every 3 months, 49% of patients had excellent pigment clearing and 31% had good pigment clearing. Postinflammatory hyperpigmentation

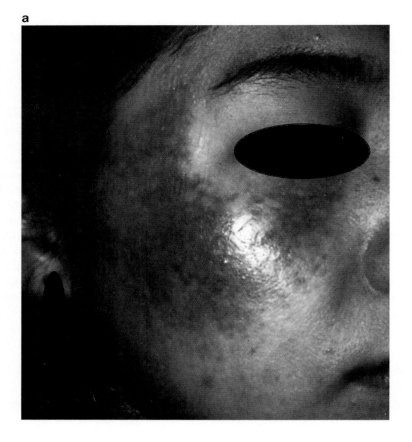

Fig. 7.3 (**a**) Nevus of Ota initial treatment. (**b**) Status post-Q-switched laser treatments

developed in 55% of patients which resolved within 4 months.[23] Chan et al compared the use of the QS alexandrite and the QS Nd:YAG for nevi of Ota in 40 Asian women, noting both to be effective, with the Nd:YAG slightly preferred when evaluated by two independent clinicians. However, scores by only one clinician was found to be statistically significant.[24] Our personal experience in Los Angeles with both lasers has shown the alexandrite to be more effective in our Latino and Asian population.

Although excellent clearing of nevus of Ota can be achieved with multiple laser treatment sessions, patients should be counseled on the potential for incomplete clearing, erythema, postinflammatory hyper- and hypopigmentation, recurrence of the condition, and permanent scarring. In a retrospective study of 211 QS alexandrite and Nd:YAG laser-treated sites, Chan et al noted the following complications: 15.3% had hypopigmentation, 2.9% had hyperpigmentation, 2.9% had textural changes, and 1.9% had scarring.[25] Recurrence after laser clearance of nevi of Ota was approximately 0.6–1.2%.[26]

b

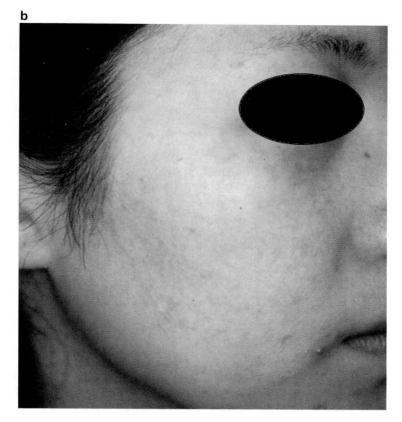

Fig. 7.3   (b) (continued)

7.1.4   Hori's Nevus or Acquired Bilateral Nevus of Ota-Like Macules

Hori's nevus is an acquired bilateral nevus of Ota-like lesion that usually presents symmetrically on the face. It is seen most commonly in middle-aged women of Asian descent. Unlike nevus of Ota, it does not have mucosal involvement. Histologically, irregular-shaped melanocytes are seen in the middle and upper dermis similar to that seen in nevus of Ota. Electron microscopy demonstrates dermal melanocytes that contain many singly dispersed melanosomes in stages II–IV of melanization.[27]

As in treatment of Ota's nevi, QS lasers have been successfully used to treat Hori's nevi. Multiple treatments are typically required. A study evaluated the QS alexandrite laser for the treatment of Hori's nevi in 32 Chinese women, noting more than 50% clearing in over 80% of patients after a mean of seven treatment sessions every 4 weeks. Temporary erythema was seen in 41% of patients and transient hypopigmentation in up to 50% of patients. Hyperpigmentation occurred in 12.5% of patients. This was treated with topical bleaching agents.[28] In a study of 66 Asian patients treated up to seven times with the QS Nd:YAG laser, Polnikorn et al found 50% of patients had good to excellent clearing.[29] Another study using the QS Nd:YAG laser (fluence of 8–10 J/cm^2, spot size 2 or 4 mm) demonstrated 100% clearance of Mori's nevi after two to five sessions in 68 of 70 patients. Fifty percent of patients had temporary hyperpigmentation. The results persisted at 3–4 years follow-up.[30]

Combination treatment with lasers has also been used to treat Hori's nevi. A scanned CO$_2$ laser followed by a QS ruby laser was found to be effective in 13 Thai patients with skin types III–IV. However, all patients had posttreatment erythema at 1-month follow-up which persisted in two patients at 3-month follow-up.[31] Recently, in a split-face study of ten Asian women with Hori's nevi, combination treatment using the QS 532 nm Nd:YAG laser followed by the QS 1,064 nm laser showed a greater degree of lightening compared with the 1,064 nm alone at 6 months follow-up. However, this combination had a higher incidence of mild postinflammatory adverse effects which lasted for 2 months.[32]

7.1.5 Melasma

Melasma is an acquired form of hyperpigmentation that is more prevalent in darker skinned women. It typically manifests as brown to gray patches on the face that worsen with sun exposure. Melasma may occur during pregnancy or oral contraceptive use but commonly arises de novo. Histologically, melanin can be found in the epidermis, dermis, or both.

The treatment of melasma is challenging and is best approached with combination treatment and preventative measures. Although the condition may resolve after termination of pregnancy, ceasing oral contraceptive use, or sun avoidance, it commonly persists indefinitely. The use of topical bleaching agents alone in conjunction with sun-protective measures may provide an adequate cosmetic outcome. Both phenolic and nonphenolic depigmenting agents have been shown to improve melasma in darker skin types.[33] In evaluating combination treatments, Pathak et al reported optimal results with the application of 2% hydroquinone, 0.05–0.1% retinoic acid, and a broad-spectrum sunscreen for the treatment of melasma in Latino women.[34] Chemical peels and lasers can be utilized alone or in conjunction with topical bleaching agents in an effort to expedite results, prevent relapse, or treat recalcitrant cases. The concurrent use of topical bleaching agents with these procedures may also minimize the risk of postinflammmatory hyperpigmentation.

The use of lasers for the treatment of melasma has yielded suboptimal results. Earlier studies with the 510 nm pigmented lesion dye laser revealed minimal improvement and even darkening of treatment areas.[35,36] Results with the QS ruby laser were inconsistent.[37,38] Ablative lasers such as the Erbium:YAG and CO$_2$ lasers carry a high risk of dyspigmentation especially in darker skin types. In a study using the Erbium:YAG laser to treat ten patients with melasma recalcitrant to bleaching creams and chemical peels, all patients developed postinflammatory hyperpigmentation 3–6 weeks postoperatively.[39] Combination laser treatment with a QS alexandrite and CO_2 laser in a split-face study in six Thai women revealed greater improvement in MASI scores on the combination treated side as opposed to the side treated by the alexandrite laser alone.[40] However, two patients developed severe hyperpigmentation and one patient had transient hypopigmentation.

A relatively new nonablative technology, FP, has shown promise for the treatment of melasma (Fig. 7.4). FP produces a pixilated pattern of multiple columns of thermal damage on the skin.[41,42] FP can control the pattern density and depth of thermal damage. In this way, different 3-dimensional column sizes of thermal damage can be created. This thermal damage extends into the reticular dermis, while producing

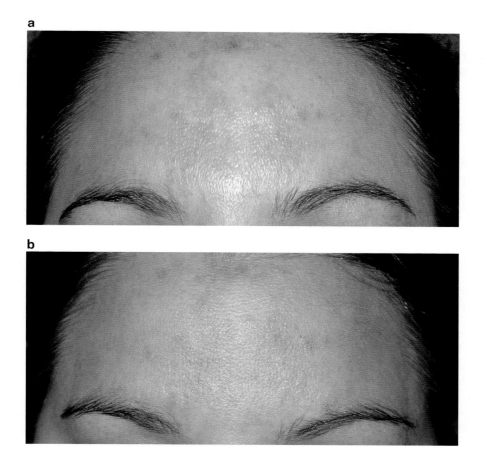

Fig. 7.4 (**a**) Baseline. (**b**) Status post fractional photothermolysis with Fraxel®

photocoagulation of the epidermis. Importantly, FP only minimally affects the tissue surrounding these columns. Thus, the remaining viable cells support a rapid healing time, with reepithelialization achieved in as little as one day. With the extrusion and replacement of damaged tissue, a "fractionalized resurfacing" occurs. The procedure is repeated four to five times at 2- to 4-week intervals. Postprocedure side effects are typically mild and include erythema and edema. Because there is no dermal or epidermal ablation, there is none of the significant recovery time associated with ablative laser therapy.[41] Lasers incorporating this technique include Erbium:YAG, CO_2, and diode, with an increasing number of choices coming to market each year.

Preliminary studies have shown improvement of melasma after a series of fractional resurfacing treatments.[43,44] In a study of ten patients with skin types III–V treated for recalcitrant melasma, 60% had more than 75% clearing after four to six fractional resurfacing treatments at 1- to 2-week intervals.[43] The precise mechanism leading to clinical improvement of melasma is unclear. Increased absorption of the concurrent bleaching agents through the microthermal treatment zones and/or increased elimination of epidermal and dermal pigment are proposed theories. Further investigations are necessary to assess the efficacy and safety of this technology in Fitzpatrick skin types V–VI.

7.1.6   Medication-Induced Hyperpigmentation

Some medications such as amiodarone, minocycline, tricyclic antidepressants, phenothiazine, antimalarials, clofazamine, gold, silver, bismuth, and arsenic may induce dyspigmentation over sun-exposed areas, varying from blue-gray to red-brown. Chemotherapy-induced hyperpigmentation may appear as a localized eruption such as the flagellate pigmentation of bleomycin or the flexural hyperpigmentation of topical carmustine, or as generalized hyperpigmentation as with busulfan, cyclophosphamide, or methotrexate.

Removal of the offending agent can lead to the resolution of the pigmentation over time; however, some medication-induced pigmentation may persist for years despite cessation of therapy.

QS lasers can be useful in the treatment of certain medication-related hyperpigmentation. The QS ruby and alexandrite lasers have been reported to be effective in the resolution of the imipramine-induced blue-gray pigmentation without discontinuing the medication.[45] Another report described the successful treatment of amiodarone-induced hyperpigmentation with the QS ruby laser.[46]

Minocycline-induced hyperpigmentation[47–49] can be treated safely and effectively with QS lasers. Alster and Gupta reported complete pigment resolution in six patients with minocycline-induced hyperpigmentation after an average of four bimonthly sessions using the QS alexandrite laser.[50] Clearance of minocycline-induced hyperpigmentation has also been reported with the QS ruby and Nd:YAG lasers. In darker skinned individuals, the use of the longer wavelength 1,064 nm QS

Nd:YAG laser would be preferable over the shorter wavelength lasers to minimize the risk of posttreatment dyspigmentation.

References

1. Ortonne JP, Pandya AG, Lui H, Hexsel D. Treatment of solar lentigines. *J Am Acad Dermatol.* 2006;54(5 Suppl 2):S262–S271.
2. Stern RS, Dover JS, Levin JA, Arndt KA. Laser therapy versus cryotherapy of lentigines: a comparative trial. *J Am Acad Dermatol.* 1994;30(6):985–987.
3. Farris PK. Combination therapy for solar lentigines. *J Drugs Dermatol.* 2004;3(5 Suppl):S23–S26.
4. Chan HH. Effective and safe use of lasers, light sources, and radiofrequency devices in the clinical management of Asian patients with selected dermatoses. *Lasers Surg Med.* 2005;37(3):179–185.
5. Chan HH, Kono T. The use of lasers and intense pulsed light sources for the treatment of pigmentary lesions. *Skin Therapy Lett.* 2004;9(8):5–7.
6. Chan H. The use of lasers and intense pulsed light sources for the treatment of acquired pigmentary lesions in Asians. In: *J Cosmet Laser Ther.* 2003:198-200.
7. Lee PK, Rosenberg CN, Tsao H, Sober AJ. Failure of Q-switched ruby laser to eradicate atypical-appearing solar lentigo: report of two cases. *J Am Acad Dermatol.* 1998;38(2 Pt 2):314–317.
8. Downs AM, Rickard A, Palmer J. Laser treatment of benign pigmented lesions in children: effective long-term benefits of the Q-switched frequency-doubled Nd:YAG and long-pulsed alexandrite lasers. *Pediatr Dermatol.* 2004;21(1):88–90.
9. Shimbashi T, Kamide R, Hashimoto T. Long-term follow-up in treatment of solar lentigo and cafe-au-lait macules with Q-switched ruby laser. *Aesthetic Plast Surg.* 1997;21(6):445–458.
10. Kono T, Manstein D, Chan HH, Nozaki M, Anderson RR. Q-switched ruby versus long-pulsed dye laser delivered with compression for treatment of facial lentigines in Asians. *Lasers Surg Med.* 2005;38(2):94–97.
11. Kono T, Chan HH, Groff WF, et al. Long-pulse pulsed dye laser delivered with compression for treatment of facial lentigines. *Dermatol Surg.* 2007;33(8):945–950.
12. Chan HH, Fung WK, Ying SY, Kono T. An in vivo trial comparing the use of different types of 532 nm Nd:YAG lasers in the treatment of facial lentigines in Oriental patients. *Dermatol Surg.* 2000;26(8):743–749.
13. Kawada A, Shiraishi H, Asai M, et al. Clinical improvement of solar lentigines and ephelides with an intense pulsed light source. *Dermatol Surg.* 2002;28(6):504–508.
14. Kono T, Groff WF, Sakurai H, et al. Comparison study of intense pulsed light versus a long-pulse pulsed dye laser in the treatment of facial skin rejuvenation. *Ann Plast Surg.* 2007;59(5):479–483.
15. Li YT, Yang KC. Comparison of the frequency-doubled Q-switched Nd:YAG laser and 35% trichloroacetic acid for the treatment of face lentigines. *Dermatol Surg.* 1999;25(3):202–204.
16. Grossman MC, Anderson RR, Farinelli W, Flotte TJ, Grevelink JM. Treatment of cafe au lait macules with lasers. A clinicopathologic correlation. *Arch Dermatol.* 1995;131(12):1416–1420.
17. Kilmer SL, Garden JM. Laser treatment of pigmented lesions and tattoos. *Semin Cutan Med Surg.* 2000;19(4):232–244.
18. Carpo BG, Grevelink JM, Grevelink SV. Laser treatment of pigmented lesions in children. *Semin Cutan Med Surg.* 1999;18(3):233–243.
19. Acland KM, Barlow RJ. Lasers for the dermatologist. *Br J Dermatol.* 2000;143(2):244–255.
20. Alster TS, Williams CM. Cafe-au-lait macule in type V skin: successful treatment with a 510 nm pulsed dye laser. *J Am Acad Dermatol.* 1995;33(6):1042–1043.
21. Watanabe S, Takahashi H. Treatment of nevus of Ota with the Q-switched ruby laser. *N Engl J Med.* 1994;331(26):1745–1750.

22. Kono T, Chan HH, Ercocen AR, et al. Use of Q-switched ruby laser in the treatment of nevus of ota in different age groups. *Lasers Surg Med*. 2003;32(5):391–395.

23. Kang W, Lee E, Choi GS. Treatment of Ota's nevus by Q-switched alexandrite laser: therapeutic outcome in relation to clinical and histopathological findings. *Eur J Dermatol*. 1999;9(8):639–643.

24. Chan HH, Ying SY, Ho WS, Kono T, King WW. An in vivo trial comparing the clinical efficacy and complications of Q-switched 755 nm alexandrite and Q-switched 1064 nm Nd:YAG lasers in the treatment of nevus of Ota. *Dermatol Surg*. 2000;26(10):919–922.

25. Chan HH, Leung RS, Ying SY, et al. A retrospective analysis of complications in the treatment of nevus of Ota with the Q-switched alexandrite and Q-switched Nd:YAG lasers. *Dermatol Surg*. 2000;26(11):1000–1006.

26. Chan HH, Leung RS, Ying SY, Lai CF, Chua J, Kono T. Recurrence of nevus of Ota after successful treatment with Q-switched lasers. *Arch Dermatol*. 2000;136(9):1175–1176.

27. Hori Y, Takayama O. Circumscribed dermal melanoses. Classification and histologic features. *Dermatol Clin*. 1988;6(2):315–326.

28. Lam AY, Wong DS, Lam LK, Ho WS, Chan HH. A retrospective study on the efficacy and complications of Q-switched alexandrite laser in the treatment of acquired bilateral nevus of Ota-like macules. *Dermatol Surg*. 2001;27(11):937–941; discussion 41-42.

29. Polnikorn N, Tanrattanakorn S, Goldberg DJ. Treatment of Hori's nevus with the Q-switched Nd:YAG laser. *Dermatol Surg*. 2000;26(5):477–480.

30. Kunachak S, Leelaudomlipi P. Q-switched Nd:YAG laser treatment for acquired bilateral nevus of ota-like maculae: a long-term follow-up. *Lasers Surg Med*. 2000;26(4):376–379.

31. Manuskiatti W, Sivayathorn A, Leelaudomlipi P, Fitzpatrick RE. Treatment of acquired bilateral nevus of Ota-like macules (Hori's nevus) using a combination of scanned carbon dioxide laser followed by Q-switched ruby laser. *J Am Acad Dermatol*. 2003;48(4):584–591.

32. Ee HL, Goh CL, Khoo LS, Chan ES, Ang P. Treatment of acquired bilateral nevus of ota-like macules (Hori's nevus) with a combination of the 532 nm Q-Switched Nd:YAG laser followed by the 1,064 nm Q-switched Nd:YAG is more effective: prospective study. *Dermatol Surg*. 2006;32(1):34–40.

33. Grimes PE. Melasma. Etiologic and therapeutic considerations. *Arch Dermatol*. 1995;131(12):1453–1457.

34. Pathak MA, Fitzpatrick TB, Kraus EW. Usefulness of retinoic acid in the treatment of melasma. *J Am Acad Dermatol*. 1986;15(4 Pt 2):894–899.

35. Fitzpatrick RE, Goldman MP, Ruiz-Esparza J. Laser treatment of benign pigmented epidermal lesions using a 300 nsecond pulse and 510 nm wavelength. *J Dermatol Surg Oncol*. 1993;19(4):341–347.

36. Grekin RC, Shelton RM, Geisse JK, Frieden I. 510-nm pigmented lesion dye laser. Its characteristics and clinical uses. *J Dermatol Surg Oncol*. 1993;19(4):380–387.

37. Goldberg DJ. Benign pigmented lesions of the skin. Treatment with the Q-switched ruby laser. *J Dermatol Surg Oncol*. 1993;19(4):376–379.

38. Taylor CR, Anderson RR. Ineffective treatment of refractory melasma and postinflammatory hyperpigmentation by Q-switched ruby laser. *J Dermatol Surg Oncol*. 1994;20(9):592–597.

39. Manaloto RM, Alster T. Erbium:YAG laser resurfacing for refractory melasma. *Dermatol Surg*. 1999;25(2):121–123.

40. Angsuwarangsee S, Polnikorn N. Combined ultrapulse CO_2 laser and Q-switched alexandrite laser compared with Q-switched alexandrite laser alone for refractory melasma: split-face design. *Dermatol Surg*. 2003;29(1):59–64.

41. Fisher GH, Geronemus RG. Short-term side effects of fractional photothermolysis. *Dermatol Surg*. 2005;31(9 Pt 2):1245–1249; discussion 9.

42. Manstein D, Herron GS, Sink RK, Tanner H, Anderson RR. Fractional photothermolysis: a new concept for cutaneous remodeling using microscopic patterns of thermal injury. *Lasers Surg Med*. 2004;34(5):426–438.

43. Rokhsar CK, Fitzpatrick RE. The treatment of melasma with fractional photothermolysis: a pilot study. *Dermatol Surg*. 2005;31(12):1645–1650.

44. Tannous ZS, Astner S. Utilizing fractional resurfacing in the treatment of therapy-resistant melasma. *J Cosmet Laser Ther.* 2005;7(1):39–43.
45. Atkin DH, Fitzpatrick RE. Laser treatment of imipramine-induced hyperpigmentation. *J Am Acad Dermatol.* 2000;43(1 Pt 1):77–80.
46. Karrer S, Hohenleutner U, Szeimies RM, Landthaler M. Amiodarone-induced pigmentation resolves after treatment with the Q-switched ruby laser. *Arch Dermatol.* 1999;135(3):251–253.
47. Green D, Friedman KJ. Treatment of minocycline-induced cutaneous pigmentation with the Q-switched Alexandrite laser and a review of the literature. *J Am Acad Dermatol.* 2001;44(2 Suppl):342–347.
48. Becker-Wegerich PM, Kuhn A, Malek L, Lehmann P, Megahed M, Ruzicka T. Treatment of nonmelanotic hyperpigmentation with the Q-switched ruby laser. *J Am Acad Dermatol.* 2000;43(2 Pt 1):272–274.
49. Friedman IS, Shelton RM, Phelps RG. Minocycline-induced hyperpigmentation of the tongue: successful treatment with the Q-switched ruby laser. *Dermatol Surg.* 2002;28(3):205–209.
50. Alster TS, Gupta SN. Minocycline-induced hyperpigmentation treated with a 755-nm Q-switched alexandrite laser. *Dermatol Surg.* 2004;30(9):1201–1204.

Chapter 8
Light Therapies for Cutaneous T-Cell Lymphoma

Katalin Ferenczi and Elma D. Baron

8.1 Introduction/Definition

Cutaneous T-cell lymphomas (CTCL) represent a broad group of non-Hodgkin's lymphomas with considerable heterogeneity with respect to clinical presentation, histology, immunophenotype, and prognosis. The preferential localization of the malignant T-cell clone to the skin is a hallmark feature characteristic of all primary CTCL.[1,2]

Mycosis fungoides (MF) and the Sézary syndrome (SS) make up the majority of cases of CTCL. The term MF was originally coined by Alibert and Bazin 200 years ago because of the mushroom-like appearance of the tumors. SS is the leukemic variant of CTCL, classically described by the triad of erythroderma, lymphadenopathy, and the presence of the malignant T-cell clone in the blood. SS was previously categorized as a subtype of MF; however, the new WHO-European Organization of Research and Treatment of Cancer (EORTC) classification system scheme lists MF and SS as separate entities (Table 8.1). Given the heterogeneity in clinical, pathological, and prognostic features of cutaneous lymphomas, it is important to distinguish MF from other forms of primary CTCL (Table 8.1).[3] Also, distinction between primary and secondary/nodal CTCL is very important as primary cutaneous lymphomas have a slow and indolent clinical course as opposed to their systemic counterparts when systemic manifestations and internal organ involvement are present from the time of diagnosis, and skin involvement is a secondary phenomenon[2] (for review, see Ferenczi and Kupper [4]).

K. Ferenczi (✉) and E.D. Baron
Department of Dermatology, University Hospitals Case Medical Center and Case Western Reserve University, Veterans Affairs Medical Center, Cleveland, OH
e-mail: katalin.ferenczi@uhhospitals.org

E.D. Baron (ed.), *Light-Based Therapies for Skin of Color*,
DOI: 10.1007/ 978-1-84882-328-0_8, © Springer-Verlag London Limited 2009

Table 8.1 WHO-EORTC classification of primary cutaneous T-cell lymphomas

Mycosis fungoides (*MF*)
Variants of MF:
  • Folliculotropic MF
  • Pagetoid reticulosis
  • Granulomatous slack skin
Sézary syndrome
Adult T-cell leukemia/lymphoma
Primary cutaneous CD30+ lymphoproliferative disorders
  • Primary cutaneous anaplastic large-cell lymphoma
  • Lymphomatoid papulosis
Subcutaneous panniculitis-like T-cell lymphoma
Extranodal NK/T-cell lymphoma, nasal type
Primary cutaneous peripheral T-cell lymphoma, unspecified
  • Primary cutaneous aggressive epidermotropic CD8+ T-cell lymphoma[a]
  • Cutaneous γ/δ T-cell lymphoma[a]
  • Primary cutaneous CD4+ small-/medium-sized pleomorphic T-cell lymphoma[a]

[a]Provisional entities

8.2 Incidence/Prevalence

The incidence of CTCL among whites is estimated at 6.1 per million persons per year and it has risen dramatically since 1973.[5] Higher annual incidence of CTCL has been reported among African-American patients (nine per million), which translates into an approximately 50% greater incidence in black as compared to white patients.[6] In contrast, the incidence of SS appears to be higher among white than in African-American patients.[5] CTCL is less common in Asians and Hispanics.

8.2.1 Pathogenesis

While much progress has been made in recent years in understanding the immunology of the disease, the exact pathogenesis of MF is not completely understood.

The malignant T-cell clone in CTCL has a skin homing memory phenotype (CD4+CD45RO+CLA+CCR4+),[4,7,8] explaining the strikingly increased affinity of the malignant T cells for the skin, in particular the epidermis. These epidermotropic neoplastic lymphocytes frequently form aggregates in proximity to Langerhans cells and form the so-called Pautrier's microabscesses in MF skin. Epidermal Langerhans cells have been suggested to play a role in constitutive antigenic stimulation of malignant T cells and subsequent proliferation and clonal expansion.[9]

In early stages of the disease, malignant T cells are – in most part – confined to the skin.

Accumulation of progressive mutations with disease progression is often associated with diminished clonal T-cell dependence on the skin and results in accumulation of malignant T cells in the peripheral blood and lymph node, such as in SS, extra-cutaneous disease, and disseminated lymphoma.

A significant reduction in the entire T-cell receptor (TCR) repertoire complexity is most notable in advanced stages of the disease.[10] Disrupted TCR repertoire complexity as well as the recent findings showing that MF/CTCL is a tumor of regulatory T cells (Tregs, CD25+CD4+), a group of lymphocytes that actively inhibit immune responses[9] provides partial explanation for the immunosuppression and susceptibility to infections noted in advanced CTCL. Immunosuppression has also been linked with a Th2 predominant cytokine pattern, frequently noted in advanced disease, along with a decline in the level of IL-12 and IFN-α.[11] Diminished levels of these cytokines are paralleled by a decrease in peripheral blood dendritic cell (DC) numbers.[11] Expansion of the malignant T-cell clone in the peripheral blood also results in concomitant decrease in cytotoxic CD8+ T-cell and NK cell populations (for review, see Kim et al[12]).

Disease progression in CTCL has been associated with several genetic abnormalities, such as p53, p16/p15 alterations, and deletion of NAV3 tumor suppressor gene (for review, see Hwang et al[13] and Karenko et al[14]). JUNB, a transcription factor responsible for regulating cell proliferation, differentiation, transformation, but also promotion of a Th2 phenotype is overexpressed in SS.[15] Dysregulation of STAT (signal transducers and activator of transcription) proteins and, most importantly, constitutive STAT3 activation in SS patients could contribute to CD25 expression by tumor cells.[16]

The chronic and indolent nature of primary CTCL has been postulated to be mediated by the slow accumulation of the malignant T-cell clone in the skin and/or intrinsic resistance of the malignant T cells to apoptosis. Defective Fas/Fas-L expression and increased expression of the antiapoptotic protein bcl-2[17-20] have been hypothesized to be part of the mechanisms underlying dysregulation of apoptosis in CTCL.

8.2.2   Clinical Findings and CTCL Variants

MF presents in mid-to-late adulthood with erythematous scaly patches (Fig. 8.1a), plaques (Fig. 8.1b), tumors (Fig. 8.2), or generalized erythema (erythroderma). The rare, poikilodermatous variant of MF presents as atrophic and dyspigmented patches (Fig. 8.3). MF lesions tend to localize to non-sun-exposed areas, such as trunk, buttocks, and this clinical observation was originally the rationale for treating the disease with light therapy.[21] Preferential facial localization can be seen in tumor stage (Fig. 8.2) and the folliculotropic variant of MF. There is considerable heterogeneity in the clinical presentation of MF and other primary CTCL variants (Table 8.1).[3]

Hypopigmented MF is a variant of MF seen almost exclusively in dark-skinned patients, predominantly children and younger individuals.[22] Hypopigmented MF presents with hypopigmented patches and plaques (Fig. 8.4) and can easily be confused with hypopigmentation due to other etiologies, such as pityriasis alba, tinea versicolor, or postinflammatory hypopigmentation. CD30+ primary cutaneous

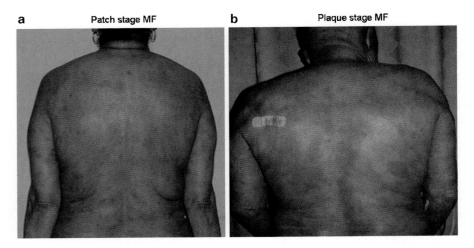

Fig. 8.1 Clinical presentation of mycosis fungoides in patch (**a**) and plaque (**b**) stage

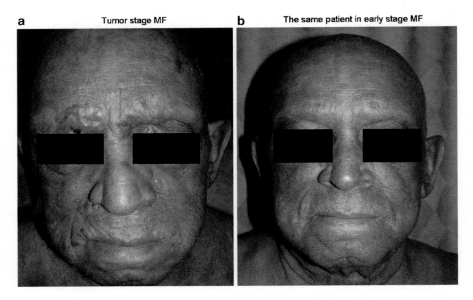

Fig. 8.2 Clinical manifestations in advanced, tumor stage mycosis fungoides (*MF*) (**a**). Note the absence of tumors in the same patient in earlier stages of the disease (**b**)

analplastic large-cell lymphomas present as solitary or localized skin lesions, nodules that have a tendency for ulceration. Lymphomatoid papulosis (LyP) is another (frequently CD30+) variant of CTCL which typically presents as waxing and waning papulovesicular, hemorrhagic, then necrotic papules.

Poikilodermatous MF

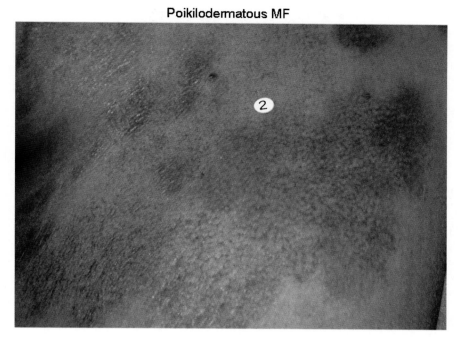

Fig. 8.3 Poikilodermatous mycosis fungoides. Note the atrophic, mottled erythematous patches on the breast of an African-American woman

Hypopigmented mycosis fungoides

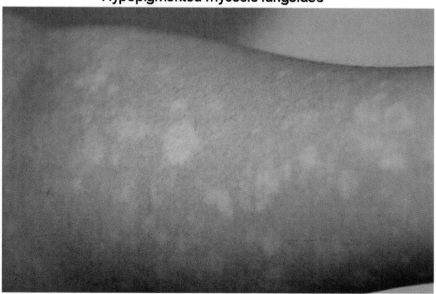

Fig. 8.4 Clinical presentation of hypopigmented mycosis fungoides

Pagetoid reticulosis, also known as Woringer-Kolopp disease, is a form of CTCL that most frequently presents as a solitary erythematous plaque involving the distal extremities.

Granulomatous slack skin is an extremely rare subtype of CTCL characterized by the slow development of folds of lax skin in the axillae and groin.

Erythroderma and generalized lymphadenopathy are features almost invariably present in SS, the leukemic variant of CTCL. Erythroderma in SS may be associated with marked exfoliation, edema, lichenification, and intense pruritus. Lymphadenopathy, alopecia, onychodystrophy, and palmoplantar hyperkeratosis are common findings.

8.2.3   Diagnosis/Histology/Workup

The clinical and histological features of cutaneous lymphomas often tend to be nonspecific for many years or even decades; therefore, establishing the diagnosis can be challenging. The diagnosis is dependent on integration of a combination of clinical features, histopathological, immunohistochemical, flow cytometry, imaging, and molecular studies.

The histology of a biopsy from MF lesion often shows a psoriasiform and/or patchy lichenoid or band-like lymphocytic infiltrate in the upper dermis (Fig. 8.5). Epidermotropism of the atypical large T cells with cerebriform nuclei is a highly characteristic feature (Fig. 8.5), although this may become less prominent in advanced disease, such as in tumor stage MF. Pautrier's microabscesses, a collection/aggregate of malignant T lymphocytes (in the presence or absence of Langerhans cells) in the epidermis, although very specific for MF, are seen only in a minority of the cases.[23] Malignant lymphocytes frequently line up along the epidermal basal layer, resembling a string of pearls. Histological findings in MF are frequently nondiagnostic and serial repeated biopsies are often necessary for a definitive diagnosis.

Immunohistochemical stains are an important adjunctive in the histological diagnosis of MF. The neoplastic T cells in MF have a CD3+CD4+ and CD45RO+ (memory) phenotype. In rare cases, such as in pagetoid reticulosis and hypopigmented MF, a CD8+ phenotype can be seen, which may be associated with an improved prognosis.[24,25] The presence of increased numbers of CD8+ T cells in CTCL lesions might indicate host antitumor response against malignant CD4+ T cells.[26] Aggressive cases of cutaneous lymphoma with a CD8+ phenotype have been reported.[27] Loss of pan-T-cell antigens such as CD2, CD3, CD5, CD7 but also CD26 is often observed, of which loss of CD7 and CD26 are the most frequently reported phenotypic aberration. Expression of the CD30 antigen is observed in primary cutaneous anaplastic large-cell lymphomas and LyP. A CD30+ phenotype is also seen in MF lesions undergoing large-cell transformation. Large-cell transformation is defined by the presence of large cells (CD30 positive or negative) in 25% or more of the dermal infiltrate and is a poor prognostic sign.[28-30]

Clonal TCR gene rearrangements are detected in most cases of CTCL.[31] Evidence for the presence of clonality can be very helpful but not very specific, as it can be

Histopathology of mycosis fungoides

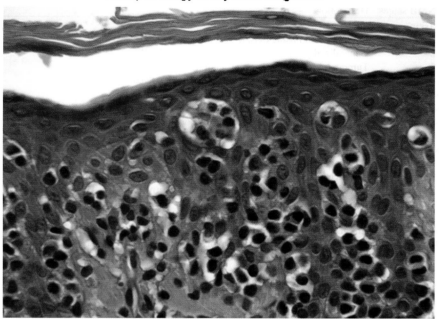

Fig. 8.5 Histopathology of classical mycosis fungoides. The skin biopsy shows an atypical lymphocytic infiltrate with prominent epidermotropism in the absence of spongiosis. The presence of Pautrier's microabscesses, a collection of atypical lymphocytes around a Langerhans cell, in the epidermis is a hallmark feature

detected in approximately 2.3% of benign dermatoses.[32] T-cell clonality can be a useful tool for assessment of minimal residual disease after treatment.[33]

The diagnosis of SS is dependent on the presence of erythroderma and molecular or flow cytometric evidence of peripheral blood involvement by clonal T cells (*see* Tables 8.2 and 8.3). Lymphadenopathy, previously described as criteria in the SS triad, although frequently present, is no longer essential for the diagnosis of SS. The current guidelines recommended by the International Society for Cutaneous Lymphomas and EORTC for evaluation and workup of a patient with suspected MF or SS are summarized in Table 8.4.[34]

8.2.4   Classification/Staging/Prognosis

The clinical behavior of cutaneous lymphomas can range from an indolent, protracted course seen in early-stage CTCL to highly aggressive clinical behavior, characteristic of advanced disease, such as tumor stage MF and SS.

8.3   CTCL Treatment

Management of CTCL starts with thorough assessment to establish accurate diagnosis, staging, and classification and should be carried out by a multidisciplinary team including a dermatologist, hematologist/oncologist, and pathologist.

Treatment of primary CTCL depends on the stage of the disease. The extent of skin involvement affects prognosis and guides therapeutic decisions: skin-directed therapies utilized in early-stage CTCL (IA and IIB) typically result in durable remission and cures may be achieved, whereas advanced stages of CTCL require systemic therapy (for review, see Naeem and Kupper[40]).

In early stages of CTCL, the malignant T cells are confined to the skin and are accessible for local treatments, such as topical steroids, bexarotene gel, photochemotherapy with psoralen plus ultraviolet A (PUVA), topical nitrogen mustard (mechlorethamine) or chlormustine (BCNU), or radiotherapy, including total skin electron beam irradiation (Table 8.5).

In advanced disease, expansion of the malignant T-cell clone in the peripheral blood and extracutaneous disease occurs, therefore skin-directed therapies are no longer sufficient and combination therapies are warranted. Biologics such as interferon-α (IFN-α) and other cytokines, such as interleukin-12 (IL-12), traditional and new retinoids such as bexarotene, and receptor-targeted cytotoxic fusion proteins such as denileukin diftitox (DAB$_{389}$IL-2) are used either as single-agent therapy or in combination with other therapies (e.g. PUVA) in the treatment of MF (*see* Table 8.5).

Table 8.5 Summary of treatment modalities employed in CTCL

Early-stage CTCL (stages IA, IB, IIA):
- Topical mechlorethamine (nitrogen mustard)
- Topical carmustine (1,3-bis(2-chloroethyl)-I-nitrosourea; BCNU)
- Topical bexarotene 1% gel (Targretin, retinoid X receptor agonist)
- Oral bexarotene
- Topical peldesine (BCX-34) (purine nucleoside phosphorylase inhibitor)
- Phototherapy (PUVA, UVB)
- Radiotherapy

Advanced disease (stages IIB, III, IV):
- Extracorporeal photopheresis ± IFN-α ± bexarotene
- Immunotherapy: IFN-α (2a most frequently, 2b) ± PUVA, ECP, IL-12
- Monoclonal antibody: anti-CD4, anti-CD52 (Campath)
- DAB389-IL2 fusion toxin
- Retinoids and rexinoids (bexarotene[b])
- Radiation: total skin electron beam irradiation
- Single agent chemotherapy: alkylating agents, methotrexate, gemcytabine, pentostatin
- Combination chemotherapy: CHOP or EPOCH[a]
- Bone marrow transplantation
- Histone deacetylase inhibitors (HDACs, e.g., Vorinostat)

[a]*CHOP* cyclophosphamide, doxorubicin, vincristine, prednisone; *EPOCH* etoposide, prednisone, doxorubicin, and cyclophosphamide
[b]Bexarotene targets retinoid X receptor

Multiagent chemotherapy is generally used in cutaneous lymphoma with evidence of extracutaneous disease and/or systemic involvement, or in widespread tumor-stage MF refractory to skin-targeted therapies, under the supervision of a multidisciplinary team. Studies have failed to show a survival benefit in patients with MF with the use of aggressive chemotherapy.

8.4   Phototherapy in CTCL

Light therapy is probably the most widely used first-line skin-directed treatment for early-stage CTCL (for review, see Baron and Stevens[41]). Most CTCL patients with early disease can achieve durable remission of their disease by employing phototherapy alone. It is increasingly used in the outpatient management of CTCL and it can be administered at a dermatologist's office or home.

Phototherapy comprises a variety of different regimens including broadband UVB (BB-UVB; 290–320 nm), narrowband UVB (NB-UVB; 311–312 nm), UVA (320–400 nm)/PUVA, UVA1 (340–400 nm), extracorporeal photopheresis (ECP, combines photosensitizer with UVA), excimer laser (308 nm), photodynamic therapy (PDT), which consists of a combination of photosensitizer treatment followed by exposure to visible light (*see* Fig. 8.6). The most frequently used light

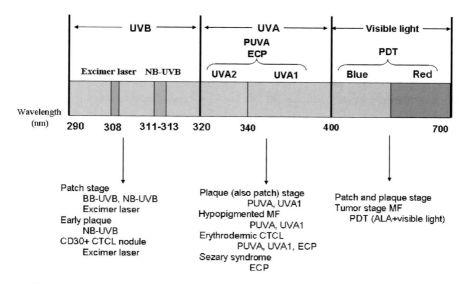

Fig. 8.6   Spectra of ultraviolet light sources in the treatment of cutaneous T-cell lymphomas (*CTCL*). *NB-UVB* narrow band UVB, *UVA* ultraviolet A, *PUVA* psoralen plus UVA, *ECP* extracorporeal photopheresis, *PDT* photodynamic therapy

Table 8.6 Skin phototype classification system based on a person's sensitivity to sunlight (A) and classification of Japanese skin phototypes (B)

A. Skin phototypes (*SPT*)
SPT I – Always burns, never tans
SPT II – Burns easily, tans minimally
SPT III – Burns moderately, tans gradually to light brown
SPT IV – Burns minimally, always tans well to moderately brown
SPT V – Rarely burns, tans profusely to dark
SPT VI – Never burns, deeply pigmented
B. Japanese phototypes
Type I – Always burns, never tans
Type II – Burns sometimes, moderately tans
Type III – Never burns, always tans

treatment in the management of MF is PUVA, which combines a photosensitizer, such as oral methoxypsoralen (MOP) with UVA and UVB light, especially NB-UVB (*see* Fig. 8.6).

All of these light therapy options have advantages and disadvantages and the choice among these options depends on multiple factors, one of the most important ones are: extent of skin involvement, presence of patches or plaques, thickness of the plaques, the presence or absence of erythroderma, and blood involvement. While UVB treatment does not require the use of a photosensitizer and is associated with fewer side effects, PUVA treatment due to longer wavelengths has a deeper penetration (approximately 1–2 cm into the mid-dermis), leads to longer remission times, and is therefore more effective in CTCL patients with thick plaques. The presence of erythroderma and peripheral blood involvement such as seen in SS warrants more than just skin-directed therapy. Such patients are good candidates for ECP treatment.

The focus of this chapter is light treatment of patients with CTCL with emphasis on phototherapy of individuals with darker skin types, such as African-American patients and races of intermediate pigmentation, such as Hispanics and Asians, which share epidemiological and clinical features of dark-skinned ethnic groups and Caucasians.

There are some fundamental differences between light and dark skin, therefore when it comes to treating CTCL using light therapy, the ethnic background must be considered. When compared with light skin, dark skin has higher melanin content in the epidermis, larger and more melanized melanosomes, and slower degradation of melanosomes in the keratinocytes.

Assessment of skin type according to Fitzpatrick's phototype classification is based on self-reported erythema sensitivity and tanning ability (Table 8.6A). This classification is an imperfect but useful guide to help adjust the parameters in a way that suits dark skin. This skin phototype classification proved to have limited value in evaluation of Asian skin, therefore a separate classification scheme exists to assess Japanese skin type. The Japanese skin type has been classified into three categories (Table 8.6B). Among the Japanese skin types, type I patients are more susceptible to skin cancer development.[42,43]

Special considerations confront clinicians when treating patients with skin of color using light treatment. One of the most important factors that must be considered when treating dark-skinned patients is the selection of the correct minimal erythema dose (MED) if treatment with UVB is considered. MED is the dose of UV radiation required to produce a minimally perceptible erythema 24 h after exposure. Selection of the appropriate MED is key for achieving effective therapeutic outcome as the MED value is usually higher in dark-skinned patients compared to patients with lighter skin color.[44,45] An MED that is approximately 6–33 times higher has been reported in blacks compared to Caucasians.[46] A gradual decrease in the MED value secondary to photoadaptation due to acquired pigmentation during repetitive UV exposures is another consideration that the clinician needs to be aware of when escalating the dose of UV light when treating CTCL in a patient with darker complexion.[47]

The starting dose of UVA is also based on the patient's skin type. Assessment of the minimal phototoxic dose (MPD) 72 h following ingestion of 8-MOP is helpful prior to initiation of PUVA treatment.

While it is believed that UV light treatment is safer for dark-skinned patients because of the lower risk of adverse effects, it has been shown that dark skin is as easily irritated as Caucasian skin.[48] Also, erythema is difficult to detect in darker skin due to its greater melanin content, therefore it is not a great indicator as an index of skin sensitivity. Reflectance spectroscopy is a useful research tool in quantification of the degree of erythema and melanin content of the skin.[49] Dark-skinned patients may be at risk for pigmentary alterations: hypo-, hyper-, and depigmentation. If the correct parameters are used, dark-skinned CTCL patients can be safely and effectively treated with UV light.

8.4.1 Phototherapy and Its Mechanism of Action

The effect of UV therapy in general is mediated via induction of apoptosis and/or immune suppression. T-cell apoptosis has been documented with most UV therapies employed in the management of CTCL, such as NB-UVB, PUVA but also UVA1 and ECP.[41,50–54]

An increase in the expression of TNF-α and IL-10 release has been suggested to play an important role in UV-induced immune suppression.[55,56] More recently, reports have shown that UV light induces regulatory T cells (Tregs), lymphocytes that inhibit immune responses, and these regulatory T cells specifically induced by UV (UV-Treg) suppress immune functions via IL-10. Platelet-activating factor binding, a potent phospholipid mediator, appears to be crucial for both PUVA- and UVB-induced immune suppression.[57,58] Platelet-activating factor has been reported to be involved in other PUVA-induced effects, including IL-10 production, apoptosis, and p53 upregulation.[58] UV treatment also results in a decrease in IL-7, a cytokine that has been shown to act as a growth factor for Sézary cells.[59,60]

Both UVB and PUVA downregulate the expression of surface molecules such as major histocompatibility complex II and intercellular adhesion molecule-1, further dampening antigen-presenting functions and other cell–cell interactions. Decreased numbers and/or diminished antigen-presenting capacity of Langerhans cells have been reported to occur in association with both UVB and PUVA.[61]

The mechanism of action of UVB in cutaneous lymphomas is postulated to be mediated by a decrease in the antigen-presenting capacity of Langerhans cells, an increase in IL-2 and -6 and TNF production by keratinocytes,[62,63] as well as induction of apoptosis.

UVB causes deoxyribonucleic acid (DNA) damage and is able to inhibit keratinocyte and T-cell proliferation.

PUVA inhibits clonal lymphocyte proliferation[64,65] and leads to induction of T-cell apoptosis.[50,51] Novel apoptogenic molecules have been recently identified to play a relevant role in PUVA therapy-associated apoptosis induced by the production of photoproducts of psoralen.[66]

The mechanism of action of UVA1 is comparable to broad-spectrum UVA, induction of lymphocyte apoptosis and decrease in the number of Langerhans cells has been reported. However, unlike PUVA and UVB, which induce one apoptotic mechanism, UVA1 seems to trigger lymphocyte apoptosis via two apoptotic pathways.[67]

8.4.2 Relationship Between Phototherapy and Skin Cancer Risk

Phototherapy within the UVB and UVA spectra has both beneficial and harmful effects on skin. UV radiation is both immunosuppressive but also highly carcinogenic. Formation of DNA adducts with activated psoralen and thymine dimers in association with PUVA and UVB treatment respectively are associated with an increased risk of skin cancer.

UV radiation induces DNA damage in epidermal cells. If the DNA damage is not repaired or the damaged cells are not eliminated by apoptosis, the consequence can be cell transformation and eventually skin tumor formation. An important "repair" gene is the p53 suppressor gene. Excessive UVB exposure can lead to mutation of the tumor suppressor p53 gene, causing specific "UV-signature mutations" in the p53 gene leading to the loss of its repair function and apoptosis resistance of the DNA-damaged cell. UV-signature mutations in the p53 gene are the most common event in the development of squamous cell carcinoma (SCC). UVB radiation-induced point mutations in the p53 gene are found in SCC and occasional basal cell carcinomas (BCCs). UVB in general is more carcinogenic than UVA in induction of SCC and NB-UVB phototherapy (311–312 nm) is considered to be less carcinogenic than BB-UVB (290–320 nm).

In contrast to UVB radiation, much of the mutagenic and carcinogenic action of UVA radiation appears to be mediated through reactive oxygen species and long-wave UVA1 (340–400 nm) exposure has been shown to result in development of SCC without the characteristic point mutations in p53 (for review, see de Gruijl[68])

A large study including 1,380 psoriasis patients who had undergone long-term PUVA treatment reported by Stern and coworkers showed a modest trend of increased risk of melanoma, small but significantly increased risk of BCC, and a significantly increased risk of SCC.[69,70] The results from this study showed a correlation between the cumulative dose received and the degree of SCC risk.[69] An approximately 14-fold higher risk of SCC was reported after more than 200 sessions of PUVA.[71] Risk of basal cell cancer was substantially increased only in patients exposed to very high levels of PUVA.[72]

The risk of malignant melanoma associated with UV therapy has been controversial. In one study published by Stern and coworkers, an increased risk of malignant melanoma was observed approximately 15 years after the first treatment with PUVA, especially among patients who received 250 treatments or more.[73]

Patients at a particularly high risk for UV-induced skin cancers are those with skin types I and II. Increasing skin pigmentation has been shown to be associated with a diminished sensitivity to UV-induced DNA damage as dark skin absorbs and scatters more energy and the thicker dermis and larger melanosomes provide better photoprotection.

UV light exposure may be a risk factor for skin cancer in Asians.[38] Low incidence of nonmelanoma skin cancer was reported in Japanese patients.[74]

Dark-skinned ethnic patients have a lower risk of cutaneous malignancies and UV radiation is not considered to be an important etiological factor for skin cancer in black patients, with the exception of basal cell cancer (for review, see Gloster and Neal[38]).

Still, potentially increased skin cancer risk associated with phototherapy regardless of skin color mandates careful monitoring and regular skin examination for cancer screening in patients undergoing such therapy. Therefore, prior to initiation of light therapy, careful consideration of other treatment options is advised for patients with a history of melanoma or nonmelanoma skin cancer. It is important to stress to these patients the importance of avoiding sun exposure, indoor tanning, and the use of sunscreens after treatment.

8.5 Psoralen Plus UVA

The preferential occurrence of MF lesions on covered areas and the relative sparing of sun-exposed skin led to the application of PUVA in the treatment of CTCL, first reported by Gilchrest and coworkers in 1976. PUVA has been widely used now for more than three decades in the management of MF, in particular plaque-stage disease.[21]

PUVA photochemotherapy is a well-established and effective treatment widely used for the treatment of early, patch-, and plaque-stage MF (stage IB/IIA), which fails to respond to topical therapies.

PUVA therapy consists of oral ingestion of a photosensitizing agent, such as 8-MOP followed by total body UVA (320–400 nm) light exposure.

Psoralens are phototoxic furocoumarin compounds that, when activated by UVA light, bind covalently to pyrimidine bases in the DNA leading to formation of monoadducts and/or interstrand cross-links.[75] They are inactivated in the liver, with a plasma half-life of 1 h, and are cleared by the kidney 24 h after administration.

Patients take an oral dose of 8-MOP (0.65 mg/kg) 1.5–2 h prior to each UVA (320–400 nm; peak emission wavelength between 350 and 360 nm) treatment. Optimally, an individual's MPD should be measured prior to the initiation of the actual light treatment course. PUVA therapy is then started with an initial dose that is equal to half or two-thirds of the individual's MPD. The initial dose is 0.5–2 J/cm^2, depending on the skin type and it is increased by 0.5–1 J/cm^2. Another alternative is to start at 70% of MPD and increase by 0–20% depending on the erythemal response.[41] Subsequent increments in the dose depend on the presence or absence of phototoxic reaction/burning. Escalating doses of UVA are administered three times weekly until complete remission or best partial response is achieved. Treatment schedules have varied in reported studies, from two to four times weekly. At this point, the frequency (but not the UVA dose) is decreased gradually, and the patient may be maintained on once-monthly therapy for more than a year after remission. Because of the risk of nonmelanoma skin cancer with high cumulative doses, an effort should be made to restrict the total PUVA dose to less than 200 treatment sessions or a total cumulative dose between 1,000 and 1,500 J/cm^2.[76]

8-MOP is the most frequently used psoralen in PUVA (Fig. 8.7). 5-MOP (Fig. 8.7) is an alternative to 8-MOP with fewer side effects, especially less nausea, and phototoxicity. Comparable therapeutic efficacy was reported in a study assessing the safety and efficacy of 8-MOP and 5-MOP in PUVA therapy for MF.[77]

Topical or paint PUVA is a modified PUVA protocol in which 8-MOP is used in form of a lotion (between 0.1% and 0.3%) applied 30 min prior to UVA exposure. Bath PUVA is another version of PUVA protocol in which the affected skin is

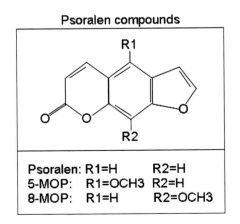

Fig. 8.7 Psoralen compounds used in PUVA therapy

soaked in a solution of 3 mg/liter of 8-MOP for 30 min before UVA exposure. In these modified PUVA protocols, the incremental dose of UVA is lower when compared to oral PUVA. Paint and bath PUVA are most frequently used in the treatment of vitiligo, psoriasis, and eczema and their use is not well established in the treatment of MF.

8.5.1 PUVA Monotherapy

PUVA therapy is highly effective in clearing early-stage disease and prolonging remissions with maintenance therapy. Overall response rates of 79–88% in stage IA and 52–59% in stage IB disease have been reported.[78,79]

In a study of 82 patients, Herrmann et al reported complete clearance of lesions and mean duration of remission of 13 months in 88% of patients with limited plaque disease and complete clearance and mean duration of remission of 11 months in 51.9% of patients with extensive plaque disease.[78] The overall complete response (CR) rate was 65% (79% for stage IA, 59% for stage IB, and 83% for stage IIA). The median time to complete remission was 3 months. Maintenance PUVA was given to most patients. The survival rates at 5 years in this study were 89% for stage IA, 78% in stage IB, and 100% in stage IIA. Clearing of the skin lesions and a durable remission were found to be much more likely with earlier stages of disease.[78]

In another study published by Roenigk in 1990, CR was observed in 88% of patients with stage IA, 52% in stage IB, and 46% in stage III. Interestingly, no response was seen in patients with stage IIB disease.[79] In this study, 38% of the complete responders relapsed despite maintenance treatment but responded to additional PUVA therapy.

Querfeld et al reported that of MF patients with stage IA/IIA who achieve a CR, 50% remain disease-free for 10 years and 50% will relapse regardless of maintenance therapy.[80] Patients that experienced a relapse responded when PUVA treatment was resumed and 36% remained disease-free. In this study, 66 patients were followed, including 2 African-American and 3 Hispanic patients. Relapse was noted in 49% of Caucasian patients, both African-American and one Hispanic patient. Interestingly, nonrelapsing patients required higher cumulative dose of PUVA and longer treatment to achieve CR than patients who later relapsed.

Another study of 44 patients reported by Honigsmann et al showed that 56% of stage IA and 39% of stage IB patients with CR had no recurrence during a period of 44 months follow-up without maintenance therapy.[81] This study also suggested that maintenance therapy is rarely effective at preventing relapse.

There appears to be no difference in clinical response to PUVA treatment in light and dark-skinned individuals as similar efficacy was reported in a study that included early-stage MF patients from Egypt showing a 70% clearance rate.[82] PUVA is also a proven and effective treatment option for the treatment of Asian patients with MF.[83] Benefit form PUVA therapy has been reported in the management of hypopigmented MF.[84]

8.5.2 PUVA Side Effects

The most frequently reported acute adverse effects of PUVA are mostly due to oral psoralen intake and include phototoxic reaction (similar to sunburn), nausea, vomiting, and pruritus. Treatment of the erythema and pruritus with emollients and other agents is usually satisfactory, and most patients eventually tolerate the therapy well. To prevent PUVA-induced cataracts, patients must wear UV-blocking goggles and protective eyewear during the day of their treatment. Shielding of the genital area is also recommended to prevent development of skin cancer in this location.

High cumulative PUVA doses can result in solar elastosis, solar lentigines, and other manifestations of photoaging and may be associated with higher risk of non-melanoma skin cancer. Patients with underlying photosensitive conditions such as lupus erythematosus, porphyria, and xeroderma pigmentosum, as well as patients with severe hepatic and renal impairment and pregnant patients should not receive PUVA therapy. Patients on PUVA are advised to avoid sunlight and apply sunscreens. Special sun avoidance precautions are needed in patients on medications associated with increased photosensitivity, such as diuretics, anticonvulsants, and certain antibiotics.

Since psoralens are metabolized by the liver, periodic hepatic function monitoring is required, especially in patients on hepatotoxic medications.

Another disadvantage of PUVA treatment is that lesions in the UV-shielded nonexposed areas (sanctuary sites), such as the flexures, are often not cleared or difficult to clear.

Patients may be refractory or become resistant to PUVA monotherapy, necessitating combination treatment. In such cases, combination treatment modalities can be attempted, such as IFN-α, systemic retinoids. Combination of PUVA therapy and topical chemotherapy such as nitrogen mustard should be avoided due to the increased incidence of skin cancer (for review, see Kim et al[85] and Guitart[86]).

8.5.3 PUVA Treatment as Part of Combination Therapy

The benefit of PUVA in combination with a number of agents, notably IFN-α, oral retinoids, and rexinoids in the management of CTCL patients resistant to mono-therapy has been reported in several studies. Such combination therapy for MF has the potential to be synergistic, improve therapeutic efficacy, and reduce toxicities.

8.5.4 PUVA Plus IFN-α

Several studies reported additional clinical benefit when PUVA was combined with IFN-α. IFN-α has been shown to have a proapoptotic effect and induce a shift in cytokine profile from Th2 to Th1,[87,88] potentiating the effect of PUVA. Such combination was reported to be safe, tolerable, and confers increased effectiveness in the management of CTCL.[89–92]

Kuzel and coworkers in a study of 39 patients with MF and SS combined PUVA treatment (three times weekly) with the maximum tolerated dose of IFN-α of 12 MU/m² three times weekly and reported an overall RR of 100%, CR was noted in 62% of the patients: 79% in stage IB patients, 80% in stage II, 33% in stage IIB, 63% in stage III, and 40% in stage IV patients.[89] PUVA was continued as maintenance therapy indefinitely while IFN-α was continued for 2 years. The median duration of remission was 28 months with a median survival of 62 months.[89]

Rupoli et al conducted a study assessing the effectiveness of PUVA plus IFN-α2b (6–18 MU weekly) combination treatment for 14 months in patients with early MF (stage IA–IIA). CR was noted in 84% of patients with stage IA, 87% in stage IB, and 73% in stage IIA.[91]

Chiarion-Sileni et al. treated 63 patients in all disease stages with escalating doses of IFN-α2a plus PUVA for 1 year, followed by PUVA maintenance in patients who experienced CR. Of the 63 patients, 74.6% achieved CR. Median response duration was 32 months and the 5-year survival rate was 75%.[90]

Roenigk et al treated 15 patients with PUVA and IFN at doses ranging from 6 to 30 MU three times weekly, 12 achieved CR and 2 had PR.[79] The median duration of response was 23 months.[79]

IFN-γ has also been reported to be effective in combination with PUVA in the management of CTCL.[93,94]

Potentially dose-limiting toxicities associated with IFN-α are fevers, malaise, leukopenia, mental status changes consisting of depression, and confusion.[79] Most of the side effects such as fever, myalgias, chills, fatigue, malaise, anorexia, weight loss and metallic taste tend to be dose-related. Initiation of therapy with a lower dose of IFN-α and gradual escalation over weeks until the desired dose is reached reduce flu-like symptoms.[89,95]

8.5.5   PUVA Plus IFN-α and/or Retinoids

The clinical efficacy of PUVA in MF can be further improved and toxicity is minimized by using it in combination with retinoids (acitretin or isotretinoin) plus/minus IFNs.

Stadler et al reported on 98 patients enrolled in a randomized controlled trial comparing PUVA (two to five times weekly) plus IFN-α (9 MU three times weekly) or PUVA and IFN-α plus a retinoid (acitretin).[96] In 82 patients with stage I/II disease, CR rates were 70% in the PUVA/IFN group compared with 38% in the IFN/acitretin group. Time to response was 18.6 weeks in the PUVA/IFN group, compared with 21.8 weeks in the IFN/acitretin group.[96]

The use of re-PUVA, a combination treatment consisting of PUVA given in conjunction with systemic retinoids was first reported by the Scandinavian Mycosis Fungoides Group.[97] A study of 69 patients with plaque-stage MF reported by Thomsen investigated the effects of PUVA alone as compared to the combination of PUVA and acitretin. Although RR in the re-PUVA group was equal to that of the PUVA (73% and 72%, respectively), in the re-PUVA group, remissions were obtained with fewer PUVA sessions and with a lower UVA dose. Also, the duration of remission was longer when maintenance retinoids were given.[97]

Studies also suggest that combined PUVA and IFN-α are more effective than combination of IFN-α and acitretin in early-stage I/II disease.[98]

8.5   PUVA Plus Rexinoids

Bexarotene is a synthetic retinoid that selectively binds the retinoid X-receptor. It has been shown to induce selective apoptosis of the malignant T-cell population.[99] Bexarotene can be used as monotherapy in CTCL and it has been shown to be safe and effective in combination with PUVA plus IFN-α2a.[100]

Combination therapy of PUVA with both high- and low-dose bexarotene (300 and 150 mg daily dose, respectively) has been shown to be effective in the treatment of MF patients.[101–103] Bexarotene given as a daily dose of 150 mg in combination with PUVA also resulted in durable remission in three of four cases of patients with SS.[104]

Side effects of bexarotene include hypertrigiceridemia and hypothyroidism, frequently requiring the addition of lipid-lowering agents and occasionally thyroid hormone replacement. Lipid-lowering agents that have been used in patients on bexarotene are atorvastatin or atorvastatin plus fenofibrate. Interestingly, patients on bexarotene taking two lipid-lowering agents have a significantly higher response rates than those taking one or no lipid-lowering agents (90% atorvastatin and fenofibrate vs 43% atorvastatin alone).[100]

In summary, deeper penetration and high efficacy in early plaque-stage MF is one of the advantages of PUVA therapy.

Although PUVA is a highly effective treatment for plaque-stage MF, the majority of patients subsequently relapse.[81,105] Its use in tumor stage (IIB) is controversial and as monotherapy it is not suitable for the management of erythrodermic CTCL/SS (for review, see Baron and Stevens[41]).

8.6   Ultraviolet A1 Therapy

Favorable clinical response in cutaneous lymphoma has been reported with the use of UVA1 therapy, a new and promising approach that uses selective long-wave UVA1 radiation (340–400 nm), while eliminating the erythemogenic UVA2 wavelengths (320–340 nm) (Fig. 8.6). It has been reported to be very effective in the treatment of several inflammatory dermatoses, such as atopic dermatitis, localized scleroderma/systemic sclerosis, urticaria pigmentosa, graft versus host disease, and psoriasis in HIV-infected patients. UVA1 has a deep penetration, therefore is effective in more advanced stages of cutaneous lymphoma, including nodular lesions of CTCL.

Zane et al reported complete clearance of cutaneous lymphoma lesions in 11 of 13 patients with widespread plaque and tumor-stage MF using high-dose UVA1 irradiation (100 J/cm^2 daily 5 days a week).[106]

Good clinical results were reported in another study conducted by Rombold et al in seven CTCL patients treated with UVA1 therapy using doses ranging between 40 and 70 J/cm².[107] UVA1 has also been used successfully in the treatment of hypopigmented MF.[108]

UVA1 treatment is generally well tolerated and it does not have the psoralen-associated gastrointestinal side effects and phototoxic reactions. Inability to clear sanctuary sites, such as the flexures, is a disadvantage. Adverse effects reported in association with UVA1 are erythema, hyperpigmentation, polymorphic light eruption, pruritus, skin dryness, photoaging, and skin cancer.[109]

8.7   Extracorporeal Photopheresis

ECP is a method developed by Edelson in 1987 to treat patients with SS.[110] It was FDA approved for use in advanced CTCL in 1988 and is now considered first-line treatment for CTCL stages III and IV either as monotherapy or as part of combination regimen.

ECP is a leukapheresis-based therapy[111] that targets apoptosis of malignant T cells in the circulation, therefore it is more likely to be effective in patients with peripheral blood involvement, such as SS but its efficacy has been reported in erythrodermic CTCL (with no peripheral blood involvement) as well. The technique consists of blood collection by apheresis, exposure of the peripheral blood mononuclear cells (PBMCs) to 8-MOP, and UVA light, followed by reinfusion of the treated cells (Fig. 8.8). Whole blood is removed from the patient via a peripheral or central venous line and centrifuged to separate the leukocyte-rich fraction. 8-MOP is then incorporated into the leukocyte-rich fraction and followed by irradiation with UVA light (320–400 nm) at a dose of 1.5–2 J/cm².[112,113]

8-MOP photosensitization of the leukocytes can be achieved either by oral administration or by extracorporeal exposure of the leukocyte-rich fraction to 8-MOP. In the past, 8-MOP was administered orally 2 h prior to the extracorporeal UVA exposure in a dose ranging between 60 and 200 ng/ml with the goal to achieve a minimum plasma concentration of 60 µg/ml as treatment efficacy was dependent on sufficient 8-MOP plasma levels. In order to circumvent the need for drug level monitoring, problems in obtaining consistent psoralen levels, and to eliminate or minimize systemic toxicity that may accompany oral psoralen ingestion, the technique was later on modified to direct methoxsalen exposure of the leukocyte-rich fraction. Liquid psoralen (methoxsalen) is added directly to the buffy coat bag at a concentration of 340 ng/ml (Uvadex®, Therakos), followed by UVA irradiation in a photoactivation chamber and the treated cells are subsequently returned to the patient. The entire procedure takes approximately 3–4 h. The procedure is performed monthly on two consecutive days every 3–4 weeks. Shortening the interval in nonresponding patients does not appear to lead to increase in the efficacy.[114]

ECP treatment is very well tolerated and has a very low side effect profile. It is available in approximately 150 medical centers worldwide.[115]

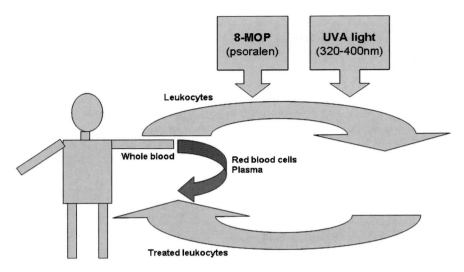

Fig. 8.8 Extracorporeal photopheresis (*ECP*) procedure consists of three major steps: collection and separation of the peripheral blood mononuclear cells, direct addition of the photosensitizer 8-MOP to the leukocyte-rich fraction, followed by reinfusion of the treated cells to the patient

ECP, although originally designed for the management of SS, has proven effective in a wide variety of inflammatory and autoimmune conditions, such as rheumatoid arthritis, acute and chronic graft versus host disease, systemic sclerosis, lupus erythematosus, and inflammatory bowel disease.[115] Clinical response to ECP in a variety of diseases is suggestive of multiple mechanisms of action.

8.7.1 ECP Mechanism of Action

Significant progress has been recently achieved in the therapy and understanding of the mechanism of action of ECP in CTCL. It has been well appreciated that induction of *lymphocyte apoptosis* and *monocyte-to-DC differentiation* are two key cellular events involved in ECP-induced antitumor immunity.

The exact mechanisms whereby ECP destroys malignant T cells are not completely understood. Combination treatment of 8-MOP and UVA causes the formation of DNA photoadducts with activated psoralens leading to DNA damage and inhibition of DNA synthesis.[51] Mechanisms other than cross-link formation have also been reported to be involved in DNA damage. UVA irradiation can induce apoptosis in CD4+ T cells through the Fas/Fas-ligand system, activated as a consequence of singlet oxygen generation,[116] suggesting that increase in Fas expression following photopheresis could be an important additional mechanism of action. An increase in the death receptor CD95 (Fas) has been observed on lymphocytes, with some studies reporting upregulation of Fas ligand.[117,118,119,120] Activation of the CD95 pathway induces apoptosis through the activation of the caspases.[121] Multiple other mechanisms have been shown to be involved in ECP-mediated lymphocyte apoptosis, such as changes to mitochondrial function observed very early in the ECP process, such as downregulation of the antiapoptotic protein bcl-2, upregulation of the proa-poptotic bax, and leading to a reversal in the Bax/Bcl-2 ratio,[122] some of which has been attributed to the effects of white blood cell collection process or UVA alone.[67,118] The time necessary to complete lymphocyte apoptosis is about 48 h, and by 72 h, 80% of the ECP-treated lymphocytes are apoptotic.[53,123,124] While malig-nant T-cell apoptosis plays a major role in the mechanism underlying ECP-effectiveness, only approximately 5–10% of pathogenic T cells are treated during one cycle, suggesting that apoptosis by itself is not sufficient to induce clinical response.

Activation of monocytes to immature DCs capable of phagocytosing apoptotic tumor cells is another process linked to ECP-induced antitumor mechanism. Monocytes appear to be relatively resistant to apoptosis induction by ECP treatment.[125] Contact with the plastic during the ECP procedure is sufficient to induce activation of monocytoid DC precursors into immature DCs capable of phagocytosing apoptotic cells.[131]

Phosphatidyl serine externalization is an important component of apoptosis as it is a potent target recognition site for phagocytosis by antigen-presenting cells (APCs).[126] Soon after the induction of T-cell apoptosis, phosphatidylserine (PS) residues, normally present on the inner cell membrane, are translocated from the inner (cytoplasmic) leaflet to the outer (cell surface) leaflet of the plasma membrane. ECP treatment could lead to enhanced lymphocyte immunogenicity by an increase in the expression of tumor antigens on malignant CTCL lymphocytes.[127,128] Apoptotic lymphocytes are then phagocytosed by DCs.[129] An increase in phagocytosis of apoptotic lymphocytes by macrophages has been reported to occur 4 h following externalization of PS.[130] This is followed by antigen presentation of apoptotic bodies and induction of a class I-restricted CD8+ cytotoxic T-cell response directed against untreated clonal T cells[131,132] (Fig. 8.9).

Reinfusion of the DCs loaded with apoptotic CTCL cells can increase CD8+ T-cell numbers and induce a potent antitumor cytotoxic T lymphocyte response with enhanced cytolytic ability.

ECP treatment-induced antitumor reaction in CTCL has also been linked with post-ECP cytokine changes. In advanced stages of CTCL, a deficiency of IFN-γ and IL12 has been reported with a predominance of Th2 cytokines. A study reported by Di Renzo et al showed that 12 months of ECP therapy resulted in correction of the Th1/Th2 imbalance/ratio.[133–135]

ECP has also been demonstrated to increase and even reverse the aberrant CD8 to CD4 ratio that is often observed, enhancing cytotoxic responses against tumor cells.

ECP has immune modulatory function possibly via enhancing the immune tolerance rather than by inducing immunosuppression. It is not thought to induce generalized immunosuppression as increased rates of infection or immunosuppression are not typically observed in ECP-treated patients.[112,115]

Extracorporeal photopheresis mechanism of action

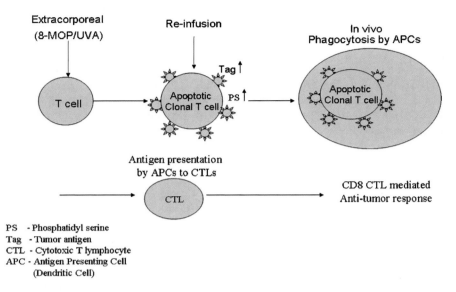

PS   - Phosphatidyl serine
Tag - Tumor antigen
CTL - Cytotoxic T lymphocyte
APC - Antigen Presenting Cell
        (Dendritic Cell)

Fig. 8.9 Extracorporeal photopheresis (*ECP*) mechanism of action. Irradiation of white blood cells in the presence of 8-MOP leads to malignant T-cell apoptosis, simultaneous externalization of phosphatidylserine (*PS*) on the cell membrane, and upregulation of tumor-specific antigens (*Tag*) on the cell surface of the malignant T-cell clone. This is followed by phagocytosis and internalization of the apoptotic T cell by antigen-presenting cells (*APC*). Reinfusion of these dendritic cells with apoptotic T cells induces a class I-restricted CD8+ cytotoxic T-cell response against untreated malignant T cells[131]

8.7.2   ECP Monotherapy

ECP is recommended first-line therapy for erythrodermic CTCL and SS by the EORTC and the joint British Association of Dermatologists and UK Cutaneous Lymphoma Group guidelines.[136,137] ECP has a significant impact on overall survival and quality of life of patients with advanced stage CTCL.[138–141] ECP when used as monotherapy in patients with erythrodermic CTCL/SS is associated with a good overall response rate between 50% and 65% and CR rates between 18% and 23%.[114,142] There are several advantages to the use of ECP in CTCL, one of them being its very low side effect profile. Another advantage is that patients undergoing long-term ECP therapy do not appear to develop infections or secondary malignancies that are typically associated with immunosuppressive therapies.[143,144] ECP can be safely used in CTCL patients of all ages, including children and elderly.[145] The results from larger studies of ECP in the treatment of erythrodermic CTCL and Sezary syndrome are summarized in Table 8.7 (for review, see Knobler and Jantschitsch[146]).

Edelson's study published in 1987 included 37 erythrodermic CTCL patients and reported a 73% response rate with a mean time to development of a response between 4 and 5 months.[110]

In the study by Gottlieb and coworkers, 71% of patients responded to ECP, 25% had partial remission as defined by more than 50% clearing of the lesions.[142] In their study, Gottlieb et al report a median survival from initiation of therapy and from the time of diagnosis of 77 and over 100 months, respectively.[142]

Less impressive clinical response was reported by Duvic et al. in a study published in 1996.[114] In this study, 18% of patients achieved a CR, 32% partial response, and a 50% overall response rate including CR and PR.

Jiang et al observed 25 patients with stages III and IV disease who had failed multiple previous modalities and noted a 20% CR, 60% PR rate after 10–13 months of treatment, and 20% were nonresponders.[147]

Response rates appear to vary widely between different study groups. Different patient selection, the presence or absence of the peripheral blood T-cell clone, stage of disease, duration of ECP might account – at least in part – for these differences between various ECP centers (for review, see Scarisbrick et al[148]). Several parameters have been identified as indicators of favorable response to ECP therapy. Patients with a normal CD4/CD8 ratio, normal CD8 cell number, and short disease duration are considered the best responders (for review, see Miller et al[113] and Knobler and Jantschitsch[146]). Table 8.8 summarizes few of the criteria and variables reported to have a positive influence on response to ECP therapy.

While most studies have been reported in the treatment of advanced stage CTCL, a benefit of ECP in early stages of the disease, such as stage IA, IB, or IIA,

Table 8.7 Summary of larger studies using ECP in the treatment of erythrodermic cutaneous T-cell lymphomas or Sézary syndrome

Authors	Year	No. of patients	OR (%)	Complete response (%)
Edelson et al[a]	1987	37	73	24
Heald et al[b]	1989	32	53	14
Dall' Amico et al[c]	1991	37	73	24
Koh et al[d]	1994	34	53	15
Duvic et al[e]	1996	34	50	18
Vonderheid et al[f]	1998	32	31	13
Bisaccia et al[g]	2000	37	54	14
Bouwhuis et al[h]	2002	55	80	62
Suchin et al[i]	2002	47	79	26

[a]Edelson. *N Engl J Med.* 1987
[b]Heald Yale. *J Biol Med.* 1989
[c]Dall'Amico. *Recenti Prog Med.* 1991
[d]Koh. *JID.* 1994
[e]Duvic. *JAAD.* 1996
[f]Vonderheid. *JAAD.* 1988
[g]Bissacia. *JAAD.* 2000
[h]Bouwhuis. *Int J Dermatol.* 2002
[i]Suchin. *Arch Dermatol.* 2002

Table 8.8 ECP response criteria

Criteria and variables that predict positive response to ECP
1. Absence of internal organ involvement or bulky lymphadenopathy
2. Decreased numbers of Sezary cells (10–20% of mononuclear cells)
3. Short duration of the disease (<2 years)
4. Close to normal CD4/CD8 ratio and %CD8+ >15%
5. White blood cell count less than 20,000/mm³
6. Response within 5 months of treatment
7. Natural killer cell activity close to normal
8. Absence of prior intensive chemotherapy
9. Presence of erythroderma

has also been reported (for review, see Miller et al,[113] Gottlieb et al,[142] Vonderheid et al,[149] and Heald et al[150]).

8.7.3   ECP Side Effects

In general, ECP is a very safe procedure and adverse effects associated with ECP are minimal. Mild side effects from ECP include headaches and transient fever (4–12 h after reinfusion of treated cells), chills, nausea, and transient increase in erythroderma.[142] Anemia secondary to inadequate return of red blood cells during the procedure may be rarely seen. Hypotension and vasovagal syncope can occur and can be corrected with infusion of normal saline. Because of volume shifts during the treatment, cardiovascular instability, severe liver or renal failure, and low weight of less than 40 kg are contraindication to ECP treatment. A history of heparin-induced thrombocytopenia is a contraindication as heparin is used to flush the ECP machine. Catheter-related infections and septicemia are infrequent. Patients undergoing long-term ECP therapy do not appear to have an increased rate of infections that are typically associated with immunosuppressive therapies.[143,144] An apparent increase in secondary neoplasms observed in patients treated with photopheresis is considered to be a CTCL-related and rather than ECP-associated phenomenon.[142]

8.7.4   Patient Selection

The best candidates for ECP treatment have erythrodermic CTCL or SS (stage III or IVA) with peripheral blood involvement (proven by molecular analysis, CD4/CD8 ratio > 10 or circulating Sézary cells >10%; see Table 8.2). ECP is performed monthly on two consecutive days and this schedule is continued for up to 6 months to assess response. Periodic reevaluation every 3 months is recommended and should include physical examination, extent of skin involvement using the SWAT score (Severity Weighted Assessment Tool),[151] hematology, chemistry, and lymphocyte markers. Tumor burden in the circulation should be measured by monitoring total leukocyte and absolute T-cell number, CD4/CD8 ratio, or Sézary cell count. Response to ECP treatment in patients with advanced CTCL may be quantitatively followed by monitoring the percentage of the malignant T-cell clone (when identifiable) by flow cytometry.[152]

The 3-monthly clinical assessment helps identify patients with good response, those who are refractory to ECP and patients with progressive disease, such as those who develop new palpable nodes >15 mm. If clinical response is suboptimal, the frequency of treatment may be increased to one cycle every 2–3 weeks but no benefit has been reported by increasing the frequency to more than one cycle every 2 weeks. If adequate and sustained response is achieved, the frequency of the treatment schedule in responders may be tapered to maintenance therapy with one cycle at 6- to 8-week intervals for 6 months, followed by one cycle every 3 months for 9 months after which the treatment can be stopped.[148] The treatment is typically continued for 6 months before declaring treatment failure and combination or alternative therapy is considered.[148] Most patients who will respond do so in the first 6 months of treatment and early response was reported to be a predictor of survival in ECP-treated patients with SS.[151]

8.7.5 Transimmunization: A Novel Modified ECP Procedure

Transimmunization ECP is an innovative alternative to conventional ECP developed by Berger et al.[131] Berger et al have shown that in the presence of malignant apoptotic T cells, monocytes are induced to undergo maturation to DCs and that overnight incubation of the ECP-treated cells can enhance contact between apoptotic cells and DCs, a process called transimmunization.

Transimmunization involves incubation of the white blood cells exposed to ECP overnight prior to reinfusion which allows more interaction between the immature DCs and apoptotic lymphocytes, more efficient phagocytosis, and processing of the apoptotic malignant T cells before final reinfusion. This procedure results in transfer of tumor antigens to newly formed DCs, capable of initiating immunization against the tumor cells. Engulfment of apoptotic cells by the APCs followed by subsequent presentation of tumor antigens results in stimulation of the equivalent of a vaccine response with the production and proliferation of the effector cells (cytotoxic cells and natural killer cells).[131]

8.7.6 ECP as Part of Combination Treatment

Response rate to photopheresis in partial responders or patients refractory to ECP may be increased with the addition of adjuvant immunomodulatory therapy, such as IFNα, IL-2 or -12, bexarotene, or methothrexate.

Bexarotene has been shown to be safe and effective in combination with ECP (75% RR), ECP/IFN-α2a (50% RR), and ECP/IFN-α2a/PUVA (100% RR).[100]

8.7.7   ECP and IFN-α and/or Systemic Retinoids

The most common adjuvant therapy added to photopheresis treatment is low dose of IFN-α (1.5–5.0×10^6 U three to five times weekly) and/or systemic retinoids (etretinate, 10–50 mg daily or bexarotene 150 mg daily). Gottlieb et al report synergistic effect in five of the nine patients treated with ECP and IFNα combination therapy.[142]

Suchin et al reported an 84% overall and 20% CR of 51 patients treated with IFN-α ($n = 30$) and systemic retinoids ($n = 21$).[112]

In a study reported by Duvic et al, 54 patients received ECP monotherapy and 32 patients received ECP in combination with IFN-α ($n = 14$) and bexarotene ($n = 15$). The response rate was slightly higher in the combination group (56%) compared with the monotherapy group (43%).[141]

Combination therapy with the addition of IFN-γ to bexarotene plus ECP therapy can be attempted in patients who are partial responders on IFN-α/bexarotene/ECP combination regimen. Substitution of IFN-γ given subcutaneously (dose between 40 and 100 μg) three times weekly for IFN-α2b in a patient with inadequate response to IFN-α/bexarotene/ECP combination resulted in complete clearing of erythroderma.[153] IFN-γ treatment was associated with increased natural killer cell activity and elevated IL-12 production.[153]

8.7.8   ECP and Sagramostim (GM-CSF)

Suchin et al report clinical response in erythrodermic CTCL patients treated with ECP and sagramostim or granulocyte/macrophage colony stimulating factor (GM-CSF) combination therapy.[112] Duvic et al reported clinical improvement in three patients treated with ECP-GM-CSF combination treatment.

8.7.9   ECP and Fludarabine

In a study conducted by Quaglino et al, 17 patient with SS and 22 patients with MF stages IIB–IV and/or peripheral blood involvement were treated with fludarabine monophosphate, a purine analogue. ECP was performed in 19 patients after chemotherapy was discontinued. After a median follow-up of 4.2 years, significantly higher response rate was seen in the FAMP-ECP group (63.2%) compared with RR in the fludarabine monophosphate monotherapy group (24%).[154] The response rate was higher in SS than that in MF patients.

8.7.10   ECP and Total Skin Electron Beam

A retrospective study of 44 patients with erythrodermic CTCL/SS carried out by Wilson et al report an 81% three-year disease-free survival among the 21 patients receiving TSEB/ECP combination compared with 49% disease-free survival in patients on TSEB therapy only.[155]

8.8   Ultraviolet B Phototherapy

UVB therapy is another light treatment approach used to treat early-stage CTCL. It has been shown that BB-UVB (290–320 nm), NB-UVB (311–313 nm), and even "natural UVB"[156] have well-documented efficacy in the management of early stages of the disease (IB and IIA), particularly in patch-stage MF. UVB treatment does not involve the ingestion of psoralen as photosensitizer and therefore has decreased toxicity compared with PUVA treatment.

8.8.1   Broadband Ultraviolet B Phototherapy

BB-UVB (290–320 nm) was the first artificial UV light source used in the management of CTCL. Efficacy of BB-UVB is limited to early patch-stage disease since shorter wavelengths have decreased depth of penetration.

Plaque-stage patients benefit less from BB-UVB compared to patch stage, where clinical remission can be achieved in 83% of patients after a median treatment time of 5 months, lasting for a median duration of 22 months.[157]

UVB therapy has been shown to be effective in patients with darker skin types and Asian patients with early-stage CTCL (IB).[158] Given the strong erythemogenic effect of UVB, it is important to perform MED testing prior to the first treatment to avoid and minimize the occurrence of phototoxic reactions.

Common side effects of UVB treatment include burning, pruritus, exacerbation, or initiation of photoinduced dermatoses, such as polymorphous light eruption, solar urticaria, or worsening connective tissue disease and may be associated with an increased risk of skin cancer.

Resnik and Vonderheid reported that similar efficacy may be achieved by home UBV phototherapy (280–350 nm) with clinical and histological clearance reported in 74% of patch-stage cutaneous lymphoma patients after a median treatment duration of 5 months.[159] More recently, home UVB, such as UVBioTek™ Home Phototherapy System Light, therapy has gained popularity in view of its similar efficacy as office UVB therapy and convenience.

8.8.2   Narrowband Ultraviolet B Therapy

NB-UVB has been proven to be a safe and effective treatment modality in early-stage (IA, IB, and IIA) MF and it is considered first-line treatment for the management of patch-stage CTCL resistant to topical therapy.

NB-UVB (311–313 nm) was originally developed as an alternative to BB-UVB (290–320 nm) for the phototherapy of psoriasis with the goal to reduce the erythema typically associated with BB-UVB treatment and risk of carcinogenesis. It has several advantages over both BB-UVB and PUVA.

NB-UVB has relatively more immunosuppressive effects when compared with BB-UVB based on its effect on natural killer cells, T cells, and cytokine responses.[160] NB-UVB is also more effective in induction of T-cell apoptosis due to deeper penetration of this wavelength compared with BB-UVB sources.[161,162] It is associated with less irritation and less severe erythema than BB-UVB.

NB-UVB has many advantages over PUVA: shorter irradiation time improves patient compliance, there are no side effects typically associated with psoralens, such as nausea and headache and does not require the use of protective eyeglasses after treatment.

NB-UVB also causes less hyperpigmentation than PUVA, making it a more attractive therapeutic modality in dark-skinned individuals.

Narrowband phototherapy uses the Philips TL-01 lamp, which has an emission spectrum of 311–313 nm and in many centers, it has replaced traditional BB-UVB phototherapy. MED testing is typically performed prior to initiation of the treatment. The starting dose and subsequent incremental doses are decided based on skin type (0.05–0.1 J/cm^2). MED for NB-UVB is five to ten times higher than that of BB-UVB and the cumulative dose needed to achieve CR is ten times higher with NB- versus BB-UVB. Patients are treated three to four times a week. The MED is determined for each patient prior to starting therapy by irradiation of a template of eight 1×1 cm^2 apertures on the upper back with an NB-UVB source 20 cm from the patient. Two standard ranges of doses that are administered 25–390 mJ/cm^2 for phototypes I and II or 70–770 mJ/cm^2 for phototypes III and IV. The initial treatment dose is 70% of a patient's individual minimal 311 nm UVB erythema dose with 20% increment at each exposure unless modified by the erythemal dose assessed at 48 h after treatment. Successive doses are determined using the following guidelines: if the previous exposure had caused no erythema, the next exposure time is increased by 40%; if the previous exposure induced a slight erythema, the next exposure is increased by 20%; and in the case of marked erythema, the same exposure time is repeated. The dose is increased weekly by 20% if previous treatments had caused no or slight erythema. Emollients are used for topical skin care. Face and genitalia need to be shielded. NB-UVB may be given as maintenance therapy after CR is achieved by decreasing the frequency of the treatments. In the office UVB, it is administered three times a week. Phototherapy is continued until complete clinical clearance or minimal residual activity is noted.

8.8.3   NB-UVB Monotherapy

Several large studies have reported beneficial effect of NB-UVB treatment in early-stage MF (IA and IB), most of them reporting between 54% and 95% CR in patch-stage MF (see Table 8.9). Previous studies have shown NB-UVB to be at least as effective as PUVA in early-stage MF.

A large retrospective study reported by Pavlotsky et al compared the efficacy of NB- and BB-UVB therapy in 68 and 43 patients, respectively. CR in stage IA MF was achieved in 84% and 89% of patients treated with NB- and BB-UVB, respectively. CR among patients with stage IB disease was 78% and 44% in NB- and BB-UVB treated groups, respectively.[163]

In another study, Diederen et al analyzed the response to treatment, relapse-free interval, and irradiation dose in 56 patients with early-stage MF (IA and IB) treated with NB-UVB or PUVA. This study found that NB-UVB treatment led to complete remission in 81% and partial remission in 19% of the patients, whereas PUVA treatment led to complete remission in 71% and partial remission in 29% of the patients, and none showed progressive disease. The mean relapse-free interval for patients treated with UVB was 24.5 months and for patients treated with PUVA, 22.8 months.[164]

Hofer et al reported complete clearance in 83.3% of patients with early MF within a mean time of 6 weeks. However, relapses occurred within a mean time of 6 months.[165] Clark et al noted complete clearance of MF lesions in 75% of patients with early-stage CTCL after a mean treatment duration of 9 weeks or 26 treatments. The mean duration of treatment was 20 months.[162]

Other studies reported complete clinical clearance in 91.3% of patients with patch-stage CTCL and in 60% of patients with plaque-stage MF.[166]

Table 8.9 Summary of studies on NB-UVB in the treatment of early patch-stage cutaneous T-cell lymphomas

Authors	Year	No. of patients	Patient skin type	Complete response (%)
Hofer et al	1999	20	Austrian study, likely I, II	95
Clark et al	2000	8	I (3), II (3), III (2)	75
Gathers et al	2002	24	I-III (12), IV–VI (12)	54
Diederen	2003	21	?	81
Gokdemir et al	2006	23	II (5), III (14), IV (4)	91
El-Mofty et al	2005	10	III (5), IV (5)	70
Brazelli et al	2007	20	II (12), III (8)	90
Pavlotsky et al	2006	68	I, II, III, IV, V	84
Boztepe	2005	14	I, II, III	78

NB-UVB has also been found to be safe and effective in darker skin types.[166] A study reported by Gathers et al has analyzed the effect of NB-UVB in 24 patients with Fitzpatrick skin types (FSTs) I through VI, with MF stages IA and IB. CR was noted in 54.2% and partial response in 29.1% of NB-UVB-treated patients. Around 16.7% of patients showed no response. In this study, three of four nonresponders had FSTs IV-VI. CR was observed in 66.7% among those with skin phototypes I–III but only in 47.1% among patients with FSTs IV–VI. These data suggest that MF patients with higher skin phototypes may not respond as well as light-skinned individuals.[167]

No correlation between skin phototype and therapeutic response was reported by Clark, although their study included skin phototypes I, II, and III.[162]

Few studies have suggested that skin phototype does not have an influence on therapeutic response and possibility of achieving CR with UVB treatment.[163,168]

Clinical improvement using NB-UVB has been shown in follicular CTCL without mucinosis, a subtype of cutaneous lymphoma involving the hair follicles with worse prognosis than classical MF.[169]

NB-UVB is a well-tolerated and safe treatment alternative for treatment of children and adolescents with MF, in whom compliance with topical therapy is not reliable.[170]

NB-UVB can also be employed in the management of hypopigmented MF. In a study by Gathers et al, a 28.6% CR and 57.1% PR was observed among patients with hypopigmented MF.[167] In this study, it was noted that higher skin phototypes appeared to have a relatively decreased responsiveness to NB-UVB.

In contrast to PUVA, maintenance therapy does not improve the likelihood of not relapsing after the discontinuation of UVB treatment. On the basis of this observation, it was suggested that treatment be stopped after CR is achieved and maintenance treatment should only be considered in case of relapse.[163]

Adverse effects of NB-UVB include mild pruritus, burning, and erythema. These side effects have been reported to be significantly less pronounced in NB-UVB when compared to BB-UVB therapy.[163] NB-UVB has also been shown to be less carcinogenic than either BB-UVB or PUVA possibly due to lower cumulative UV doses and minimal radiation in the more mutagenic 290–310 nm range.[160,162,167,171]

In summary, a rapid and clinically significant improvement can be achieved using both NB-UVB and BB-UVB in early-stage CTCL. Because of the benefits and less side effects, NB-UVB may be the first therapeutic option in patch-stage CTCL. In case of progression or lack or response to UVB, switching to PUVA is an option.[164]

8.8.4   Combination Regimens with UVB

The advantage of combination treatments using UVB is taking advantage of distinct mechanism of action acting synergistically or at least in an additive fashion. The combination of UVB with psoralens, such as in PUVA, does not appear to be associated with beneficial effect. A study designed to analyze whether the efficacy of NB-UVB could be enhanced by addition of psoralens (NB-PUVB), previously showed to have increased efficacy in psoriasis,[172] failed to show any difference in therapeutic effectiveness in MF patients.[82]

Only a few studies assessed the role of UVB in combination with systemic agents.

8.8.5 *NB-UVB Plus Bexarotene*

If PUVA is contraindicated (e.g. for ophtalmological reasons), combination treatment with oral bexarotene and NB-UVB therapy may represent a safe alternative for the treatment of plaque-stage MF. Successful treatment of a stage IB MF patient with combination treatment using bexarotene 300 mg daily and NB-UVB therapy has been reported.[173]

8.8.6 *NB-UVB Plus IFN-γ*

In a study of 12 patients with CTCL (stages IB–III) treated with a combination of NB-UVB and IFN-γ conducted by Shimauchi et al, CR was observed in 4 of 12, including patients with erythrodermic CTCL.[174]

8.9 308-nm Excimer Laser

Excimer laser is emerging as a new therapeutic modality reported to be effective in early-stage CTCL, particularly in patients with limited patch-stage CTCL. Excimer laser is a xenon-chloride lamp with a peak emission of 308 nm. In contrast to NB-UVB, which delivers polychromatic continuous incoherent light, the excimer laser emits monochromatic short-pulse radiation through a 1.8 × 1.8 cm circular spot size. While excimer laser (308 nm) and NB-UVB (311–313 nm) have close emission spectrum, the excimer laser appears to be a stronger T-cell apoptosis inducer in vitro.[175] Another advantage of excimer laser is delivery of higher fluences to the lesion while sparing the unaffected healthy skin.

Mori et al first reported the use of excimer laser for the treatment of early-stage MF in four patients treating seven lesions. The authors delivered weekly treatments for a total number of treatments ranging from 4 to 11 with a total UVB 308-nm dose ranging from 5 to 9.3 J/cm². All patients had complete remission.[176]

In another study reported by Nistico, ten lesions from five patients with patch-stage MF were treated with excimer laser using a cumulative dose between 6 and 12 J/cm².

The number of treatments ranged from four to ten at 7- to 10-day intervals. Complete remission was achieved in all patients.[177]

Several other studies reported on the efficacy of excimer laser in patch-stage MF. Passeron et al observed good clinical response in four of five patch-stage MF patients.[178]

Two case reports showed evidence for good clinical results with the use of excimer laser in the treatment of a patient with LyP and a solitary cutaneous CD30+ lymphoproliferative nodule.[179,180] Resolution of 75% of the LyP lesions was noted after a total of 13 treatments three times weekly with a maximum fluence of 500 mJ/cm^2.[179]

Adverse effects reported in association with excimer laser treatment are erythema, pruritus, blisters, erosions, and hyperpigmentation.[179] Long-term studies are needed to assess the risk of carcinogenesis related to excimer laser therapy. Lower cumulative UV doses may be associated with a relatively decreased risk of nonmelanoma skin cancers.

8.10   Photodynamic Therapy

PDT using 5-aminolevulinic acid (ALA-PDT) is another novel approach that has been proven to be an effective and safe treatment modality for CTCL. PDT consists of either systemic or topical application of a photosensitizer, such as 5-ALA followed by irradiation using noncoherent laser light in the visible spectrum.

ALA is a hydrophilic photosensitizer, which after topical application easily penetrates the stratum corneum. 5-ALA or its esters (e.g. methyl-ALA) are not photosensitizers themselves but are precursors that are metabolized to the photosensitizer protoporphyrin IX in malignant T cells. Activation of ALA results in formation of singlet oxygens, which are cytotoxic. Selective ALA uptake by activated and malignant T cells[181] allows for direct apoptosis induction specifically targeting tumor cells. PDT has also been shown to inhibit malignant T-cell proliferation.[52]

The technique consists of topical application of 16–20% 5-ALA in a cream or ointment base under occlusion for 4–6 h. The red fluorescence of porphyrins can be visualized with Wood's light before beginning of the treatment, followed by exposure of the treated area to visible light at a dose ranging from 40 to 144 J/cm^2. The wavelengths within the visible spectrum used in most studies raged from 570 to 740 nm (for review, see Zane et al[182]). The treatment can be repeated at weekly intervals or every 2–4 weeks until complete clearing of the lesion is achieved.

Several reports have been published showing successful clearance of CTCL lesions using ALA-PDT in both early-patch and plaque-stage but also in tumor-stage MF as well as in several CTCL variants, such as CD30+ ALCL, CD8+ CTCL,[183–185] unilesional CTCL.[182]

ALA-PDT treatment is usually well tolerated. The most frequent side effects of ALA-PDT treatment are pain, burning, local erythema, and blistering.

Encouraging clinical response has been reported with the use of Pc4-PDT in the management of CTCL. Pc4 is a novel silicon phthalocyanine photosensitizer, structurally related to porphyrins developed at Case Western Reserve University with faster penetration through the basal layer of the epidermis and no side effects, such as pain (for review, see Miller et al[186]).

References

1. Mackie R. In: Burton JL, Champion RH, Burns PA, Breathnack SM, eds. *Cutaneous Lymphomas and Lymphocytic Infiltrates*. Oxford: Blackwell Science; 1998:2373–2402.
2. Willemze R, Meijer CJ. Classification of cutaneous T-cell lymphoma: from Alibert to WHO-EORTC. *J Cutan Pathol*. 2006;33(Suppl 1):18–26.
3. Willemze R, Jaffe ES, Burg G, et al. WHO-EORTC classification for cutaneous lymphomas. *Blood*. 2005;105(10):3768–3785.
4. Ferenczi K, McKee P, Kupper TS, Cutaneous lymphoma. In: Sober H, ed. Atlas of Clinical Oncology. Hamilton, Ontario: BC Decker;2000:85–117.
5. Criscione VD, Weinstock MA. Incidence of cutaneous T-cell lymphoma in the United States, 1973-2002. *Arch Dermatol*. 2007;143(7):854–859.
6. Keehn CA, Belongie IP, Shistik G, et al. The diagnosis, staging, and treatment options for mycosis fungoides. *Cancer Control*. 2007;14(2):102–111.
7. Ferenczi K, Fuhlbrigge RC, Pinkus J, Pinkus GS, Kupper TS. Increased CCR4 expression in cutaneous T cell lymphoma. *J Invest Dermatol*. 2002;119(6):1405–1410.
8. Kupper TS, Fuhlbrigge RC. Immune surveillance in the skin: mechanisms and clinical consequences. *Nat Rev Immunol*. 2004;4(3):211–222.
9. Berger CL, Hanlon D, Kanada D, et al. The growth of cutaneous T-cell lymphoma is stimulated by immature dendritic cells. *Blood*. 2002;99(8):2929–2939.
10. Yawalkar N, Ferenczi K, Jones DA, et al. Profound loss of T-cell receptor repertoire complexity in cutaneous T-cell lymphoma. *Blood*. 2003;102(12):4059–4066.
11. Wysocka M, Zaki MH, French LE, et al. Sezary syndrome patients demonstrate a defect in dendritic cell populations: effects of CD40 ligand and treatment with GM-CSF on dendritic cell numbers and the production of cytokines. *Blood*. 2002;100(9):3287–3294.
12. Kim EJ, Hess S, Richardson SK, et al. Immunopathogenesis and therapy of cutaneous T cell lymphoma. *J Clin Invest*., 2005;115(4):798–812.
13. Hwang ST, Janik JE, Jaffe ES, Wilson WH. Mycosis fungoides and Sezary syndrome. *Lancet*. 2008;371(9616):945–957.
14. Karenko L, Hahtola S, Päivinen S et al. Primary cutaneous T-cell lymphomas show a deletion or translocation affecting NAV3, the human UNC-53 homologue. *Cancer Res*. 2005;65(18):8101–8110.
15. Mao X, Orchard G, Lillington DM, Russell-Jones R, Young BD, Whittaker SJ. Amplification and overexpression of JUNB is associated with primary cutaneous T-cell lymphomas. *Blood*. 2003;101(4):1513–1519.
16. Eriksen KW, Kaltoft K, Mikkelsen G et al. Constitutive STAT3-activation in Sezary syndrome: tyrphostin AG490 inhibits STAT3-activation, interleukin-2 receptor expression and growth of leukemic Sezary cells. *Leukemia*. 2001;15(5):787–793.
17. Dereure O, Levi E, Vonderheid EC, Kadin ME. Infrequent Fas mutations but no Bax or p53 mutations in early mycosis fungoides: a possible mechanism for the accumulation of malignant T lymphocytes in the skin. *J Invest Dermatol*. 2002;118(6):949–956.
18. Nagasawa T, Takakuwa T, Takayama H et al. Fas gene mutations in mycosis fungoides: analysis of laser capture-microdissected specimens from cutaneous lesions. *Oncology*. 2004;67(2):130–134.
19. van Doorn R, Dijkman R, Vermeer MH, Starink TM, Willemze R, Tensen CP. A novel splice variant of the Fas gene in patients with cutaneous T-cell lymphoma. *Cancer Res*. 2002;62(19):5389–5392.

20. Dummer R, Michie SA, Kell D et al. Expression of bcl-2 protein and Ki-67 nuclear prolifera-
    tion antigen in benign and malignant cutaneous T-cell infiltrates. *J Cutan Pathol.*
    1995;22(1):11–17.
21. Gilchrest BA, Parrish JA, Tanenbaum L, Haynes HA, Fitzpatrick TB. Oral methoxsalen pho-
    tochemotherapy of mycosis fungoides. *Cancer.* 1976;38(2):683–689.
22. Qari MS, Li N, Demierre MF. Hypopigmented mycosis fungoides: case reports and literature
    review. *J Cutan Med Surg.* 2000;4(3):142–148.
23. Pimpinelli N, Olsen EA, Santucci M et al. Defining early mycosis fungoides. *J Am Acad
    Dermatol.* 2005;53(6):1053–1063.
24. Haghighi B, Smoller BR, LeBoit PE, Warnke RA, Sander CA, Kohler S. Pagetoid reticulosis
    (Woringer-Kolopp disease): an immunophenotypic, molecular, and clinicopathologic study.
    Mod Pathol. 2000;13(5):502–510.
25. El-Shabrawi-Caelen L, Cerroni L, Medeiros LJ, McCalmont TH. Hypopigmented mycosis
    fungoides: frequent expression of a CD8+ T-cell phenotype. *Am J Surg Pathol.*
    2002;26(4):450–457.
26. Hoppe RT, Medeiros LJ, Warnke RA, Wood GS. CD8-positive tumor-infiltrating lymphocytes
    influence the long-term survival of patients with mycosis fungoides. *J Am Acad Dermatol.*
    1995;32(3):448–453.
27. Berti E, Tomasini D, Vermeer MH, Meijer CJ, Alessi E, Willemze R. Primary cutaneous CD8-
    positive epidermotropic cytotoxic T cell lymphomas: a distinct clinicopathological entity with
    an aggressive clinical behavior. *Am J Pathol.* 1999;155(2):483–492.
28. Vergier B, de Muret A, Beylot-Barry M et al. Transformation of mycosis fungoides: clinicopatho-
    logical and prognostic features of 45 cases: French Study Group of Cutaneious Lymphomas.
    Blood. 2000;95(7):2212–2218.
29. Salhany KE, Cousar JB, Greer JP, Casey TT, Fields JP, Collins RD. Transformation of cutane-
    ous T cell lymphoma to large cell lymphoma: a clinicopathologic and immunologic study. *Am
    J Pathol.* 1988;132(2):265–277.
30. Cerroni L, Rieger E, Hödl S, Kerl H. Clinicopathologic and immunologic features associated
    with transformation of mycosis fungoides to large-cell lymphoma. *Am J Surg Pathol.*
    1992;16(6):543–552.
31. Smoller BR, Santucci M, Wood GS, Whittaker SJ. Histopathology and genetics of cutaneous
    T-cell lymphoma. *Hematol Oncol Clin North Am.* 2003;17(6):1277–1311.
32. Ponti R, Quaglino P, Novelli M et al. T-cell receptor gamma gene rearrangement by multiplex
    polymerase chain reaction/heteroduplex analysis in patients with cutaneous T-cell lymphoma
    (mycosis fungoides/Sezary syndrome) and benign inflammatory disease: correlation with
    clinical, histological and immunophenotypical findings. *Br J Dermatol.* 2005;153(3):
    565–573.
33. Poszepczynska-Guigne E, Bagot M, Wechsler J, Revuz J, Farcet JP, Delfau-Larue MH.
    Minimal residual disease in mycosis fungoides follow-up can be assessed by polymerase
    chain reaction. *Br J Dermatol.* 2003;148(2):265–271.
34. Olsen E, Vonderheid E, Pimpinelli N. et al. Revisions to the staging and classification of mycosis
    fungoides and Sezary syndrome: a proposal of the International Society for Cutaneous
    Lymphomas (ISCL) and the cutaneous lymphoma task force of the European Organization of
    Research and Treatment of Cancer (EORTC). *Blood.* 2007;110(6):1713–1722.
35. Kim YH, Liu HL, Mraz-Gernhard S, Varghese A, Hoppe RT. Long-term outcome of 525
    patients with mycosis fungoides and Sezary syndrome: clinical prognostic factors and risk for
    disease progression. *Arch Dermatol.* 2003;139(7):857–866.
36. Sausville EA, Eddy JL, Makuch RW et al. Histopathologic staging at initial diagnosis of
    mycosis fungoides and the Sezary syndrome: definition of three distinctive prognostic groups.
    Ann Intern Med. 1988;109(5):372–382.
37. Halder RM, Bang KM. Skin cancer in blacks in the United States. *Dermatol Clin.*
    1988;6(3):397–405.
38. Gloster Jr. HM, Neal K. Skin cancer in skin of color. *J Am Acad Dermatol.* 2006;55(5):741–760;
    quiz 761-764.

39. Akaraphanth R, Douglass MC, Lim HW. Hypopigmented mycosis fungoides: treatment and a 6(1/2)-year follow-up of 9 patients. *J Am Acad Dermatol*. 2000;42(1 Pt 1):33–39.
40. Naeem H, Cheng SX, Kupper TS. Treatment of Primary Cutaneous Lymphomas. In: Sober H, ed. *Atlas of Clinical Oncology*. Hamilton, Ontario: BC Decker; 2000.
41. Baron ED, Stevens SR. Phototherapy for cutaneous T-cell lymphoma. *Dermatol Ther*. 2003;16(4):303–310.
42. Kawada A. UVB-induced erythema, delayed tanning, and UVA-induced immediate tanning in Japanese skin. *Photodermatol*. 1986;3(6): p327–333.
43. Danno K. PUVA therapy: current concerns in Japan. *J Dermatol Sci*. 1999;19(2):89–105.
44. Agin PP, Desrochers DL, Sayre RM. The relationship of immediate pigment darkening to minimal erythemal dose, skin type, and eye color. *Photodermatol*. 1985;2(5):288–294.
45. Andreassi L, Simoni S, Fiorini P, Fimiani M. Phenotypic characters related to skin type and minimal erythemal dose. *Photodermatol*. 1987;4(1):43–46.
46. Kollias N, Sayre RM, Zeise L, Chedekel MR. Photoprotection by melanin. *J Photochem Photobiol B*. 1991;9(2):135–160.
47. Palmer RA, Aquilina S, Milligan PJ, Walker SL, Hawk JL, Young AR. Photoadaptation during narrowband ultraviolet-B therapy is independent of skin type: a study of 352 patients. *J Invest Dermatol*. 2006;126(6):1256–1263.
48. Stamatas GN, Kollias N. Blood stasis contributions to the perception of skin pigmentation. *J Biomed Opt*. 2004;9(2):315–322.
49. Zonios GJ, Bykowski, Kollias N. Skin melanin, hemoglobin, and light scattering properties can be quantitatively assessed in vivo using diffuse reflectance spectroscopy. *J Invest Dermatol*. 2001;117(6):1452–1457.
50. Johnson R, Staiano-Coico L, Austin L, Cardinale I, Nabeya-Tsukifuji R, Krueger JG. PUVA treatment selectively induces a cell cycle block and subsequent apoptosis in human T-lymphocytes. *Photochem Photobiol*. 1996;63(5):566–571.
51. Yoo EK, Rook AH, Elenitsas R, Gasparro FP, Vowels BR. Apoptosis induction of ultraviolet light A and photochemotherapy in cutaneous T-cell lymphoma: relevance to mechanism of therapeutic action. *J Invest Dermatol*. 1996;107(2):235–242.
52. Fox FE, Niu Z, Tobia A, Rook AH. Photoactivated hypericin is an anti-proliferative agent that induces a high rate of apoptotic death of normal, transformed, and malignant T lymphocytes: implications for the treatment of cutaneous lymphoproliferative and inflammatory disorders. *J Invest Dermatol*. 1998;111(2):327–332.
53. Bladon J, Taylor PC. Extracorporeal photopheresis induces apoptosis in the lymphocytes of cutaneous T-cell lymphoma and graft-versus-host disease patients. *Br J Haematol*. 1999;107(4):707–711.
54. Zhang C, Richon V, Ni X, Talpur R, Duvic M. Selective induction of apoptosis by histone deacetylase inhibitor SAHA in cutaneous T-cell lymphoma cells: relevance to mechanism of therapeutic action. *J Invest Dermatol*. 2005;125(5):1045–1052.
55. Rivas JM, Ullrich SE. The role of IL-4, IL-10, and TNF-alpha in the immune suppression induced by ultraviolet radiation. *J Leukoc Biol*. 1994;56(6):769–775.
56. Ullrich SE. Mechanism involved in the systemic suppression of antigen-presenting cell function by UV irradiation: keratinocyte-derived IL-10 modulates antigen-presenting cell function of splenic adherent cells. *J Immunol*. 1994;152(7):3410–3416.
57. Walterscheid JP, Ullrich SE, Nghiem DX. Platelet-activating factor, a molecular sensor for cellular damage, activates systemic immune suppression. *J Exp Med*. 2002;195(2):171–179.
58. Wolf P, Nghiem DX, Walterscheid JP. et al. Platelet-activating factor is crucial in psoralen and ultraviolet A-induced immune suppression, inflammation, and apoptosis. *Am J Pathol*. 2006;169(3):795–805.
59. Takashima A, Matsue H, Bergstresser PR, Ariizumi K. Interleukin-7-dependent interaction of dendritic epidermal T cells with keratinocytes. *J Invest Dermatol*. 1995;105(1 Suppl):50S–53S.
60. Dalloul A, Arock M, Fourcade C, et al. Interleukin-7 is a growth factor for Sezary lymphoma cells. *J Clin Invest*. 1992;90(3):1054–1060.

61. Bergfelt L. UV-related skin conditions and Langerhans' cell populations in human skin. *Acta Derm Venereol.* 1993;73(3):194–196.
62. Duthie MS, Kimber I, Norval M. The effects of ultraviolet radiation on the human immune system. *Br J Dermatol.* 1999;140(6):995–1009.
63. Simon JC, Tigelaar RE, Bergstresser PR, Edelbaum D, Cruz PD Jr. Ultraviolet B radiation converts Langerhans cells from immunogenic to tolerogenic antigen-presenting cells:Induction of specific clonal anergy in CD4+ T helper 1 cells. *J Immunol.* 1991;146(2):485–491.
64. Cox NH, Turbitt ML, Ashworth J, Mackie RM. Distribution of T cell subsets and Langerhans cells in mycosis fungoides, and the effect of PUVA therapy. *Clin Exp Dermatol.* 1986;11(6):564–568.
65. Gasparro FP, Berger CL, Edelson RL. Effect of monochromatic UVA light and 8-methoxypsoralen on human lymphocyte response to mitogen. *Photodermatol.* 1984;1(1):10–17.
66. Caffieri S, Di Lisa F, Bolesani F, et al. The mitochondrial effects of novel apoptogenic molecules generated by psoralen photolysis as a crucial mechanism in PUVA therapy. *Blood.* 2007;109(11):4988–4994.
67. Godar DE. UVA1 radiation triggers two different final apoptotic pathways. *J Invest Dermatol.* 1999;112(1):3–12.
68. de Gruijl FR. Photocarcinogenesis: UVA vs. UVB radiation. *Skin Pharmacol Appl Skin Physiol.* 2002;15(5):316–320.
69. Stern RS, Laird N. The carcinogenic risk of treatments for severe psoriasis: Photochemotherapy Follow-up Study. *Cancer.* 1994;73(11):2759–2764.
70. Stern RS, Bolshakov S, Nataraj AJ, Ananthaswamy HN. p53 mutation in nonmelanoma skin cancers occurring in psoralen ultraviolet a-treated patients: evidence for heterogeneity and field cancerization. *J Invest Dermatol.* 2002;119(2):522–526.
71. Stern RS, Lunder EJ. Risk of squamous cell carcinoma and methoxsalen (psoralen) and UV-A radiation (PUVA): a meta-analysis. *Arch Dermatol.* 1998;134(12):1582–1585.
72. Stern RS, Liebman EJ, Vakeva L. Oral psoralen and ultraviolet-A light (PUVA) treatment of psoriasis and persistent risk of nonmelanoma skin cancer. PUVA Follow-up Study. *J Natl Cancer Inst.* 1998;90(17):1278–1284.
73. Stern RS, Nichols KT, Vakeva LH. Malignant melanoma in patients treated for psoriasis with methoxsalen (psoralen) and ultraviolet A radiation (PUVA): the PUVA Follow-Up Study. *N Engl J Med.* 1997;336(15):1041–1045.
74. Takashima A, Matsunami E, Yamamoto K, Kitajima S, Mizuno N. Cutaneous carcinoma and 8-methoxypsoralen and ultraviolet A (PUVA) lentigines in Japanese patients with psoriasis treated with topical PUVA: a follow-up study of 214 patients. *Photodermatol Photoimmunol Photomed.* 1990;7(5):218–221.
75. Caffieri S. Furocoumarin photolysis: chemical and biological aspects. *Photochem Photobiol Sci.* 2002;1(3):149–157.
76. British Photodermatology Group. British Photodermatology Group guidelines for PUVA. *Br J Dermatol.* 1994;130(2):246–255.
77. Wackernagel A, Hofer A, Legat F, Kerl H, Wolf P. Efficacy of 8-methoxypsoralen vs. 5-methoxypsoralen plus ultraviolet A therapy in patients with mycosis fungoides. *Br J Dermatol.* 2006;154(3):519–523.
78. Herrmann JJ, Roenigk HH Jr, Hurria A, et al. Treatment of mycosis fungoides with photochemotherapy (PUVA): long-term follow-up. *J Am Acad Dermatol.* 1995;33(2 Pt 1):234–242.
79. Roenigk HH Jr. Kuzel TM, Skoutelis AP, et al. Photochemotherapy alone or combined with interferon alpha-2a in the treatment of cutaneous T-cell lymphoma. *J Invest Dermatol.* 1990;95(6 Suppl):198S–205S.
80. Querfeld C, Rosen ST, Kuzel TM, et al. Long-term follow-up of patients with early-stage cutaneous T-cell lymphoma who achieved complete remission with psoralen plus UV-A monotherapy. *Arch Dermatol.* 2005;141(3):305–311.
81. Hönigsmann H, Brenner W, Rauschmeier W, Konrad K, Wolff K. Photochemotherapy for cutaneous T cell lymphoma. A follow-up study. *J Am Acad Dermatol.* 1984;10(2 Pt 1):238–245.

82. El-Mofty M, El-Darouty M, Salonas M, et al. Narrow band UVB (311 nm), psoralen UVB (311 nm) and PUVA therapy in the treatment of early-stage mycosis fungoides: a right-left comparative study. *Photodermatol Photoimmunol Photomed.* 2005;21(6):281–286.
83. Tran D, Kwok YK, Goh CL. A retrospective review of PUVA therapy at the National Skin Centre of Singapore. *Photodermatol Photoimmunol Photomed.* 2001;17(4):164–167.
84. Neuhaus IM, Ramos-Caro FA, Hassanein AM. Hypopigmented mycosis fungoides in childhood and adolescence. *Pediatr Dermatol.* 2000;17(5):403–406.
85. Kim YH, Martinez G, Varghese A, Hoppe RT. Topical nitrogen mustard in the management of mycosis fungoides: update of the Stanford experience. *Arch Dermatol.* 2003;139(2):165–173.
86. Guitart J. Combination treatment modalities in cutaneous T-cell lymphoma (CTCL). *Semin Oncol.* 2006;33(1 Suppl 3):S17–S20.
87. Kacinski BM, Flick M. Apoptosis and cutaneous T cell lymphoma. *Ann N Y Acad Sci.* 2001;941:194–199.
88. Dummer R. Immunomodulators in the treatment of cutaneous lymphomas. *Expert Opin Biol Ther.* 2002;2(3):279–286.
89. Kuzel TM, Roenigk HH Jr, Samuelson E, et al. Effectiveness of interferon alfa-2a combined with phototherapy for mycosis fungoides and the Sezary syndrome. *J Clin Oncol.* 1995;13(1):257–263.
90. Chiarion-Sileni V, Bononi A, Fornasa CV, et al. Phase II trial of interferon-alpha-2a plus psolaren with ultraviolet light A in patients with cutaneous T-cell lymphoma. *Cancer.* 2002; 95(3):569–575.
91. Rupoli S, Goteri G, Pulini S, et al. Long-term experience with low-dose interferon-alpha and PUVA in the management of early mycosis fungoides. *Eur J Haematol.* 2005;75(2): 136–145.
92. Mostow EN, Neckel SL, Oberhelman L, Anderson TF, Cooper KD. Complete remissions in psoralen and UV-A (PUVA)-refractory mycosis fungoides-type cutaneous T-cell lymphoma with combined interferon alfa and PUVA. *Arch Dermatol.* 1993;129(6):747–752.
93. Yamamoto T. Takahashi Y, Katayama I, Nishioka K. Alteration of cytokine genes and bcl-2 expression following immunotherapy with intralesional IFN-gamma in a patient with tumor-stage mycosis fungoides. *Dermatology.* 1998;196(3):283–287.
94. Kaplan EH, Rosen ST, Norris DB, Roenigk HH Jr, Saks SR, Bunn PA Jr. Phase II study of recombinant human interferon gamma for treatment of cutaneous T-cell lymphoma. *J Natl Cancer Inst.* 1990;82(3):208–212.
95. Olsen EA, Bunn PA. Interferon in the treatment of cutaneous T-cell lymphoma. *Hematol Oncol Clin North Am.* 1995;9(5):1089–1097.
96. Stadler R, Otte HG, Luger T, et al. Prospective randomized multicenter clinical trial on the use of interferon-2a plus acitretin versus interferon-2a plus PUVA in patients with cutaneous T-cell lymphoma stages I and II. *Blood.* 1998;92(10):3578–3581.
97. Thomsen K, Hammar H, Molin L, Volden G. Retinoids plus PUVA (RePUVA) and PUVA in mycosis fungoides, plaque stage. A report from the Scandinavian Mycosis Fungoides Group. *Acta Derm Venereol.* 1989;69(6):536–538.
98. Whittaker SJ, Foss FM. Efficacy and tolerability of currently available therapies for the mycosis fungoides and Sezary syndrome variants of cutaneous T-cell lymphoma. *Cancer Treat Rev.* 2007;33(2):146–160.
99. Zhang C, Hazarika P, Ni X, Weidner DA, Duvic M. Induction of apoptosis by bexarotene in cutaneous T-cell lymphoma cells: relevance to mechanism of therapeutic action. *Clin Cancer Res.* 2002;8(5):1234–1240.
100. Talpur R, Ward S, Apisarnthanarax N, Breuer-Mcham J, Duvic M. Optimizing bexarotene therapy for cutaneous T-cell lymphoma. *J Am Acad Dermatol.* 2002;47(5):672–684.
101. Singh F, Lebwohl MG. Cutaneous T-cell lymphoma treatment using bexarotene and PUVA: a case series. *J Am Acad Dermatol.* 2004;51(4):570–573.
102. Stern DK, Lebwohl M. Treatment of mycosis fungoides with oral bexarotene combined with PUVA. *J Drugs Dermatol.* 2002;1(2):134–136.

103. Papadavid E, Antoniou C, Nikolaou V, et al. Safety and efficacy of low-dose bexarotene and PUVA in the treatment of patients with mycosis fungoides. *Am J Clin Dermatol.* 2008;9(3):169–173.
104. McGinnis KS, Shapiro M, Vittorio CC, Rook AH, Junkins-Hopkins JM. Psoralen plus long-wave UV-A (PUVA) and bexarotene therapy: an effective and synergistic combined adjunct to therapy for patients with advanced cutaneous T-cell lymphoma. *Arch Dermatol.* 2003;139(6):771–775.
105. Abel EA, Sendagorta E, Hoppe RT, Hu CH. PUVA treatment of erythrodermic and plaque-type mycosis fungoides. Ten-year follow-up study. *Arch Dermatol.* 1987;123(7):897–901.
106. Zane C, Leali C, Airò P, De Panfilis G, Pinton PC. "High-dose" UVA1 therapy of widespread plaque-type, nodular, and erythrodermic mycosis fungoides. *J Am Acad Dermatol.* 2001;44(4):629–633.
107. Rombold S, Lobisch K, Katzer K, Grazziotin TC, Ring J, Eberlein B. Efficacy of UVA1 phototherapy in 230 patients with various skin diseases. *Photodermatol Photoimmunol Photomed.* 2008;24(1):19–23.
108. Roupe G. Hypopigmented mycosis fungoides in a child successfully treated with UVA1-light. *Pediatr Dermatol.* 2005;22(1):82.
109. Dawe RS. Ultraviolet A1 phototherapy. *Br J Dermatol.* 2003;148(4):626–637.
110. Edelson R, Berger C, Gasparro F, et al. Treatment of cutaneous T-cell lymphoma by extracorporeal photochemotherapy. Preliminary results. *N Engl J Med.* 1987;316(6):297–303.
111. Knobler E, Warmuth I, Cocco C, Miller B, Mackay J. Extracorporeal photochemotherapy – the Columbia Presbyterian experience. *Photodermatol Photoimmunol Photomed.* 2002;18(5):232–237.
112. Suchin KR, Junkins-Hopkins JM, Rook AH. Treatment of cutaneous T-cell lymphoma with combined immunomodulatory therapy: a 14-year experience at a single institution. *Arch Dermatol.* 2002;138(8):1054–1060.
113. Miller JD, Kirkland EB, Domingo DS, et al. Review of extracorporeal photopheresis in early-stage (IA, IB, and IIA) cutaneous T-cell lymphoma. *Photodermatol Photoimmunol Photomed.* 2007;23(5):163–171.
114. Duvic M, Hester JP, Lemak NA. Photopheresis therapy for cutaneous T-cell lymphoma. *J Am Acad Dermatol.* 1996;35(4):573–579.
115. Rook AH, Suchin KR, Kao DM, et al. Photopheresis: clinical applications and mechanism of action. *J Investig Dermatol Symp Proc.* 1999;4(1):85–90.
116. Morita A, Werfel T, Stege H, Evidence that singlet oxygen-induced human T helper cell apoptosis is the basic mechanism of ultraviolet-A radiation phototherapy. *J Exp Med,* 1997; 186(10):1763–1768.
117. Aringer M, Graninger WB, Smolen JS, et al. Photopheresis treatment enhances CD95 (fas) expression in circulating lymphocytes of patients with systemic sclerosis and induces apoptosis. *Br J Rheumatol.* 1997;36(12):1276–1282.
118. Di Renzo M, Rubegni P, Sbano P, et al. ECP-treated lymphocytes of chronic graft-versus-host disease patients undergo apoptosis which involves both the Fas/FasL system and the Bcl-2 protein family. *Arch Dermatol Res.* 2003;295(5):175–182.
119. Bladon J, Taylor PC. Treatment of cutaneous T cell lymphoma with extracorporeal photopheresis induces Fas-ligand expression on treated T cells, but does not suppress the expression of co-stimulatory molecules on monocytes. *J Photochem Photobiol B.* 2003;69(2):129–138.
120. Tambur AR, Ortegel JW, Morales A, Klingemann H, Gebel HM, Tharp MD. Extracorporeal photopheresis induces lymphocyte but not monocyte apoptosis. *Transplant Proc.* 2000;32(4):747–748.
121. Medema JP, Scaffidi C, Kischkel FC, et al. FLICE is activated by association with the CD95 death-inducing signaling complex (DISC). *Embo J.* 1997;16(10):2794–2804.
122. Bladon J, Taylor PC. Lymphocytes treated by extracorporeal photopheresis demonstrate a drop in the Bcl-2/Bax ratio: a possible mechanism involved in extracorporeal-photopheresis-induced apoptosis. *Dermatology.* 2002;204(2):104–107.

123. Morison WL, Parrish JA, McAuliffe DJ, Bloch KJ. Sensitivity of mononuclear cells to PUVA: effect on subsequent stimulation with mitogens and on exclusion of trypan blue dye. *Clin Exp Dermatol.* 1981;6(3):273–277.
124. Gerber A, Bohne M, Rasch J, Struy H, Ansorge S, Gollnick H. Investigation of annexin V binding to lymphocytes after extracorporeal photoimmunotherapy as an early marker of apoptosis. *Dermatology.* 2000;201(2):111–117.
125. Maeda A, Schwarz A, Kernebeck K, et al. Intravenous infusion of syngeneic apoptotic cells by photopheresis induces antigen-specific regulatory T cells. *J Immunol.* 2005;174(10):5968–5976.
126. Fadok VA, de Cathelineau A, Daleke DL, Henson PM, Bratton DL. Loss of phospholipid asymmetry and surface exposure of phosphatidylserine is required for phagocytosis of apoptotic cells by macrophages and fibroblasts. *J Biol Chem.* 2001;276(2):1071–1077.
127. Hanlon DJ, Berger CL, Edelson RL. Photoactivated 8-methoxypsoralen treatment causes a peptide-dependent increase in antigen display by transformed lymphocytes. *Int J Cancer.* 1998;78(1):70–75.
128. Moor AC, Schmitt IM, Beijersbergen van Henegouwen GM, Chimenti S, Edelson RL, Gasparro FP. Treatment with 8-MOP and UVA enhances MHC class I synthesis in RMA cells: preliminary results. *J Photochem Photobiol B.* 1995;29(2-3): p. 193–198.
129. Skoberne M, Beignon AS, Larsson M, Bhardwaj N. Apoptotic cells at the crossroads of tolerance and immunity. *Curr Top Microbiol Immunol.* 2005;289:259–292.
130. Verhoven B, Krahling S, Schlegel RA, Williamson P. Regulation of phosphatidylserine exposure and phagocytosis of apoptotic T lymphocytes. *Cell Death Differ.* 1999;6(3):262–270.
131. Berger CL, Xu AL, Hanlon D, et al. Induction of human tumor-loaded dendritic cells. *Int J Cancer.* 2001;91(4):438–447.
132. Bladon J, Taylor PC. Extracorporeal photopheresis: a focus on apoptosis and cytokines. *J Dermatol Sci.* 2006;43(2):85–94.
133. Di Renzo M, Rubegni P, De Aloe G, et al. Extracorporeal photochemotherapy restores Th1/Th2 imbalance in patients with early stage cutaneous T-cell lymphoma. *Immunology.* 1997;92(1):99–103.
134. Rook AH, et al. IL-12 reverses cytokine and immune abnormalities in Sezary syndrome. *J Immunol.* 1995;154(3):1491–1498.
135. Rook AH, Wood GS, Yoo EK, et al. Interleukin-12 therapy of cutaneous T-cell lymphoma induces lesion regression and cytotoxic T-cell responses. *Blood.* 1999;94(3):902–908.
136. Trautinger F, Knobler R, Willemze R, et al. EORTC consensus recommendations for the treatment of mycosis fungoides/Sezary syndrome. *Eur J Cancer.* 2006;42(8):1014–1030.
137. Whittaker SJ, Marsden JR, Spittle M, et al. Joint British Association of Dermatologists and U.K. Cutaneous Lymphoma Group guidelines for the management of primary cutaneous T-cell lymphomas. *Br J Dermatol.* 2003;149(6):1095–1107.
138. Zic JA. The treatment of cutaneous T-cell lymphoma with photopheresis. *Dermatol Ther.* 2003;16(4):337–346.
139. Demierre MF, Kim YH, Zackheim HS. Prognosis, clinical outcomes and quality of life issues in cutaneous T-cell lymphoma. *Hematol Oncol Clin North Am.* 2003;17(6):1485–1507.
140. Zic JA, Stricklin GP, Greer JP, et al. Long-term follow-up of patients with cutaneous T-cell lymphoma treated with extracorporeal photochemotherapy. *J Am Acad Dermatol.* 1996;35(6):935–945.
141. Duvic M, Chiao N, Talpur R. Extracorporeal photopheresis for the treatment of cutaneous T-cell lymphoma. *J Cutan Med Surg.* 2003;7(4 Suppl):3–7.
142. Gottlieb SL, Wolfe JT, Fox FE, et al. Treatment of cutaneous T-cell lymphoma with extracorporeal photopheresis monotherapy and in combination with recombinant interferon alfa: a 10-year experience at a single institution. *J Am Acad Dermatol.* 1996;35(6):946–957.
143. Lim HW, Edelson RL. Photopheresis for the treatment of cutaneous T-cell lymphoma. *Hematol Oncol Clin North Am.* 1995;9(5):1117–1126.

144. Suchin KR, Cassin M, Washko R, et al. Extracorporeal photochemotherapy does not suppress T- or B-cell responses to novel or recall antigens. *J Am Acad Dermatol*. 1999;41(6):980–986.
145. Geskin L. ECP versus PUVA for the treatment of cutaneous T-cell lymphoma. *Skin Therapy Lett*. 2007;12(5):1–4.
146. Knobler R, Jantschitsch C. Extracorporeal photochemoimmunotherapy in cutaneous T-cell lymphoma. *Transfus Apher Sci*. 2003;28(1):81–89.
147. Jiang SB, Dietz SB, Kim M, Lim HW. Extracorporeal photochemotherapy for cutaneous T-cell lymphoma: a 9.7-year experience. *Photodermatol Photoimmunol Photomed*. 1999;15(5):161–165.
148. Scarisbrick JJ, Taylor P, Holtick U, et al. U.K. consensus statement on the use of extracorporeal photopheresis for treatment of cutaneous T-cell lymphoma and chronic graft-versus-host disease. *Br J Dermatol*. 2008;158(4):659–678.
149. Vonderheid EC, Zhang Q, Lessin SR, et al. Use of serum soluble interleukin-2 receptor levels to monitor the progression of cutaneous T-cell lymphoma. *J Am Acad Dermatol*. 1998;38(2 Pt 1):207–220.
150. Heald P, Rook A, Perez M, et al. Treatment of erythrodermic cutaneous T-cell lymphoma with extracorporeal photochemotherapy. *J Am Acad Dermatol*. 1992;27(3):427–433.
151. Stevens SR, Ke MS, Parry EJ, Mark J, Cooper KD. Quantifying skin disease burden in mycosis fungoides-type cutaneous T-cell lymphomas: the severity-weighted assessment tool (SWAT). *Arch Dermatol*. 2002;138(1):42–48.
152. Ferenczi K, Yawalkar N, Jones D, Kupper TS. Monitoring the decrease of circulating malignant T cells in cutaneous T-cell lymphoma during photopheresis and interferon therapy. *Arch Dermatol*. 2003;139(7):909–913.
153. McGinnis KS, Ubriani R, Newton S, et al. The addition of interferon gamma to oral bexarotene therapy with photopheresis for Sezary syndrome. *Arch Dermatol*. 2005;141(9):1176–1178.
154. Quaglino P, Fierro MT, Rossotto GL, Savoia P, Bernengo MG. Treatment of advanced mycosis fungoides/Sezary syndrome with fludarabine and potential adjunctive benefit to subsequent extracorporeal photochemotherapy. *Br J Dermatol*. 2004;150(2):327–336.
155. Wilson LD, Jones GW, Kim D, et al. Experience with total skin electron beam therapy in combination with extracorporeal photopheresis in the management of patients with erythrodermic (T4) mycosis fungoides. *J Am Acad Dermatol*. 2000;43(1 Pt 1):54–60.
156. Tippel H, Engst R. Mycosis fungoides. Results of helioclimate therapy in high mountains (Davos, 1,560). *Hautarzt*. 1986;37(8):450–453.
157. Ramsay DL, Lish KM, Yalowitz CB, Soter NA. Ultraviolet-B phototherapy for early-stage cutaneous T-cell lymphoma. *Arch Dermatol*. 1992;128(7):931–933.
158. Abe M, Ohnishi K, Kan C, Ishikawa O. Ultraviolet-B phototherapy is successful in Japanese patients with early-stage mycosis fungoides. *J Dermatol*. 2003;30(11):789–796.
159. Resnik KS, Vonderheid EC. Home UV phototherapy of early mycosis fungoides: long-term follow-up observations in thirty-one patients. *J Am Acad Dermatol*. 1993;29(1):73–77.
160. el-Ghorr AA, Norval M. The effect of chronic treatment of mice with urocanic acid isomers. *Photochem Photobiol*. 1997;65(5):866–872.
161. Ozawa M, Ferenczi K, Kikuchi T, et al. 312-Nanometer ultraviolet B light (narrow-band UVB) induces apoptosis of T cells within psoriatic lesions. *J Exp Med*. 1999;189(4):711–718.
162. Clark C, Dawe RS, Evans AT, Lowe G, Ferguson J. Narrowband TL-01 phototherapy for patch-stage mycosis fungoides. *Arch Dermatol*. 2000;136(6):748–752.
163. Pavlotsky F, Barzilai A, Kasem R, Shpiro D, Trau H. UVB in the management of early stage mycosis fungoides. *J Eur Acad Dermatol Venereol*. 2006;20(5):565–572.
164. Diederen PV, van Weelden H, Sanders CJ, Toonstra J, van Vloten WA. Narrowband UVB and psoralen-UVA in the treatment of early-stage mycosis fungoides: a retrospective study. *J Am Acad Dermatol*. 2003;48(2):215–219.
165. Hofer A, Cerroni L, Kerl H, Wolf P. Narrowband (311-nm) UV-B therapy for small plaque parapsoriasis and early-stage mycosis fungoides. *Arch Dermatol*. 1999;135(11):1377–1380.
166. Gökdemir G, Barutcuoglu B, Sakiz D, Köşlü A. Narrowband UVB phototherapy for early-stage mycosis fungoides: evaluation of clinical and histopathological changes. *J Eur Acad Dermatol Venereol*. 2006;20(7):804–809.

167. Gathers RC, Scherschun L, Malick F, Fivenson DP, Lim HW. Narrowband UVB phototherapy for early-stage mycosis fungoides. *J Am Acad Dermatol.* 2002;47(2):191–197.
168. Brazzelli V, Antoninetti M, Palazzini S, Prestinari F, Borroni G. Narrow-band ultraviolet therapy in early-stage mycosis fungoides: study on 20 patients. *Photodermatol Photoimmunol Photomed.* 2007;23(6):229–233.
169. Matsuoka Y, Yoneda K, Katsuura J, et al. Successful treatment of follicular cutaneous T-cell lymphoma without mucinosis with narrow-band UVB irradiation. J Eur Acad Dermatol Venereol., 2007;. 21(8): p. 1121-1122.
170. Ferahbas A, Utas S, Ulas Y, Kontas O, Karakukcu M, Arseven V. Narrow band UVB treatment for a child with mycosis fungoides. *Pediatr Dermatol.* 2006;23(3):302–303.
171. Man I, Crombie IK, Dawe RS, Ibbotson SH, Ferguson J. The photocarcinogenic risk of narrowband UVB (TL-01) phototherapy: early follow-up data. *Br J Dermatol.* 2005;152(4):755–757.
172. Sakuntabhai A, Diffey BL, Farr PM. Response of psoriasis to psoralen-UVB photochemotherapy. *Br J Dermatol.* 1993;128(3):296–300.
173. Lokitz ML, Wong HK. Bexarotene and narrowband ultraviolet B phototherapy combination treatment for mycosis fungoides. *Photodermatol Photoimmunol Photomed.* 2007;23(6):255–257.
174. Shimauchi T, Sugita K, Nishio D, et al. Alterations of serum Th1 and Th2 chemokines by combination therapy of interferon-gamma and narrowband UVB in patients with mycosis fungoides. *J Dermatol Sci.* 2008;50(3):217–225.
175. Novak Z, Bónis B, Baltás E, et al. Xenon chloride ultraviolet B laser is more effective in treating psoriasis and in inducing T cell apoptosis than narrow-band ultraviolet B. *J Photochem Photobiol B.* 2002;67(1):32–38.
176. Mori M, Campolmi P, Mavilia L, Rossi R, Cappugi P, Pimpinelli N. Monochromatic excimer light (308 nm) in patch-stage IA mycosis fungoides. *J Am Acad Dermatol.* 2004;50(6):943–945.
177. Nistico S, Costanzo A, Saraceno R, Chimenti S. Efficacy of monochromatic excimer laser radiation (308 nm) in the treatment of early stage mycosis fungoides. *Br J Dermatol.* 2004;151(4):877–879.
178. Passeron T, Zakaria W, Ostovari N, et al. Efficacy of the 308-nm excimer laser in the treatment of mycosis fungoides. *Arch Dermatol.* 2004;140(10):1291–1293.
179. Kontos AP, Kerr HA, Malick F, Fivenson DP, Lim HW, Wong HK. 308-nm excimer laser for the treatment of lymphomatoid papulosis and stage IA mycosis fungoides. *Photodermatol Photoimmunol Photomed.* 2006;22(3):168–171.
180. Meisenheimer JL. Novel use of 308-nm excimer laser to treat a primary cutaneous CD30+ lymphoproliferative nodule. *J Drugs Dermatol.* 2007;6(4):440–442.
181. Boehncke WH, König K, Rück A, Kaufmann R, Sterry W. In vitro and in vivo effects of photodynamic therapy in cutaneous T cell lymphoma. *Acta Derm Venereol.* 1994;74(3):201–205.
182. Zane C, Venturini M, Sala R, Calzavara-Pinton P. Photodynamic therapy with methylaminolevulinate as a valuable treatment option for unilesional cutaneous T-cell lymphoma. *Photodermatol Photoimmunol Photomed.* 2006;22(5):254–258.
183. Coors EA, von den Driesch P. Topical photodynamic therapy for patients with therapy-resistant lesions of cutaneous T-cell lymphoma. *J Am Acad Dermatol.* 2004;50(3):363–367.
184. Markham T, Sheahan K, Collins P. Topical 5-aminolaevulinic acid photodynamic therapy for tumour-stage mycosis fungoides. *Br J Dermatol.* 2001;144(6):1262–1263.
185. Edstrom DW, Porwit A, Ros AM. Photodynamic therapy with topical 5-aminolevulinic acid for mycosis fungoides: clinical and histological response. *Acta Derm Venereol.* 2001;81(3):184–188.
186. Miller JD, Baron ED, Scull H, et al. Photodynamic therapy with the phthalocyanine photosensitizer Pc 4: the case experience with preclinical mechanistic and early clinical-translational studies. *Toxicol Appl Pharmacol.* 2007;224(3):290–299.

Chapter 9
Light Treatment and Photodynamic Therapy in Acne Patients with Pigmented Skin

Vicente Torres and Luis Torezan

9.1 Introduction

Acne vulgaris is one of the most common dermatological disorders encountered in everyday practice. It is routinely treated with a variety of topical and systemic medications; however, factors such as antibiotic resistance, patient needs for faster results, and adverse effects associated with some drugs have led researchers to seek out alternative therapies.

Newer technologies have recently emerged to aid physicians in their treatment of patients with acne. A variety of lasers and light sources have been shown to be useful as therapy for a variety of conditions including moderate-to-severe acne vulgaris. Light sources including blue light and intense pulsed lights are becoming regular in addition to routine medical management in order to enhance the therapeutic response in these patients. Photodynamic therapy (PDT) may change many of the acne vulgaris paradigms as its place in the therapeutic armamentarium becomes cemented in the treatment of moderate-to-severe inflammatory acne vulgaris, with increasing numbers of clinical studies around the world showing the effectiveness of using external photosensitizers like 5-aminolevulinic acid (5-ALA) or methyl aminolevulinate in combination with light (PDT) in this patient group.

The use of these techniques may have different outcomes and clinical results in different skin types and, in particular, in patients with non-Caucasian, ethnic pigmented skin; however, the experience with these devices in Latin America is limited because the cost of both the technologies and photosensitizers are prohibitive.

In this chapter, we will summarize the limited experience with light and PDT in the treatment of acne in Latin-American patients with pigmented skin, based on limited protocols performed in small groups of patients with acne, personal communications, and anecdotal recommendations from colleagues who are using these procedures for acne treatment.

V. Torres and L. Torezán
Department of Dermatology Juárez Hospital México City.
Photodinamic Group, Hospital de las Clínicas, Facultad de Medicina,
Universidade de São Paulo, Brazil
e-mail: drvicente_2006@yahoo.com.mx

E.D. Baron (ed.), *Light-Based Therapies for Skin of Color*,
DOI: 10.1007/ 978-1-84882-328-0_9, © Springer-Verlag London Limited 2009

9.2   Acne Epidemiology in Latin America

In Latin America, the genetic mixture between Europeans and native Indians has resulted in a "mestiza" skin type that is prone to the development of pigment disorders. It should also be noted that in many countries of South America, there exists an important Afro-American patient population.

It is known that acne is most frequent and severe in Caucasian population than in other racial groups; however, in the American continent, acne vulgaris is still often the most common dermatological disorder in daily practice in either private practice or public hospitals.[1]

Most patients who seek light-based treatments for their acne have been on isotretinoin in the past and are unwilling to be retreated with systemic retinoids. In many cases, they do not have severe acne but present with cyclical relapsing moderate acne and a sense of frustration with the "typical" therapies. This motivation to try new treatments is the primary driver for the development of alternative treatments for acne, such as lights, lasers, and PDT globally, including those Latin patients with pigmented skin.

9.3   Pigmented Skin

All human ethnic groups have the same number of melanocytes, but in patients with pigmented skin, more melanin is produced and is packaged into larger and more numerous melanosomes. In Caucasian skin, the melanosomes are small and packaged together in membranes and remain around the basal layer of the epidermis. However, pigmented skin demonstrates melanosome dispersal throughout the layers of the epidermis. These patients tan more easily, retain tan longer, have a thicker stratum corneum, larger and more numerous fibroblast cells (More keloids), larger macrophages, and larger oil glands.[2]

All these features contribute to the altered biological response of pigmented skin to light including treatment with lasers, other light sources, and PDT. The most common complication after light or PDT therapy is postinflammatory hyperpigmentation (PIH).

Darker racial group represents a wide range of ethnic groups including black, Asian, Latino, American-Indian, and pacific islanders, most of them included in the Fitzpatrick skin types IV to VI.[3]

PIH is a reaction observed after injury or mechanical trauma to the skin. It is manifested by macules or pigment patches at the site of a previous inflammation response. Lesions usually persist for months or longer, depending of the intensity of pigmentation and its location.

The use of PDT involves physician choice on the type of photosensitizer, incubation time, light potency, and wave length exposure, with great care being taken when treating skin types IV to VI to avoid the development of PIH. Some authors have recommended application of bleaching agents 2 weeks before any aggressive treatment and compliance with strict sun protection after procedures.[4]

9.4   Mechanism of Action of Light and PDT in the Acne Treatment

In general, light-based treatments have two therapeutic approaches; the first one is the reduction of *Propionibacterium acnes* levels, and the second one is the disruption of sebaceous gland function.[5] Light may also have anti-inflammatory properties via action on inflammatory cytokines.[6,7]

9.4.1   Endogenous Porphyrins

The production of porphyrins by *P. acnes* (protoporphyrin, uroporphyrin, and coproporphyrin III) established the scientific basis for the treatment of acne using PDT. This substance acts as a photophore and mediates a PDT response following exposure to light. These porphyrins absorb visible light at several wavelengths, including blue and red light wavelengths, between 400 and 700 nm. Absorption of light excites the porphyrin compound causing formation of singlet oxygen and reactive free radicals. Theoretically, the oxygen radicals destroy lipids in the cell wall of *P. acnes* destroying the organism.[8]

9.4.2   Different Wavelengths and Light Treatments in Acne

Similar to the effect of antibacterial agents, reduction in *P. acnes* levels by light therapy may play a role in improving acne lesions. Many light sources may affect *P. acnes*, including narrow-band light sources, intense pulse light (IPL) devices (broadband light), KTP lasers (532 nm), pulse dye lasers (585–595 nm), and various orange/red light lasers, or light sources (610–635 nm); these light sources have wavelengths that correspond to an absorption peak of *P. acnes* porphyrins.

Longer wavelengths penetrate more deeply into the skin, but are less effective in activating porphyrins.

The most used wavelength in acne treatment has been the blue light (415 nm) because it cause photoactivation of the coproporphyrin III produced by *P. acnes*.

The different protocols using blue light in different patient populations have been mildly to moderately effective in clinical trials, presumably due to the poor skin penetration by blue light.[9]

There is one report comparing blue light therapy with topical 1% clindamycin solution for inflammatory acne in which lesions were reduced 34% after blue light therapy, compared with 14% with clindamycin.[10]

One poster from a Japanese study in the *J Am Acad Dermatol* in 2005 confirms the efficacy of phototherapy with a newly developed, high-intensity enhanced, narrowband blue light source in patients with mild-to-moderate acne that was performed in 42 acne patients who were treated twice a week up to 5 weeks. Acne lesions were reduced by 60%. No patient discontinued treatment because of adverse effects. In vitro investigation revealed that irradiation from this light source reduced the number of *P. acnes*, but not *Staphylococcus epidermidis* that were isolated from the patients.

Phototherapy using this blue light source was effective and well tolerated in acne patients, and had an ability to decrease numbers of *P. acnes* in vitro like an antibiotic.

The importance of this study is that Japanese patients have a highly pigmented skin compared with some other racial groups, and yet the use of high-intensity enhanced narrowband blue light source did not result in reported side effects such as PIH. Furthermore, the use of blue light avoids the usage of liquid nitrogen that may be a cause itself of PIH.

The red light (635 nm) is less effective than blue light at porphyrin activation; however, it penetrates deeper. There are some protocols that have shown that the combination of red light plus blue light increase effectiveness in the treatment of acne patients.[11]

Another poster showed a pilot study of the efficacy and safety of infrared (IR) light in the treatment of inflammatory acne vulgaris. An intense IR light pulse device was used to treat the acne lesions of 20 patients with inflammatory acne using an IR-pulsed light hand piece. The treatment parameters were wavelength range of 850–1,350 nm, fluence of 46–52 J/cm^2, and a pulse width of 3–4 s. Ten of 11 patients who had more than one IR treatment had improvement in their conditions, ranging from "fewer blemishes" to "no acne lesions remaining." One patient (1/11) was still experiencing flare-ups. Two to three monthly IR treatments produced favorable outcomes in nine of ten patients. There is also evidence that IR treatment reduces skin oiliness. In summary, the use of IR treatment shows good efficacy and safety for inflammatory acne in this pilot trial. The authors established that this technique is particularly advantageous for females of childbearing age who may prefer not to use oral isotretinoin because of teratogenic effects. No adverse effects were reported.[12]

In some Latin-American countries, empirically, some dermatologists use IPL in wavelengths from 430 to 1,100 nm like complement of acne standard therapy. As a result of this technique, a clearing effect of the pigmented skin and postinflammatory melanosis is produced. This technique is used for the treatment of melasma patients too.

Treatments that affect *P. acnes*, including antibacterial agents and light-sources, generally are effective only when used frequently; relapse typically occurs soon after cessation of use. In acne, therefore, light-based treatments that primarily target *P. acnes* probably should be combined with agents that affect comedogenesis, such as topical retinoids, which inhibit formation of both comedones and microcomedo (precursor of all acne lesions).

Theoretically, the 1,450-nm wavelength Smoothbeam may be the ideal wavelength for treating acne because it produces peak heating right at the level of the sebaceous gland; this is a diode laser that probably targets and withers the sebaceous glands.

In a study using a diode laser 1,450-nm wavelength performed by Uebelhoer, 22 subjects were randomized to receive four laser treatments, 3–4 weeks apart, on one side of the face, with the other side serving as the control. They were treated with about 10 J/cm² initially, with skin surface cooling, but this was increased subsequently to 14–16 J/cm². In the 15 subjects who received four treatments and had assessments 6 weeks after the final treatment, the reduction in lesion counts on the treated side was 40% greater than that on the no treated side. The reductions occurred in both papular and comedonal lesions. Erythema following the treatment generally resolved within 15 min. Although there is discomfort, most of the patients rated their discomfort as "less than moderate."[13]

The Smoothbeam (1,450 nm) laser targets the sebaceous glands and causes a reduction in acne lesion counts documented in a study of 27 people with back acne treated with this device and it was "likely due to a slight functional impairment of the glands secondary to mild thermal damage created at the time of irradiation." Treatment has a secondary effect on the rate of sebum production and the *P. acnes* population, both of which are associated with acne.[14]

The lead author of this study was Dilip Paithankar, PhD of Candela; two authors were from the Naval Medical Center in San Diego, where the study was done. The 27 subjects had acne of similar severity on both sides of the upper back, which were treated with laser and cryogen spray; control areas were treated with cryogen spray only. Four treatments were administered, with 3 weeks in between treatments. The average radiant exposure was 18 J/cm², ranging from 14 to 22 J/cm².

A significant reduction in inflammatory and noninflammatory lesion counts was seen after the first treatment and 3 weeks after the first, second, and third treatments, compared with the control sides. Three weeks after the first treatment, the mean lesion count fell from 7.22 to 2.67 in 27 patients. Three weeks after the second treatment, the mean lesion count had dropped to 1.04 in 23 patients. Control sides had small, statistically nonsignificant changes. Statistically and clinically significant reductions in lesion counts also were seen at the 6-, 12-, and 24-week follow-up visits, compared with control areas. No acne lesions were seen on the treated sides of the backs in 14 of the 15 study participants who completed the 24-week follow-up.

Biopsies obtained at 2 and 6 months after treatment found that sebaceous glands and associated ductal structures were not different from control areas, so "on routine microscopy, there appeared to be no long-term alteration in adnexal structure architecture," the investigators concluded.

There were no unusual side effects or adverse reactions. Erythema, which was expected, was the most common side effect, but it resolved.

Hyperpigmentation in three patients resolved by the 6-week follow-up visit.

At this point seems that the disruption of sebaceous gland function may be associated with a longer duration of action versus reduction of *P. acnes*. But since there are very few data about the long-term effects of light-based therapies in clinical practice, validation of this theory awaits controlled clinical trials. Additional factors to consider with treatments that target the sebaceous gland include the degree of damage to the gland and the extent to which it recovers. Likely, PDT using external photosensitizers is the best option for the sebaceous gland disruption.

9.5   Some Protocols for Light Acne Treatment in USA

Based in the idea that light and PDT appears to be the next frontier in acne treatment. In the USA, three devices have either been approved or cleared by the Food and Drug Administration for light-based treatment of acne: the clear light blue-light therapy, which uses a noncoherent light source (405–420 nm), the cool touch Nd:YAG laser (1,320 nm), and the Smoothbeam diode laser (1,450 nm).

9.5.1   Mild Acne

To treat mild acne that has not responded well to topical or medical therapy, the use of clear light device, a noncoherent light source (405–420 nm), or some device emitting blue light is recommended because it is perhaps the safest and most convenient procedure.

9.5.2   Moderate Acne

For moderate acne, any one of the three devices approved by FDA is an option. If the patient has any acne scarring, the lasers are probably better because they may improve the scarring.

If the patient has a darker complexion, blue light is better because such patients run the risk of pigmentation changes from the cryogen spray used with lasers.

9.5.3   Severe Acne

Severe acne probably requires laser treatment because the lasers may go deeper and damage sebaceous glands. Cystic acne needs isotretinoin, however, and even the lasers probably do not penetrate deep enough to be of use.

9.6   External Photosensitizers for PDT in Acne

The external photosensitizers available in Latin America are Levulan (Kerastick) 5-ALA in many countries of the continent (Stiefel laboratories) and in Brazil methyl aminolevulinate (Metvix, Galderma laboratories).

Bacterial destruction may also be enhanced by the use of a photosensitizer with light therapy. Ashkenazi and coworkers showed that addition of ALA dramatically reduced bacterial viability in vitro compared with untreated cultures (seven orders of magnitude versus two orders of magnitude).[15]

However, Horfelt et al reported no reduction in *P. acnes* measurements in skin surface biopsies after PDT treatment of 15 patients with acne.[16]

The latter group speculated that PDT may have a mechanism of action in acne other than eradication of *P. acnes.*

While it is known that light sources can target bacteria, a robust bactericidal action has not been shown with *P. acnes* either in vitro or in vivo.[17]

In a comparative study of IPL alone and IPL combined with PDT for the treatment of facial acne in Asian skin, Yeung et al did not reach significant improvement of inflammatory acne when compared to control group. In this study, the authors applied MAL for 30 min only, and patients were submitted to four treatments at 3-week interval. After 12 weeks, mean reduction of inflammatory lesions was 65% in PDT group, 23% in IPL, and 88% in control group. Crusting and PIH were seen in 10% of IPL and PDT groups, and subsided within a week after treatment. It must be commented that a 30-min MAL incubation time may be considered too short to provide enough PpIX concentration on the skin. Therefore, PDT reaction (i.e. edema, erythema) is reduced and final results are expected to be less effective.[18]

Has been other reports using a pulsed dye laser instead of blue light combined with topical ALA reducing acne lesions by 62% by 1 month, following a single session in a series of ten patients, reported by Alexiades-Armenakas.[19]

In her study, patients had ALA applied 45 min prior to laser treatment. Two lasers were used, one a long-pulsed 595-nm laser and the other a 585-nm laser. Very low fluences were used: 3 J/cm^2 for the long-pulsed laser and 2 J/cm^2 for the other laser. The improvement with the laser treatment occurred very rapidly, on the order of a few days. In this study, the improvement tended to last for about 3 weeks, after which, most of the patients began reporting the appearance of new lesions. Some patients developed new lesions in previously uninvolved areas adjacent to the treated areas.

With a treatment like PDT, the evidence of efficacy in treating acne is much less strong, but there is the trade-off of the process being a negative experience for the patient. "Photochemicals [used in PDT] cause cell membrane damage, and with the process, there is pain. The outcome may be positive, but this is not a positive event in the life of the patient. For some authors when PDT is used to treat something like cancerous lesions, the process is entirely justified, but as a repetitive treatment for acne, it is far more questionable.

Light-based therapies can also target sebocytes and the sebaceous glands. Destruction of the sebaceous gland is possible, but is toxic to the epidermis.[20]

The concern, along with pain, currently limits treatments that target the sebaceous gland. If a painless, nontoxic treatment that disrupts sebaceous gland function can be found, it should provide significant benefit in acne.

Free oxygen radicals generated by application of photosensitizers may damage the gland and eliminate or reduce sebum excretion.

The general sense everywhere in relation with this new area of the acne treatment in this moment is that light therapies don't work very well for acne, because a photochemical effect should prevail over any photothermal effect to excite endogenous porphyrins produced by *P. acnes.*

In addition, the only studies to show microscopic damage to the sebaceous glands have been those using an external photosensitizer like 5-ALA with long incubation times, continuous wave light sources, and red light only. Some acne patients may respond to various light-based treatments, but most of the time the improvement is modest and short-lived, and the therapy should be at this moment only a complement of the standard therapy used in acne.

The informal protocols used in countries like Mexico using blue light alone, blue light plus 5-ALA, IPL plus 5-ALA, and red light plus ALA have not been published yet, and the study groups are to little.

9.7 Outcomes and Complications of PDT in Pigmented Skin Patients with NMSC and Applications for PDT Treatment in Acne Patients

The use of PDT in patients with nonmelanoma skin cancer with Fitzpatrick skin type III to V has, in our hands, shown excellent outcomes in terms of cure and recurrence rates and have been a good lobby for calculating the outcomes and complications in patients with acne treated by PDT; however, it is true that more pigmentary changes are expected. PIH is one of the major complications seen in patients with skin types over III, and the more inflammatory reaction induced by PDT, the more PIH is observed, especially when we treat large NMSC that are located in the lower limbs. Although PIH is a concern, it improves in up to 4 weeks after last PDT session.

Bleaching creams with hydroquinone may be used for those who still show PIH or complain of pigmentary changes after PDT.

9.8 PIH in Acne Patients Treated with PDT

When treating inflammatory acne with topical PDT, using either ALA or MAL, it is true that some patients do experience transient PIH between sessions.

In Brazil, one of the authors of this chapter has been treating acne patients with MAL-PDT for up to 1 year. The protocol includes patients with skin types I to IV and inflammatory acne, unresponsive to other treatment options such as oral antibiotics and isotretinoin, or patients with proved no adherence to treatment who chose PDT like a therapeutic option.

MAL is applied on the face and occluded for 90 min and is then illuminated with a LED (light emission diode) device of 635 nm at total dose of 37 J/cm^2 (Fig. 9.1, 9.2, and 9.3).

Three treatment sessions are performed one month apart. All patients experience pain during illumination which lasts for up to 6 h after treatment, although an air cooling device is used during the treatment session.

Topical MAL-PDT shows good result for inflammatory acne with a mean reduction of about 60% in inflammatory lesions, and no effect on noninflammatory lesions are observed. The results in general show maintained response up to 6 months after

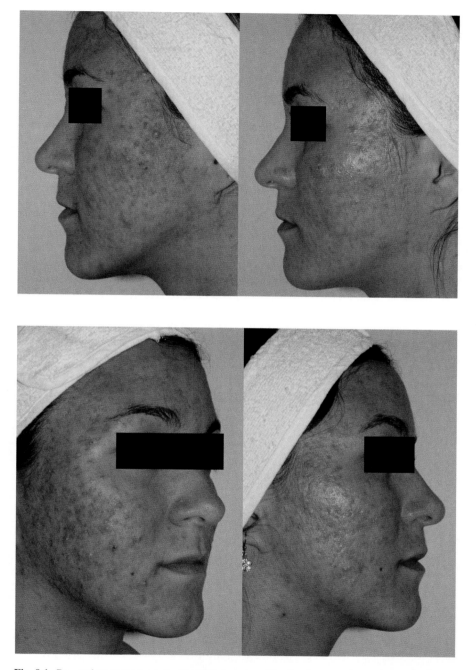

Fig. 9.1 Pre- and postacne treated with PDT phototype III, after three treatments 1-month apart 90 min incubation of MAL and illuminated with LED of 635 nm at dose of 37 J/cm². No PIH was seen

the last treatment session. PIH is not a really frequent problem and is expected to be most common in patients skin type IV with severe inflammatory lesions of acne.

At least in our experience in Brazil, no patient required topical bleaching creams before or after PDT in all cases.

In our hands, either ALA or MAL PDT for acne treatment shows similar results, and may be considered a treatment option for severe inflammatory acne unresponsive to standard antiacne therapy.

Some darker skinned patients had transient hyperpigmentation, presumably not related with the light itself but related to the cryogen spray used for cooling with the laser.[21]

For example, the Japanese skin is biologically similar to the American-Indians. One example of this is that melasma and postinflammatory melanosis are frequent in both populations.

Hyperpigmentation and epidermal exfoliation after PDT is a very frequent complication in some protocols in Japanese patients. Pigmentation change persisted over 1 week to 2 months. Epidermal exfoliation lasted from fourth to tenth day. That is why, in Japan exist some PDT protocols to avoid pigmentation and epidermal exfoliation using 5-ALA administered orally in patients with skin phototypes IV and V that can be an option for the treatment of Latin patients with dark skin (Fig. 9.2).

Pigmentation after topically applied ALA-PDT is caused by melanogenesis, which is a photodynamic reaction to the accumulation of PpIX in the epidermis. Other adverse effects and complications are erythema, swelling, reactive acne, reactive sebum, and herpes simplex.

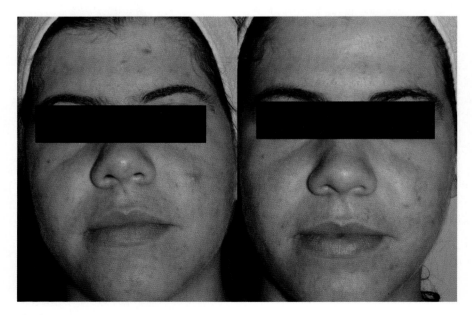

Fig. 9.2 Same protocol phototypes III

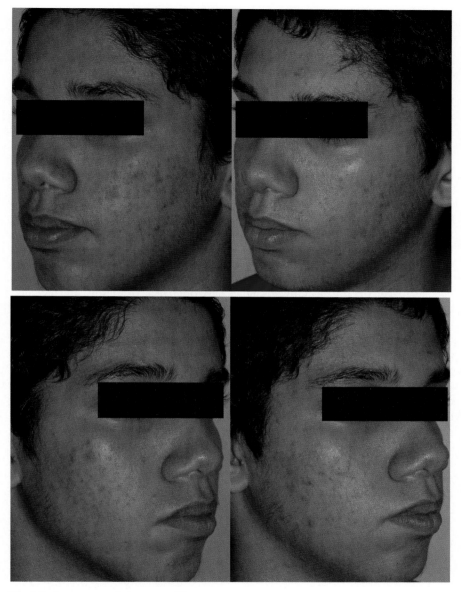

Fig. 9.3 Same protocol phototypes IV

Lower levels of radiation are recommended for initial treatments in pigmented skin. At subsequent PDT treatments, a step-by-step increase of the light energy is recommended.[22,23]

9.9 Experience Using Light and PDT for Acne Treatment in Latin America

Procedures and protocols using Light and PDT for the acne treatment in Latin America for patients with pigmented skin are under way, and are not defined yet; however, we are running some trials like the one done recently in the Barcelona meeting about PDT in a group of acne patients using MAL, 90 min of incubation, and illuminated with LED 635 nm at a total dose of 37 J/cm^2.[24]

9.10 Conclusions

Clinical data on the use of laser and light-based therapies is still emerging but suggests that both may offer benefit in acne; however, more data are needed to define their role in acne treatment. Optimal strategies, frequencies, and device settings remain to be clarified.

While meaningful progress has been made in the study of light-based treatment of acne, to date the existing clinical studies have often lacked controls, and included only small numbers of patients.

In addition, very few studies have compared light-based treatments with standard and well-validated pharmaceutical treatments, and none with the current recommended therapy for most types of acne – combination therapy with a topical retinoid plus antimicrobial agent(s). Further, little information is available about long-term effects of therapy. In recent times, a number of controlled studies utilizing split-face designs and randomization have been published (most with relatively small numbers of patients); however, much remains to be determined about the optimal device, dosing, and frequency of administration for these procedures in active acne.

Hyperpigmentation and epidermal exfoliation after some PDT procedures is a relatively frequent complication in Latin patients and there is not a consensus about the use or not of bleaching agents before or after the procedure. Other factor to keep in mind is the high dose of solar radiation in many countries of Latin America that can be an additional factor for complications after PDT.

In this moment, the recommendation about the empiric use of hydroquinone either before or after PDT for acne treatment is an irregular behavior in patients with pigmented skin in Latin America.

References

1. Torres V. Primer Consenso Mexicano para el Manejo del Acné. *Dermatol Rev Mex.* 2003;47(2):95–97.
2. Sanchez MR. Cutaneous diseases in Latinos. *Dermatol Clin.* 2003;21:689–697.
3. Taylor SC. Epidemiology of skin diseases in ethnic populations. *Dermatol Clin.* 2003;21: 601–607.

4. Stratigos AJ, Katsambas AD. Optimal management of recalcitrant disorders of hyperpigmentation in dark-skinned patients. *Am J Clin Dermatol.* 2004;5:161–168.

5. Mariwalla K, Rohrer TE. Use of lasers and light-based therapy for treatment of acne vulgaris. *Lasers Surg Med.* 2005;37(5):333–342.

6. W.J. Cunliffe V. Goulden phototherapy and acne vulgaris. *Br J Dermatol.* 2000;142:855–856.

7. Taub AF. Procedural treatments for acne vulgaris. *Dermatol Surg.* 2007;33:1005–1026.

8. Elman M, Lebzelter I. Light therapy in the treatment of acne vulgaris. *Dermatol Surg.* 2004;30: 139–146.

9. Phototherapy in the treatment of acne vulgaris: what is its role? In: Charakida A, Seaton ED, Charakida M, Mouser P, Avgerinos A, Chu AC. *Am J Clin Dermatol.* 2004;5:211–216.

10. Gold MH, Rao J, Goldman MP, Bridges TM, Bradshaw VL, Boring MM, Guider AN. A multicenter clinical evaluation of the treatment of mild to moderate inflammatory acne vulgaris of the face with visible blue light in comparison to topical 1% clindamycin antibiotic solution. *J Drugs Dermatol.* Jan–Feb 2005.

11. Fukao M, Kawada A, Aragane Y, Endo H. An Open study and in vitro investigation of acne phototherapy with a high intensity enhanced narrowband blue light source. J Am Acad Dermatol. March 2005:14.

12. Gupta A, Vasily D. A pilot study of the efficacy and safety of infrared light in the treatment of inflammatory acne vulgaris. *J Am Acad Dermatol.* February 2007:AB23.

13. Uebelhoer NS, Bogle MA, Dover JS, Arndt KA, Rohrer TE. Comparison of stacked pulses versus double-pass treatments of facial acne with a 1,450-nm laser. *Dermatol Surg.* May 2007; 33(5):552–559.

14. Paithankar DY, Ross EV, Saleh BA, Blair MA, Graham BS. Acne treatment with a 1,450 nm wavelength laser and cryogen spray cooling. *Lasers Surg Med.* 2002;31(2):106–114.

15. Ashkenazi H, Malik Z, Harth Y, Nitzan Y. Eradication of Propionibacterium acnes by its endogenic porphyrins after illumination with high intensity blue light. *FEMS Immunology and Medical Microbiology* 2006;35(1):17–24.

16. Hörfelt C, Stenquist B, Larkö O, Faergemann J, Wennberg AM. Photodynamic therapy for acne vulgaris: a pilot study of the dose-response and mechanism of action. *Acta Derm Venereol.* 2007;87(4):325–329.

17. Seaton ED, Mouser PE, Charakida A, Alam S, Seldon PE, Chu AC. Investigation of the mechanism of action of nonablative pulsed-dye laser therapy in photorejuvenation and inflammatory acne vulgaris. *Brit J Dermatol.* 2006;155(4):748–755.

18. Yeung CK, Shek SY, Bjerring P, et al. A comparative study of IPL alone and its combination with PDT for the treatment of face acne in Asian skin. *Lasers Surg Med.* 2007;39:1–6.

19. Macrene A-A. New and emerging treatments for acne and photoaging. *J Drugs Dermatol.* January 1, 2006;5(1):85.

20. Hongcharu W, Taylor CR, Chang Y, et al. Topical ALA-photodynamic therapy for the treatment of acne vulgaris. *J Invest Dermatol.* 2000;115:183–192.

21. Manuskiatti W, Eimpunth S, Wanitphakdeedecha R. Effect of cold air cooling on the incidence of postinflammatory hyperpigmentation after Q-switched Nd:YAG laser treatment of acquired bilateral nevus of ota-like macules. *Arch Fac Plast Surg.* 2007;143(9):1139–1143.

22. Horfelt C, et al. Topical methyl aminolevulinate PDT for the treatment of facial acne vulgaris: results of a randomized, controlled study. *Br J Dermatol.* 2006;155:608–613.

23. Wiegell SR, Wulf HC. Photodynamic therapy of acne vulgaris using 5-ALA versus methyl aminolevulintate. *J Am Acad Dermatol.* 2006;54:647–651.

24. Torezan L, Niwa A, Festa-Neto C, Sanches Jr. JA. Photodynamic therapy for facial acne vulgaris using methyl aminolevulinate: six month follow up. Poster presented at the PDT annual Congress – Euro-PDT Meeting, Barcelona, 7–8th March, 2008.

Chapter 10
Clinical Application of Intense Pulsed Light in Asian Patients

Yuan-Hong Li, Yan Wu, and Hong-Duo Chen

Asian skin is quite different from Caucasian skin in a variety of aspects. Asian skin is relatively darker than Caucasian skin. They are prone to get sun tanning, instead of sun burning, which are very common in Caucasian people with Fitzpatrick phototype I to III. Most Asian skin belongs to Fitzpatrick phototype III or more. Asian skin is more apt to develop postinflammatory hyperpigmentation (PIH) and hypopigmentation following any procedure that induces inflammation. Asians are far more likely than Caucasians to develop keloid. Thus, more cautions should be given to Asian skin to avoid any damage to the integrity of the epidermis. Furthermore, photoaging in Asians tends to occur at a later age and has more pigmentary problems but less wrinkling than in Caucasians.[1] This difference is partially due to the higher epidermal melanin content.

As has already been well documented, there are larger and more melanized melanosomes in Asian skin than in Caucasian skin. In order to avoid the overdamage to the epidermal melanin, lower energy and mild treatment parameters of IPL therapy are proposed for Asian skin.

10.1 Pigmented Disorders

10.1.1 Ephelides and Lentigines

Ephelides, or freckles, are small, usually less than 0.5 cm in diameter, discrete brown macules that appear on sun-exposed skin. Histologically they demonstrate as melanocyte proliferation without nest formation along the basement membrane. Intense pulsed light (IPL) sources that emit a broad band of visible light (400–1,200 nm) from a noncoherent filtered flashlamp affect pigmentation via photothermal effects. IPL has

Y-H. Li (✉), Y. Wu, and H-D. Chen
Department of Dermatology, No. 1 Hospital of China Medical University,
Shenyang 110001, China
e-mail: liyuanhong@vip.sina.com

E.D. Baron (ed.), *Light-Based Therapies for Skin of Color,*
DOI: 10.1007/ 978-1-84882-328-0_10, © Springer-Verlag London Limited 2009

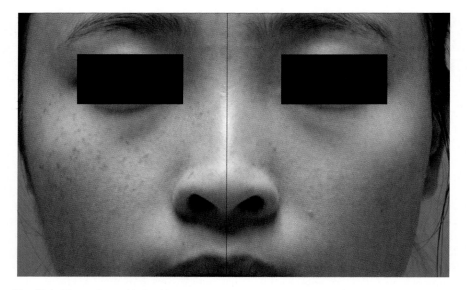

Fig. 10.1 The patient with freckles received one session of treatment on the left face (560 nm filter, single pulse, 4 ms pulse width, 14 J/cm²). The right side is spared as the self-control. This picture was taken at 1-month follow-up visit

been studied for the treatment of lentigines and ephelides with cutoff filters ranging from 550 to 590 nm, a fluence of 25–35 J/cm², and a pulse width of 4.0 ms. These studies have been performed on Asian skin with surprisingly no PIH. This lower risk of PIH and the limited postoperative downtime have made IPL a popular choice. The patient should understand, however, that multiple treatments may be necessary. In our practice, for those who do not wish to have any downtime, or for those who wish to improve not only their pigmentation but also pore size and skin texture, we offer IPL treatment combined with other laser modalities in the same treatment session to obtain a better outcome. The recommended filters are 560 and 590 nm. The recommended parameters (e.g. Lumenis One, Lumenis, Santa Clara, USA) are single pulse (pulse width: 3–4 ms) at 12–14 J/cm² for fair skin and double pulse (pulse width: 3 ms, pulse delay: 20–30 ms) at 15–17 J/cm² for dark skin. After two sessions, all the 69 freckle patients obtained over 50% clearance.[2] In a split-face study, 70% patients obtained over 50% clearance after two sessions on the treated side of face. See Fig. 10.1 for details.

10.2 Café au Lait Macules

The use of Q-switched lasers (ruby 694 nm, frequency-doubled Nd:YAG 532 nm)[3] and pulsed dye laser (PDL) (510 nm)[4] in the treatment of Café au lait macules (CALMs) has yielded variable results with a high risk of recurrence if pigment is left behind. Up to 50% of patients demonstrated a similar variable degree of repigmentation following a long-time follow-up period.

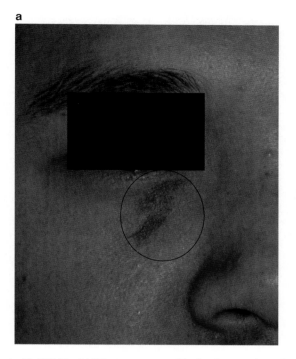

Fig. 10.2 A patient with CALMs. (**a**) Prior to treatment; (**b**) after three sessions of treatment (560 nm filter, double pulse, 3 ms pulse width, 35 ms pulse delay, 14 J/cm²)

Yoshida et al performed the treatment of pigmented lesions with neurofibromatosis 1 by intense pulsed–radio frequency in combination with topical application of vitamin D_3 ointment. Eight patients were treated in this study and the improvement was moderate to good in six cases (75%).[5]

We treated 58 Chinese patients of CALMs with Lumenis One IPL (560 nm filter, single pulse, 3–4 ms pulse width, 14 J/cm² for fair skin; 560 nm filter, double pulse, 3 ms pulse width, 30 ms pulse delay, 15–17 J/cm² for dark skin). With the succession of four treatments, 35%, 63%, 75%, and 87% patient obtained over 50% improvement.[2] See Fig. 10.2 for details.

10.3   Melasma

Melasma is commonly seen in Asian population. Traditional therapies are less effective and may cause adverse effects. We tried IPL (Lumenis One, Lumenis) in 89 women with melasma. Subjects received a total of four IPL treatments at a 3-week interval (560/590/615/640 nm filter, pulse width of 3–4 ms, pulse delay of 25–40 ms, fluence of 13–17 J/cm²). Changes in facial hyperpigmentation and telangiectasia were evaluated using a Mexameter, the melasma area and severity index (MASI), and a global evaluation by the patients and blind investigators. Sixty-nine of 89 patients (77.5%)

b

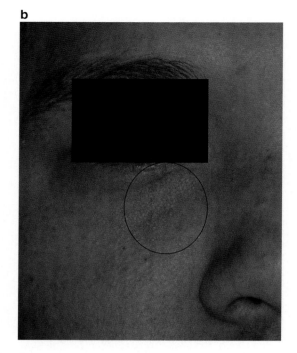

Fig. 10.2 (continued)

obtained 51–100% improvements, according to the overall evaluation by dermatologists. Self-assessment by the patients indicates that 63 of 89 patients (70.8%) considered more than 50% or more improvements. Mean MASI scores decreased substantially from 15.2 to 4.5. Mexameter results demonstrated a significant decrease in the degree of pigmentation and erythema beneath the melasma lesions. Patients with the epidermal-type melasma responded better to treatment than the mixed-type. Adverse actions were minimal.[6] See Figs. 10.3 and 10.4 for details.

10.4 Postburn Hyperpigmentation

Ho et al has tried IPL in the treatment of postburn hyperpigmentation to assess its efficacy and side effects. Multilight™ (ESC Medical Systems Ltd., Yokneam, Israel) of the IPL family was used to treat these patients at intervals of 3–4 weeks for three to seven treatments. Patients were treated with an energy fluence of 28–46 J/cm², pulse width of 1.7–4 ms, double pulse mode, and a delay of 15–40 ms. Among the 19 Chinese patients, over 78% showed more than 50% clinical clearance and nearly 32% of the patients were able to achieve more than 75% clearing. Although two patients had no clinical response, one patient had 100% clearing. Three patients developed blisters and one patient had erythema that all resolved within 1 week without leaving permanent marks. They have been followed up from 11 to 32 months and there was no recurrence of the hyperpigmentation.[7]

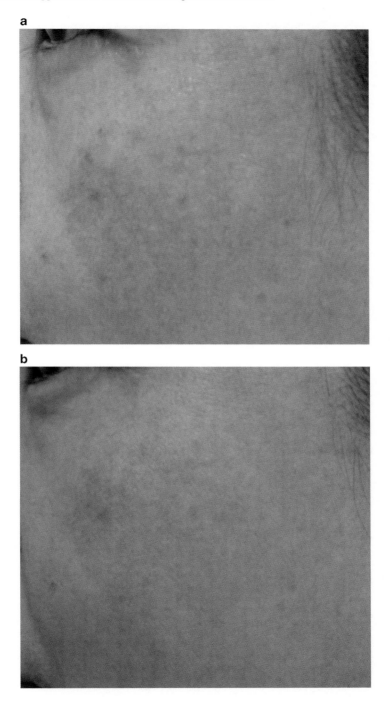

Fig. 10.3 A representative photograph of a melasma patient before and after IPL treatments. Parameters: 590 nm filter, triple pulse, 3 ms pulse width, 30 ms pulse delay, 15–17 J/cm². Left side of face

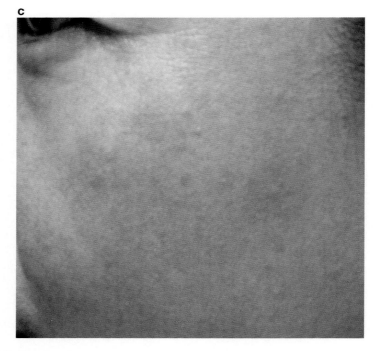

Fig. 10.3 (continued)

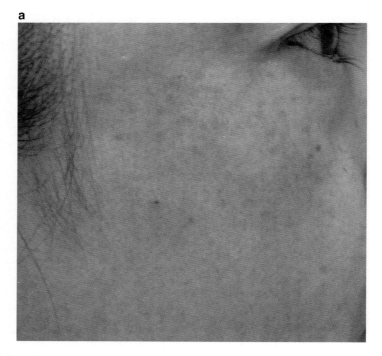

Fig. 10.4 (**a**) Pretreatment; (**b**) after four sessions; (**c**) at 3-month follow-up visit. Right side of face

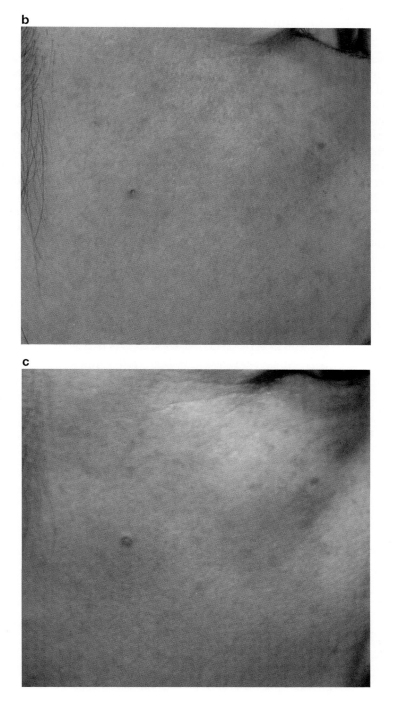

Fig. 10.4   (continued)

10.5 Port-Wine Stain

Asian patients with more melanin in the epidermis are at a higher risk of adverse effects after laser treatment of vascular diseases. Although the PDL is regarded as the gold standard in treating port-wine stain (PWS), at times patients find the results disappointing and the various side effects, such as pronounced purpura and pigmented changes, to be disturbing.

Bjerring et al used IPL system for the treatment of PWS resistant to multiple PDL treatments. Fifteen PWS patients, who were previously found to be resistant to multiple PDL treatments, were treated four times with a second-generation IPL system. Patients with dye laser-resistant PWS could be divided into two groups: responders to IPL treatments (46.7%) and nonresponders (53.3%). All responders obtained more than 50% reduction, and 85.7% of the responders obtained between 75% and 100% reduction of their lesions. The IPL treatment modality was found to be safe and efficient for the treatment of PWS, except for those located in the V2 area.[8]

We also tried IPL (Lumenis One) in treating PWS and got good results. See Fig. 10.5 for details.

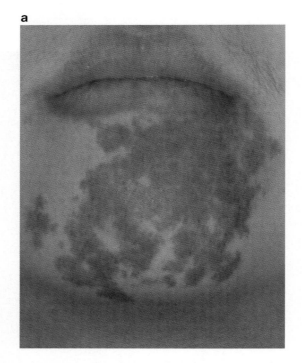

Fig. 10.5 A patient with port-wine stain (*PWS*). (**a**) Before the treatment; (**b**) after four sessions of treatment (560 nm filter, triple pulse, 3 ms pulse width, 50 ms pulse delay, 20–24 J/cm^2, 2 pass)

b

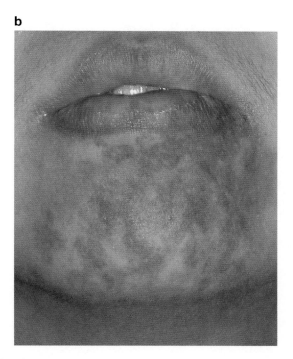

Fig. 10.5   (continued)

10.6   Acne and Rosacea

A rising number of laser- or light-based therapies are addressing the need for effective acne treatments with minimal downtime. In order to evaluate the efficacy of IPL in the treatment of acne, Chang et al performed IPL equipped with a 530- to 750-nm filter on 30 female Korean patients (mean age, 25.7 years) with mild-to-moderate acne. All patients experienced the reduction of inflammatory lesion counts in both sides of face. There was no significant difference between IPL-treated and IPL-untreated sides of the face for mean papule plus pustule counts, 3 weeks after three sessions. As to red macules, 63% were good or excellent on the laser-treated side compared with 33% on the untreated side. Improvement of irregular pigmentation and skin tone was detected on the laser-treated side than the untreated side.[9]

We have used IPL in treating acne patients and rosacea patients at a 3-week interval. It could significantly reduce the inflammatory papules, pustules, red macules, and even acne scars. See Figs. 10.6 and 10.7 for details.

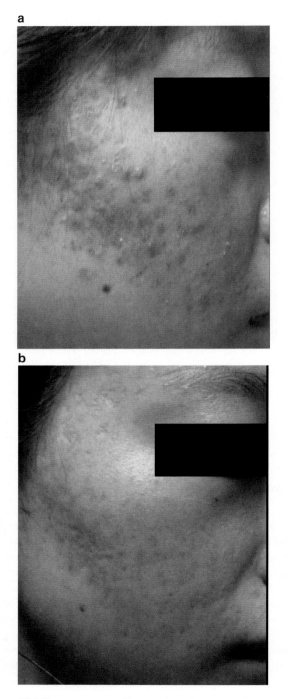

Fig. 10.6 A patient with inflammatory acne. She experienced a dramatic improvement of inflammatory papules, pustules, red macules, and acne scars. (**a**) Before the treatment; (**b**) after three sessions of treatment (590 nm filter, triple pulse, 3 ms pulse width, 30 ms pulse delay, 17–19 J/cm^2)

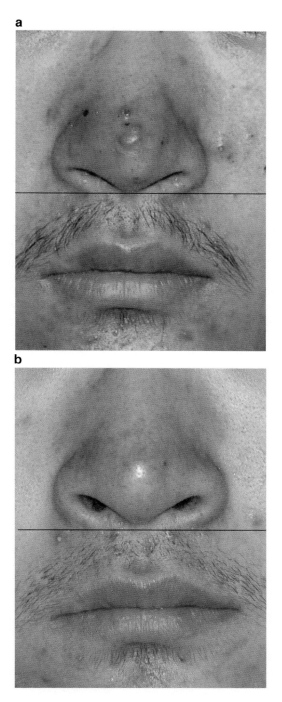

Fig. 10.7 A rosacea boy received three sessions of treatment on the nose (the perioral region was spared to avoid the damage to the moustache). (**a**) Before the treatment; (**b**) after three sessions of treatment (590 nm filter, triple pulse, pulse width 3 ms, pulse delay 35 ms, 17–20 J/cm², 2 pass)

10.7 Photoaging

Cumulative exposure to sun is the main reason for skin aging. Photoaging skin is characterized by fine and coarse wrinkles, dyspigmentation, telangiectasia, sallow color, dry and rough texture, laxity, increased pore size, and a leathery appearance in habitually sun-exposed skin. Bitter et al has reported that the noncoherent IPL device could efficiently solve all the above problems at the same time.[10]

One hundred and fifty-two Chinese women with photoaging skin were treated with IPL (Lumenis One) in our open-labeled study. Subjects received a total of four IPL treatments at a 3- to 4-week interval. One hundred and thirty-nine of 152 patients (91.44%) experienced a score decrease of 3 or 2 grade, according to the dermatologist. One hundred and thirty-six of the 152 patients (89.47%) rated their overall improvement as excellent or good. The mean melanin index and erythema index values deceased with each session. Melanin index on forehead and erythema index on cheilion decreased most significantly. Adverse effects were limited as mild pain and transient erythema. IPL treatment is a safe and effective method for photoaging skin in Asian patients. Adverse effects were minimal and acceptable.[11] See Fig. 10.8 for details.

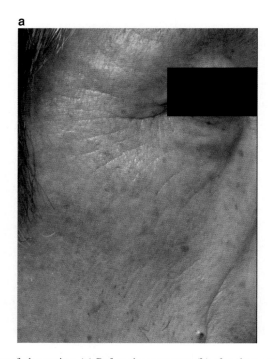

Fig. 10.8 A patient of photoaging. (**a**) Before the treatment; (**b**) after three sessions of treatment (640 nm filter, triple pulse, 3 ms pulse width, 30 ms pulse delay, 17–19 J/cm^2)

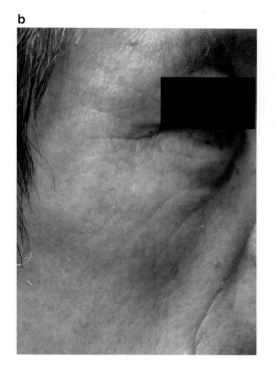

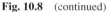

Fig. 10.8   (continued)

References

1. Chung JH. Photoaging in Asians. *Photodermatol Photoimmunol Photomed*. 2003;19:109–121.
2. Liu M, Li YH, Wu Y, et al. Efficacy of intense pulsed light on freckles, café-au-lait spots and seborrheic keratosis. *Chi J Dermatol*. 2007;40:337–339 (in Chinese).
3. Grossman MC, Anderson RR, Farinelli W, et al. Treatment of cafe au lait macules with lasers. A clinicopathologic correlation. *Arch Derm*. 1995;131:1416–1420.
4. Alster TS. Complete elimination of large café-au-lait birthmarks by the 510-nm pulsed dye laser. *Plast Reconstr Surg*. 1995;96:1660–1664.
5. Yoshida Y, Sato N, Furumura M, et al. Treatment of pigmented lesions of neurofibromatosis 1 with intense pulsed–radio frequency in combination with topical application of vitamin D3 ointment. *J Derm*. 2007;34:227–230.
6. Li YH, Chen John ZS, et al. Efficacy and safety of intense pulsed light in treatment of melasma in Chinese women. *Dermatol Surg*. 2008;34:693–701.
7. Ho WS, Chan HH, Ying SY, et al. Prospective study on the treatment of postburn hyperpigmentation by intense pulsed light. *Laser Med Surg*. 2003;32:42–45.

8. Bjerring P, Christiansen K, Troilius A. Intense pulsed light source for the treatment of dye laser resistant port-wine stains. *J Cosmet Laser Ther.* 2003;5:7–13.

9. Chang SE, Ahn SJ, Rhee DY, et al. Treatment of facial acne papules and pustules in Korean patients using an intense pulsed light device equipped with a 530- to 750-nm filter. *Dermatol Surg.* 2007;33:676–679.

10. Bitter PH. Noninvasive rejuvenation of photodamaged skin using serial, full-face intense pulsed light treatments. *Dermatol Surg.* 2000;26:835–843.

11. Li YH, Wu Y, Chen John ZS, et al. Application of a new intense pulsed light device in the treatment of photoaging skin in Asian patients. *Dermatol Surg.* 2008;34:1459–1464.

Index

A

Acne keloidalis nuchae, 155–157
Acne treatment
    endogenous porphyrins, 251
    protocols, USA, 254
    wavelengths and light treatments
        erythema, 253
        infrared (IR) treatment, 252
        laser and cryogen spray, 253
        Propionibacterium acnes,
            251–253
        sebaceous glands, 252, 253
Acquired bilateral nevus. *See* Hori's
        nevus
Acral-lentiginous melanoma (ALM), 64
African-American skin, photoaging
    facial sagging, 58, 59
    guttate hypomelanosis, 59, 60
    melanin, 57
    melanoma, 61
    pigment dyschromia, 58
    seborrheic keratoses, 59, 60
    squamous cell carcinoma (SCC), 58
Agar, N., 115, 119
Al-Arashi, M.Y., 29
Aldraibi, M.S., 149
Alster, T.S., 140
Altshuler, G.B., 17
Anbar, T.S., 180
Anderson, R.R., 16
Arad, S., 119
Arca, E., 182
Armas, L.A., 129
Ashkenazi, 254,
Asian skin, photoaging
    acral-lentiginous melanoma
        (ALM), 64
    hyperpigmentation, 62
    seborrheic keratoses, 62, 63

B

Basal cell carcinomas (BCCs), 126–127
Battle, E.F., 151
Bennett, M.F., 45
Berger, C.L., 231
Bitter, P.H., 274
Bjerring, P., 270
Black, J.F., 15
Brancaccio, R., 151
Broadband ultraviolet B (BB-UVB)
        phototherapy, 233–234

C

Café au lait macules (CALMs), 194–195,
        264–265
Calcipotriol/calcipotriene, vitiligo
        phototherapy, 182–183
Calzavara-Pinton, P.G., 83
Chang, S.E., 271
Chan, H.H., 194, 196
Chédiak-Higashi syndrome, 89
Chen, H-D., 263
Chiarion-Sileni, V., 223
Chronological aging, 47, 48
CHS. *See* Contact hypersensitivity response
Chui, C.T., 151
Clark, C., 235
Contact hypersensitivity response (CHS), 125
Cooper, K.D., 45
Cooperman, M., 151
CPDs. *See* Cyclobutane pyrimidine dimers
Cutaneous T-cell lymphomas (CTCL)
        definition, 205–206
        extracorporeal photopheresis
            combination treatment, 231–232
            fludarabine, 232–233
            interferon-α (IFN-α) and systemic
                retinoids, 232

Cutaneous T-cell lymphomas (CTCL) (*cont.*)
    mechanism of action, 226–228
    8-methoxypsoralen (8-MOP), 225
    monotherapy, 228–230
    patient selection, 230–231
    peripheral blood mononuclear cells
        (PBMCs), 225, 226
    sagramostim (GM-CSF), 232
    side effects, 230
    skin electron beam, 233
    transimmunization, 231
  incidence/prevalence
    classification/staging/prognosis,
      211–213
    clinical findings and variants, 207–210
    diagnosis/histology/workup, 210–211
    pathogenesis, 206–207
  multiagent chemotherapy, 215
  308-nm excimer laser, 237–238
  photodynamic therapy, 238–239
  phototherapy
    mechanism of action, 217–218
    skin cancer risk, relationship, 218–219
  psoralen plus UVA (PUVA)
    combination therapy, 222
    interferon-α (IFN-α), 222–224
    8-methoxypsoralen (8-MOP), 220
    monotherapy, 221
    mycosis fungoides (MF), 219
    retinoids, 223–224
    rexinoids, 224
    side effects, 222
  treatment modalities, 214
  ultraviolet A1 therapy, 224–225
  ultraviolet B phototherapy
    BB-UVB phototherapy, 233–234
    combination regimens, 236–237
    NB-UVB therapy, 234–237
Cyclobutane pyrimidine dimers (CPDs),
    116–117

D
Delayed tanning (DT), 118
Del Bino, S., 116
Dermal atrophy, 54
Dermatology, light applications
  diagnosis
    confocal microscopy, 28–29
    optical coherence tomography, 29–30
    optical spectroscopy, 28
    polarization imaging, 29
  therapeutic applications
    acne vulgaris, 31, 33

    hair removal, 31
    photodynamic therapy, 33–34
    pigmented lesions and tattoos, 30
    rejuvenation, 31–33
    vascular lesions, 30–31
Dermatosis papulosa nigra, 59
Descartes' law. *See* Snell's law
Diederen, P.V., 235
Dierickx, C.C., 137
Di Renzo, M., 227
Dissecting cellulitis, follicular disorders
  laser therapy, 159, 161
  medical therapies, 159
  Nd:YAG laser, 159–160
  scalp vertex and occiput, 157, 158
Domingo, D.S., 111
Don, P., 180
Downs, A., 163
Duvic, M., 229, 232

E
ECP. *See* Extracorporeal photopheresis (ECP)
Edelson, R., 225, 229
Eide, M.J., 128
Eller, M.S., 119
El Mofty, M., 171, 179, 181
Ephelides, 263–264
Epidermal atrophy, 54
Eumelanins
  absorption spectrum, 94
  biosynthesis, 90
  dihydroxyindole (DHI) and DHI carbolic
    acid (DHICA), 91
  laser hair removal, 96
  redox properties, 94–96
Extracorporeal photopheresis (ECP)
  combination treatment, 231–232
  fludarabine, 232–233
  interferon-α (IFN-α) and systemic
    retinoids, 232
  mechanism of action
    antitumor immunity, 226
    phosphatidylserine (PS), 227, 228
    T-cell apoptosis, 227
    white blood cells irradiation, 228
  8-methoxypsoralen (8-MOP), 225
  monotherapy
    erythrodermic CTCL, 228
    Sézary syndrome, 228–229
  patient selection, 230–231
  peripheral blood mononuclear cells
    (PBMCs), 225, 226
  sagramostim (GM-CSF), 232

side effects, 230
skin electron beam, 233
transimmunization, 231

F
Fai, D., 182
Fairchild, P., 153, 154
Ferenczi, K., 205
Fisher, G.J., 116
Fitzpatrick skin type (FST), 113–114
Follicular disorders, dark skin
  acne keloidalis nuchae, 155–157
  dissecting cellulitis
    laser therapy, 159, 161
    medical therapies, 159
    Nd:YAG laser, 159–160
    scalp vertex and occiput, 157–158
  hidradenitis suppurativa (HS)
    follicular hyperkeratosis and
      obstruction, 161
    inflammation, 162–163
    left axilla, 164–165
    Nd:YAG laser, 163–164
  hirsutism and hypertrichosis
    hair-removal system types, 138–139
    laser-induced side effects, 148–149
    laser light selection, 139–143
    laser parameters and test spots,
      143–145
    patient selection, 145–146
    preoperative discussion, 146–147
    selective photothermolysis theory,
      136–138
    treatment protocol, 147–148
  intense pulsed light (IPL), 164, 166
  light sources types, 136
  pseudofolliculitis barbae (PFB)
    absorption coefficient, 154
    African-American male, 149–150
    inflammatory papules, 151–152
    management, 150–151
    Nd:YAG laser, 152–154
  shifting demograph, statistics, 135
FST. See Fitzpatrick skin type

G
Gathers, R.C., 236
Gilchrest, B.A., 219
Glaser, D.A., 151
GM-CSF. See Granulocyte/macrophage
    colony stimulating factor
    (GM-CSF)

Goktas, E.O., 182
Goldinger, S.M., 182
Gold, M.H., 163
Gottlieb, S.L., 229, 232
Granulocyte/macrophage colony stimulating
    factor (GM-CSF), 232
Guttate hypomelanosis, 59, 60

H
Hadi, S.M., 181
Hamzavi, I.H., 135
Hennessy, A., 120
Hermansky Pudlak syndrome (HPS), 89
Herrmann, J.J., 221
Hexsel, C.L., 171
Hidradenitis suppurativa (HS)
  follicular hyperkeratosis and obstruction, 161
  inflammation in, 162–163
  left axilla, 164–165
  Nd:YAG laser, 163–164
Hill, H.Z., 115
Hirsutism and hypertrichosis
  hair-removal system types, 138–139
  laser-induced side effects, 148–149
  laser light selection
    absorption spectra, 142
    chin area, 141
    epidermal melanin absorption, 140
    Nd:YAG laser, 142–143
  laser parameters and test spots
    fluence, 143–144
    post test spots, 144–145
  patient selection, 145–146
  preoperative discussion, 146–147
  selective photothermolysis theory
    human anagen hair follicle,
      137–138
    melanin pigments, 136
    thermal relaxation time (TRT), 137
  treatment protocol, 147–148
Hispanic skin, photoaging
  dyspigmentation, 64, 65
  skin neoplasms, 64
  solar lentigines, 64–66
Hofer, A., 181, 235
Hönigsmann, H., 221
Hörfelt, C., 255
Hori's nevus, 197–198
Ho, W.S., 266
HS. See Hidradenitis suppurativa
Huggins, R.H., 171
Hyperpigmentation, non-caucasian skin,
    120–122

I

Immediate pigment darkening (IPD), 118
Immunosuppression, non-caucasian skin, 124–126
Intense pulsed light (IPL), 164, 166
  Asian patients
    acne and rosacea, 271–273
    Café au lait macules (CALMs), 264–265
    melasma, 265–266
    photoaging, 274–275
    pigmented disorders, 263–264
    port-wine stain, 270–271
    postburn hyperpigmentation, 266
  system, 189–190, 194
Iwasaki, J., 161

J

Jablonksi diagram, 7
Jacques, S.L., 151
Jiang, S.B., 229

K

Kauvar, A.N., 151
Kelly, D.A., 125
Khatri, K.A., 146
Kikuchi, A., 127
Kono, T., 190
Krahl, D., 161
Krasner, B.D., 159, 161
Kullavanijaya, P., 182
Kushimoto, T., 89

L

Lang, D., 83
Langerhans cells (LCs), 125
Lapins, J., 163
Laser therapies
  Café au lait macules (CALMs), 194–195
  lentigines, 190–194
  medication-induced hyperpigmentation, 200–201
  melasma, 198–200
  nevus of Ota, 195–197
Lee, J., 164
Lentigines, 190–194, 263–264
Liew, S.H., 166
Light–skin interaction principles
  dermatology
    acne vulgaris, 31, 33
    confocal microscopy, 28–29

hair removal, 31
optical coherence tomography, 29–30
optical spectroscopy, 28
photodynamic therapy, 33–34
pigmented lesions and tattoos, 30
polarization imaging, 29
rejuvenation, 31–33
vascular lesions, 30–31
fundamental properties, light, 2–4
medical light sources
  arc lamps, 22
  coherence and monochromaticity, 21–22
  collimated and diverging light beams, 20–21
  continuous wave and pulsed light, 21
  halogen lamps, 22
  lasers, 23–27
  light-emitting diode (LED), 22–23
  spontaneous and stimulated emission, 19–20
  superluminescent diodes, 23
optical interactions
  fluorescence and phosphorescence, 7
  internal reflection, light, 6
  light propagation, skin, 5
  light refraction, 6
  nonradiative deactivation processes, 7
  Raman scattering, 7–8
  skin chromophores, 11–15
  skin fluorophores, 15–16
  skin structure and optical properties, 8–12
  Snell's law, 6
  specular and diffuse reflection, 5–6
photochemical effects, 18–19
photomechanical effects, 18
photothermal effects, 16–18
Lim, H.W., 171
Li, Y-H., 263
Lymphomatoid papulosis (LyP), 208

M

Macrene A-A., 255
Ma, F., 129
Mahmoud, B.H., 135
MAL. *See* Methyl aminolevulinate (MAL)
Matsui, M.S., 111
Matsuoka, L.Y., 125
McAuliffe, D.J., 151
Medical light sources
  arc lamps, 22
  coherence and monochromaticity, 21–22

collimated and diverging light beams,
20–21
continuous wave and pulsed light, 21
halogen lamps, 22
lasers, 23–27
light-emitting diode (LED), 22–23
spontaneous and stimulated emission, 19–20
superluminescent diodes, 23
Medication-induced hyperpigmentation,
200–201
Melanin
melanocytes
development and homeostasis, 84–86
melanization, 86, 88–92
regulation, 96–99
pigmentation, racial differences
carotenes and hemoglobin, 100
Fontana-Masson stain, 102
hematoxylin and eosin, 101, 102
keratinocytes, 100
protection
acute and chronic effects, UVR, 92
epidermal keratinocyte apoptosis, 93
optical properties, 94
redox properties, 94–96
UV-induced erythema, 93
Melanin, non-caucasian skin, 115–117
Melanization
epidermal melanin unit, 86, 88
melanin synthesis, 90–92
melanosome
formation, 88–89
transfer, 92
Melanocytes
development and homeostasis
autosomal dominant disorder,
piebaldism, 86, 87
melanoblast migration, 86
microphthalmia transcription factor
(MITF), 85
neural crest cells, 84, 85
PAX3, 84–85
Waardenburg syndrome, 86, 87
melanization
epidermal melanin unit, 86, 88
melanin synthesis, 90–92
melanosome, 88–89, 92
regulation, 96–99
Melanosomes, 113
Melasma, 198–200, 265–266
8-Methoxypsoralen (8-MOP), 220
Methyl aminolevulinate (MAL), 256–260
Microphthalmia transcription factor
(MITF), 119

Mori, M., 237
Morison, W.L., 115
Mycosis fungoides (MF), 205, 207–213

N
Nanni, C.A., 151, 154
Narrowband ultraviolet B (NB-UVB) therapy
bexarotene and interferon-γ (IFN-γ), 237
maintenance therapy, 235
minimal erythema dose (MED), 234
monotherapy, 235–236
Narrowband UVB (NB-UVB) phototherapy
vs. BB-UVB, 180
vs. 308-nm monochromatic excimer
light, 180
pigmentation stability and predictors
response, 179–180
vs. PUVA, 174, 180
Nevus of Ota, 195–197
Nieuweboer-Krobotova, L., 179
Njoo, M.D., 180
NMSC. See Nonmelanoma skin cancer
(NMSC)
Non-caucasian skin
vs. caucasian skin
Fitzpatrick skin type (FST), 113–114
habits, 128–129
melanosomes, 113
ethnic populations, UVR and skin cancer,
126–128
hyperpigmentation
melasma, 122
PIH, 120–121
immunosuppression
inflammatory and immunomodulatory
markers, 126
skin types I–IV, 125–126
UVR-induced skin cancer, 124
long-term cumulative UV exposure,
122–124
melanin
apoptotic effect, 117
CPDs, 116–117
DNA damage, 115–116
minimal erythema dose (MED), 116
UV and pheomelanin, 115
sunlight, cutaneous effects, 112–113
tanning
ethnic skin, 118–119
IPD and DT, 118
UVR protection, epidermal thickening,
119–120
vitamin D, 129

Nonmelanoma skin cancer (NMSC), 256
Nylander, K., 98

O

Optical interactions
   fluorescence and phosphorescence, 7
   internal reflection, light, 6
   light propagation, skin, 5
   light refraction, 6
   nonradiative deactivation processes, 7
   Raman scattering, 7–8
   skin chromophores
      absorption, water and human fat
      hemoglobin derivatives, absorption, 14
      molar extinction coefficient, 12, 13
   skin fluorophores, 15–16
   skin structure and optical properties
      absorption and scattering coefficients,
        9–11
      dermis, 9, 10
      epidermis, 8–10
      subcutaneous fat, 10, 11
   Snell's law, 6
   specular and diffuse reflection, 5–6
Ortel, B., 83
Ortonne, J.P., 69

P

Pagetoid reticulosis, 210
Paithankar, D.Y., 253
Parrish, J.A., 16
Passeron, T., 181, 238
Pavlotsky, F., 235
PDT. *See* Photodynamic therapy (PDT)
PFB. *See* Pseudofolliculitis barbae
Pheomelanin
   absorption spectrum, 94
   biosynthesis, 90
   celtic skin types, 91
   redox properties, 94–96
Photoaging, 122–124
   clinical features
      African–American skin, 57–61
      Asian skin, 61–64
      Hispanic skin, 64–66
   histological features
      epidermal and dermal atrophy, 54
      melanosomes, 55, 56
      solar elastosis, 55
      stratum lucidum and stratum corneum, 55
   pathophysiology
      chronic inflammation, 51–52

      connective tissue remodeling, 50
      matrix metalloproteinases (MMPs), 47
      mitochondrial DNA, 49–50
      reactive oxygen species (ROS), 52–53
      telomeres, 48–49
      UVA and UVB, 46, 47
      UV-induced melanogenesis, 53–54
      vascular changes, 51
   prevention
      antioxidants, 67–68
      photoprotection, 66
      sunscreens, 67
   treatment
      alpha-and polyhydoroxy acids, 68
      chemical peels, 71
      lasers, 70–71
      retinoids, 68–69
      skin-lightening agents, 69–70
Photodynamic therapy (PDT)
   complications and applications, 256
   external photosensitizers
      5-aminolevulinic acid (ALA), 254
      intense pulsed light (IPL), 255
   postinflammatory hyperpigmentation (PIH)
      inflammatory acne, 256
      melanogenesis, 258
Pigmented skin acne patients
   epidemiology, Latin America, 250
   light and PDT treatment mechanism
      complications and applications, 256
      different wavelengths and light
        treatments, 251–253
      endogenous porphyrins, 251
      treatment protocols, 254
   MAL-PDT, 256–259
   PDT, external photosensitizers, 254–256
   postinflammatory hyperpigmentation
      (PIH), 250, 256–259
Poikilodermatous mycosis fungoides, 207, 209
Polypodium leucotomos, vitiligo
   phototherapy, 183
Postinflammatory hyperpigmentation (PIH),
   120–121
Pseudofolliculitis barbae (PFB)
   absorption coefficient, 154
   African-American male, 149–150
   inflammatory papules, 151–152
   management, 150–151
   Nd:YAG laser, 152–154
Psoralen plus UVA (PUVA)
   combination therapy, 222
   interferon-α (IFN-α), 222–223
   8-methoxypsoralen (8-MOP), 220
   monotherapy, 221

mycosis fungoides (MF), 219
phototherapy, 174, 179, 183–184
retinoids, 223–224
rexinoids, 224
side effects, 222

Q
Quaglino, P., 232
Querfeld, C., 221

R
Racz, M., 83
Resnik, K.S., 233
Rijken, F., 116, 117, 126
Roenigk, H.H. Jr., 221, 223
Rogers, C.J., 151
Roh, K., 123
Rombold, S., 225
Ross, E.V., 154, 161
Rupoli, S., 223

S
Sartorius, 163
Schmitz, S., 115
Seborrheic keratoses, 59, 60, 62, 63
Selgrade, M.K., 125
Sellheyer, K., 161
Se, M.S., 189
Sézary syndrome (SS), 205–207, 211–213
Sheehan, J.M., 116
Shimauchi, T., 237
Sitek, J.C., 179
Snell's law, 6
Solar elastosis, 55
Stadler, R., 223
Strauss, R.M., 163
Suchin, K.R., 232
Sun protection factor (SPF), 112
Suzuki, T., 62

T
Tacrolimus, vitiligo phototherapy, 181–182
Tadokoro, T., 118, 119
Tanning
    ethnic skin, 118–119
    IPD and DT, 118
T-oligos, 119
Torezan, L., 249
Torres, V., 249
Tuchin, V.V., 1

U
Ultraviolet A1 therapy (UVA1 therapy), 224–225
Ultraviolet B phototherapy
    broadband ultraviolet B phototherapy (BB-UVB), 233–234
    combination regimens, 236–237
    narrowband ultraviolet B (NB-UVB) therapy
        bexarotene and interferon-γ (IFN-γ), 237
        maintenance therapy, 235
        minimal erythema dose (MED), 234
        monotherapy, 234–236
Ultraviolet radiation (UVR)
    epidermal thickening, 119–120
    immunosuppression, 124–126
    skin cancer, ethnic populations, 126–128
UVA1 therapy. *See* Ultraviolet A1 therapy

V
Vermeer, M., 125
Vitamin D, 129
Vitiligo phototherapy
    broadband UVA, 181
    calcipotriol/calcipotriene, 182–183
    history, 171–172
    mechanism and rationale, 172–173
    NB-UVB
        pigmentation stability and predictors response, 179–180
        vs. BB-UVB, 180
        vs. 308-nm monochromatic excimer light, 180
        vs. PUVA, 174, 180
    photochemotherapy studies, 175–178
    Polypodium leucotomos, 183
    side effects
        acute effects, 184–185
        long-term side effects, 185
    tacrolimus combination, 181–182
    targeted UVB phototherapy, 181
    treatment protocols
        308-nm excimer laser, 184
        PUVA photochemotherapy, 183–184
Vonderheid, E.C., 233

W
Waardenburg syndrome, 86, 87
Westerhof, W., 179
Wilson, L.D., 233
Wu, Y., 263